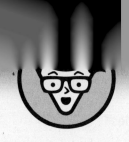

Diabetes & Keeping Fit

by Dr. Sheri R. Colberg

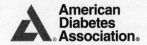
American Diabetes Association®

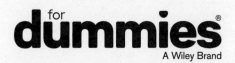
A Wiley Brand

Diabetes & Keeping Fit For Dummies®

Published by: **John Wiley & Sons, Inc.**, 111 River Street, Hoboken, NJ 07030-5774, www.wiley.com

Copyright © 2018 by John Wiley & Sons, Inc., Hoboken, New Jersey

Published simultaneously in Canada

For general information on our other products and services, please contact our Customer Care Department within the U.S. at 877-762-2974, outside the U.S. at 317-572-3993, or fax 317-572-4002. For technical support, please visit https://hub.wiley.com/community/support/dummies.

Wiley publishes in a variety of print and electronic formats and by print-on-demand. Some material included with standard print versions of this book may not be included in e-books or in print-on-demand. If this book refers to media such as a CD or DVD that is not included in the version you purchased, you may download this material at http://booksupport.wiley.com. For more information about Wiley products, visit www.wiley.com.

Library of Congress Control Number: 2017960683

ISBN 978-1-119-36324-8 (pbk); ISBN 978-1-119-36326-2 (ebk); ISBN 978-1-119-36325-5 (ebk)

Manufactured in the United States of America

10 9 8 7 6 5 4 3 2 1

Contents at a Glance

Introduction 1

Part 1: Getting Started with Diabetes 5
CHAPTER 1: Getting an Overview of Diabetes 7
CHAPTER 2: Managing Health and Diabetes Fitness 25
CHAPTER 3: Understanding Diabetes Medications 41

Part 2: Mastering Exercise and Nutrition Basics 61
CHAPTER 4: Finding Out How Exercise Works 63
CHAPTER 5: Avoiding Exercise Glucose Extremes 83
CHAPTER 6: Eating Better for Health 103
CHAPTER 7: Eating Right for Exercise 125

Part 3: Getting Up and Moving 139
CHAPTER 8: Setting the Stage for Getting Active 141
CHAPTER 9: Setting Your Workout Up for Success 161
CHAPTER 10: Including Cardio Training 181
CHAPTER 11: Building Strength through Resistance 203
CHAPTER 12: Finding Your Balance 225
CHAPTER 13: Focusing on Flexibility 239
CHAPTER 14: Mixing It Up with Cross-Training 259

Part 4: Keeping Fit at Any Age or Any Stage 265
CHAPTER 15: Training with Extra Body Weight 267
CHAPTER 16: Exercising with Health Complications 285
CHAPTER 17: Being Active and Female 299
CHAPTER 18: Taking Special Considerations for Kids and Seniors 305
CHAPTER 19: Managing Diabetes as an Athlete 323

Part 5: The Part of Tens 337
CHAPTER 20: Ten Tips to Boost Your Overall Health 339
CHAPTER 21: Ten Easy Exercises to Build a Strong Core without
Leaving the House 347
CHAPTER 22: Ten Ways to Get Motivated to Exercise (When You're Not) 357

Index 363

Table of Contents

INTRODUCTION 1

About This Book. 1

Foolish Assumptions. 2

Icons Used in This Book 2

Beyond the Book. 3

Where to Go from Here 4

PART 1: GETTING STARTED WITH DIABETES 5

CHAPTER 1: Getting an Overview of Diabetes 7

Knowing Your Risks for Diabetes 8

Understanding the Culprits: Glucose and Insulin. 8

   Glucose is the actor. 9

   Insulin is the director 9

Navigating the Types of Diabetes 11

   Taking a look at type 1 diabetes 11

   Talking about type 2 diabetes 12

   Getting a handle on gestational diabetes 13

   Previewing prediabetes 14

Diagnosing Diabetes or Prediabetes 14

   Recognizing the symptoms 14

   Testing for diabetes and prediabetes. 15

   Getting tested for gestational diabetes 17

   Being misdiagnosed with type 2 diabetes 18

Self-Monitoring Your Blood Glucose 18

Using a Blood Glucose Meter 19

   Tackling types of meters. 20

   Examining what affects meter readings. 20

   Looking ahead to other ways to measure blood glucose 21

   Exploring the pros and cons of continuous glucose monitors ... 21

Discovering Why Being Fit with Diabetes Matters 22

CHAPTER 2: Managing Health and Diabetes Fitness. 25

Knowing the Importance of Getting Moving. 26

Understanding How Exercise and Food Affect Your Body
with Diabetes. 26

   Recognizing why exercise training is critical 27

   Grasping how food affects your blood glucose 28

Uncovering More about Fitness and Aging 29

   Questioning whether aging, inactivity, or diabetes is to blame ... 29

   Slowing down aging with exercise 30

Investigating the Impact of Fitness and Other Factors on
Insulin Action 30
    Looking at what impacts how insulin works 31
    Revving up your insulin action. 31
Deciding When to Consult with Your Doctor First 33
Setting Diabetes, Health, and Fitness Goals .34
    Diabetes targets and goals. 35
    Health goals 37
    Fitness goals. 37
Surveying Cardiovascular Risks That May Limit Exercise 38
Living Long and Well with Diabetes or Prediabetes. 39

CHAPTER 3: **Understanding Diabetes Medications** 41
Knowing How Oral Diabetes Medications Work. 41
    Targeting specific tissues 42
    Identifying which pills work best to lower glucose. 42
Using (Non-Insulin) Injected Medication 45
    Amylin 45
    GLP-1 agonists 46
Changing Doses for Exercise 46
    Oral medications that may cause exercise lows. 47
    Medications unlikely to cause lows. 48
Understanding Insulin Use. 49
    Basal and bolus insulins and their actions 50
    Insulin delivery methods 52
    Insulin and exercise interactions. 53
    Lowering insulin for physical activity 54
    Exercise and insulin needs in athletes 56
Monitoring Effects of Other Medications. 57
    Non-diabetes medications with exercise effects 57
    Other medications with no exercise effects 58
    Non-diabetes medications affecting blood glucose. 59

PART 2: MASTERING EXERCISE AND
NUTRITION BASICS 61

CHAPTER 4: **Finding Out How Exercise Works** 63
Knowing How Hormones React. 64
    Directing the flow of glucose in blood 64
    Understanding why your glucose sometimes goes up
    with exercise 65
    Staying elevated too long after a workout. 65
Engaging Your Exercise Energy Systems 66
    Phosphagens system (short and powerful) 67
    Lactic acid system (fast, furious, and painful) 68
    Aerobic system (lasts longer). 68

Using Carbohydrate and Fat as Fuels...........................70
    Carbohydrate: A high-octane fuel.....................70
    Forget the "fat-burning range"......................71
Predicting Your Usual Glucose Response 71
Factoring in Exercise Variables 72
    Type (which exercises) 72
    Intensity (how hard) 73
    Duration (how long) 76
    Frequency (how often) 77
    Timing (when you work out) 77
    Training effects (how fit you are)..................79
Accounting for Other Factors 80
    Environment..80
    Insulin regimen changes 80
    Bodily concerns 81
    Hypoglycemia-associated autonomic failure (HAAF) 82

CHAPTER 5: Avoiding Exercise Glucose Extremes................ 83
Exercising with an Ideal Blood Glucose 83
Identifying Hypoglycemia (Lows)...............................84
    Exploring what causes low blood glucose 85
    Recognizing the symptoms of lows...................86
Treating and Preventing Hypoglycemia.........................88
    Examining tips for confronting hypoglycemia........88
    Preventing exercise lows if you use insulin........91
    Avoiding lows all the time.........................93
    Using exercise to prevent and treat lows...........97
    Dealing with exercise spontaneity 98
Managing Hyperglycemia (Highs) and Exercise 99
    When to wait to exercise 100
    When blood glucose is high, but exercise is okay...........100
    Reduce highs after exercise........................101

CHAPTER 6: Eating Better for Health........................103
Knowing Which Foods Make a Body Healthy 103
    Choosing foods that lower inflammation 104
    Focusing on fiber..................................106
    Taking in carbohydrates............................108
    Cutting back on sugar..............................111
    Boosting your health with protein 112
    Fitting healthy fats into your diet 113
    Eating more healthful meals and snacks.............116

Getting Your Vitamins and Minerals from Foods
or Supplements 117
B vitamins. 117
Vitamin D 118
Magnesium. 119
Deciding Whether You Need Other Supplements 120
Being cautious about supplements 120
Creatine. 121
Whey protein (essential amino acids). 121
Carnitine 122
Antioxidants 122

CHAPTER 7: **Eating Right for Exercise**. 125
Fueling Your Body with Carbohydrates 126
Carbohydrate intake during exercise. 126
Normal daily carbohydrate needs 127
Exercise carbohydrates for insulin users only. 128
Glycogen repletion and carbohydrates 130
Pumping Up with Protein. 131
Protein intake for everyone 131
Protein intake for insulin users 132
Maximizing protein for training and aging 132
Using Fat during Exercise. 133
Fat use and intake for everyone 134
Strategic fat intake for insulin users. 134
Taking Caffeine or Drinking Coffee to Power Workouts 135
Staying Hydrated with Fluids. 136
Fluids during exercise. 136
What to do if your blood glucose is high 137
Using sports drinks, juice, and more 138

PART 3: GETTING UP AND MOVING 139

CHAPTER 8: **Setting the Stage for Getting Active**. 141
Finding the Right Activities. 141
Getting "fit" according to the latest guidelines 142
Standing up more 143
Homing in on your favorite workouts 143
Choosing an activity that's a workout. 143
Tricking yourself into finishing. 143
Picking Workout Clothes and Equipment 144
Dressing right. 145
Choosing the right footwear 145
Getting the equipment you need 146

Staying Motivated to Be Active 146
    Starting (or jump-starting) your motivational engine. 146
    Tracking your progress. 147
    Using mobile technology to get fit 150
Assessing and Overcoming Barriers. 151
    Finding out what your barriers are. 151
    Getting past your unique barriers. 153
    Setting some SMART goals. 155
Debunking Common Exercise Myths 157
    No pain, no gain. 157
    Exercise makes you tired 157
    To lose fat, you have to be in a fat-burning range 157
    If you don't use your muscles, they turn into fat 158
    Lose weight first, because weight training will bulk you up 158
    Lifting weights more slowly builds larger muscles. 158
    Working on your abs will make your belly flat 159
    You can't exercise too much 159
    To gain muscle, eat more protein. 159
    If you're not sweating, you're not working out hard enough 160

CHAPTER 9: **Setting Your Workout Up for Success**...............161
Adding in Spontaneous Physical Activity 161
    Identifying the benefits of SPA time 162
    Taking a stand against being sedentary. 163
    Getting thinner by doing spontaneous activities 163
Choosing the Best Training for Diabetes. 164
    Cardio (aerobic) and interval workouts 165
    Resistance (strength) and core training....................167
    Balance exercises 168
    Flexibility training 169
    Cross-training for optimal fitness 169
Warming Up and Cooling Down 171
Carving Out a Fitness Routine 171
    Finding time every day to be active 171
    Creating a personalized workout plan to keep
    you accountable 172
    Changing up your routine with hard and easy days 172
    Getting enough beauty sleep. 173
    Progressing (slowly) over time. 173
Steering Clear of Certain Activities 173
Preventing and Managing Injuries 174
    Identifying common injuries 175
    Avoiding other acute injuries. 176
    Treating acute injuries properly 176

Common causes of all injuries. 177
Preventing and treating overuse injuries. 177
Expecting some muscle soreness from exercise 179
Dealing with muscle cramps 179

CHAPTER 10: **Including Cardio Training** 181
Getting Started with Cardio Training 182
Considering which activities you should do 182
Looking at amount, intensity, and duration 182
Remembering to warm up and cool down 184
Determining whether to see a doctor first 184
Walking Your Way to Better Health 184
Walking correctly to avoid injury. 185
Planning out your walking routine 185
Jogging or Running Indoors or Outdoors. .186
Examining outdoor jogging versus indoor treadmills 186
Perfecting your technique 187
Keeping your joints and feet healthy with footwear 187
Speeding through a workout plan 188
Gearing up for a longer event 189
Including Some Interval Training 189
Investigating more ways to do interval training 190
Hitting on whether high-intensity intervals are for you. 191
Putting Indoor Cardio Machines to Use. 191
Exploring elliptical machines 192
Surveying stair-steppers and other cross-trainers. 192
Cycling indoors as an alternative 193
Rowing to get fitter 193
Cross-country skiing indoors 194
Other Activities to Get Aerobically Fit. 194
Swimming your way to better health 194
Biking outdoors 195
Trying Easy Aerobic Activities. 196
Seated march. 197
Seated foot drill 197
Seated arm curls 198
Seated overhead punches 198
Standing march 200
Standing raise the roof. 200

CHAPTER 11: **Building Strength through Resistance**. 203
Maximizing Your Muscle Strength to Supercharge Your Health 204
Recruiting all your fibers to keep your muscle 205
Training when you're on a diet 205
Enhancing your insulin action and health 206

Getting the Most Out of Your Resistance Training................207

    Warming up 207

    Mixing it up with resistance bands, hand weights,
    weight machines, and more...................................208

    Getting in plenty of reps and sets often enough 210

    Knowing how much, how often, and how to do
    resistance training correctly.................................211

    Getting stronger and stronger over time.....................211

Working Out the Right Way 213

    Using the right technique....................................213

    Pulling your weight with the right plan 214

    Choosing the right exercises 215

Incorporating More Core Training 215

    Knowing what core training can do for you...................215

    Discovering which core exercises to do......................216

Staying Safe by Taking Precautions 217

Working Out with Easy Resistance Exercises at Home or Work.....218

    Sit-to-stand exercise 218

    Chair push-ups..219

    Chair sit-ups 220

    Wall push-ups...221

    Standing leg curls 222

    Standing calf raises 223

CHAPTER 12: Finding Your Balance 225

Examining the Effects of Aging and Diabetes on Balance.........226

    Understanding that your balance declines as you get older 226

    Recognizing that diabetes adds to loss of balance............226

    Checking your own balance..................................227

Improving Balance to Stay on Your Feet 227

    Knowing which muscles to focus on.........................228

    Like a stork: Practicing standing on one leg 228

Supercharging Your Balance with Anytime Exercises
and Activities 229

    Boost your glutes with side leg raises 229

    Kick back with toe raises....................................229

    Keep moving forward with calf raises 230

    Grab a towel with your toes.................................230

    Stand on a cushion 230

    Change the way you stand...................................230

    Get up with sit-to-stand exercises...........................230

    Walk heel-to-toe..231

    Travel backward...231

    Practice posture by tucking your chin 231

Using Yoga or Tai Chi to Boost Flexibility, Strength,
and Balance 231
Working on Balance in Your Spare Time 232
    Single leg balance 232
    Three-way leg swing 233
    Balance/reach 234
    Forward lean 234
    Toe raise 236
    Heel raise 236

CHAPTER 13: **Focusing on Flexibility** 239
Breaking Down What Stretching Does for You 240
    Figuring out why flexibility matters. 240
    Evaluating static versus dynamic stretching 241
    Considering whether dynamic moves mean fewer injuries 241
Stretching Effectively. 242
Reviewing Muscles and Basic Stretches. 242
    Arms, neck, and shoulders. 244
    Core muscles 244
    Legs, hips, and buttocks 245
Practicing Some Yoga Poses 245
    Basic and foundational poses 245
    More-advanced yoga poses. 247
Trying a Whole-Body Approach to Relax 250
    Training your body and mind to destress 250
    Using visualization to perform better. 252
Working on Flexibility with Some Stretching Exercises 252
    Neck stretch 253
    Shoulder/upper-back stretch. 253
    Chest/shoulder stretch. 254
    Upper-back/back of arm stretch 255
    Back of upper-leg stretch 256
    Calf stretch 257

CHAPTER 14: **Mixing It Up with Cross-Training**. 259
Benefiting from Doing Cross-Training 259
    Increasing blood glucose and glycogen use 260
    Experiencing fewer injuries 260
    Enjoying more variety. 261
    Staving off boredom 261
    Taking the right approach to any type of cross-training 262
Combining Cardio and Resistance Work to Combat Diabetes 263
CrossFit Training with Diabetes. 263

PART 4: KEEPING FIT AT ANY AGE OR ANY STAGE 265

CHAPTER 15: **Training with Extra Body Weight** 267

Limiting the Impact of Your Extra Weight Gain.................. 268
  Aiming to be fit and thin (if possible) 268
  Recognizing that where you store your fat matters........... 268
Keeping Active to Manage Your Weight...................... 270
  Preventing type 2 diabetes with activity.................... 270
  Choosing aerobic and resistance workouts................... 270
  Giving your backside a break............................. 271
  Starting out slowly but steadily 271
  Picking activities you enjoy.............................. 272
Dealing with Arthritis and Other Joint Problems 272
  Working out with arthritic joints 272
  Managing discomfort or pain 273
  Avoiding other joint issues............................... 273
Losing Weight and Keeping It Off 274
  Losing some weight along the way........................ 274
  Keeping the weight off 275
Avoiding Insulin Weight Gain and Using Diabetes
Medications to Lose Weight................................ 277
  Dodging weight gain from insulin use 277
  Adjusting other diabetes medications to lose weight 279
Considering Other Weight Loss Issues....................... 281
Keeping Diabetes from Making You Blue 282
Getting Enough Sleep to Get Thinner....................... 282

CHAPTER 16: **Exercising with Health Complications** 285

Dealing with Health Complications........................ 286
Exercising Safely with Nerve Damage 286
  Working around damaged feet and legs 286
  Staying on top of central nerve issues 288
Being Active with Vessel Disease.......................... 289
  Heart disease 290
  High blood pressure and stroke 291
  Peripheral artery disease (PAD)........................... 292
Eyeing Ways to Exercise with Retinopathy 293
  Mild or moderate retinopathy........................... 294
  Severe (proliferative) retinopathy 294
Staying Active with Kidney Disease........................ 295
Managing Exercise with Health Issues 296

CHAPTER 17: **Being Active and Female** 299

Understanding How Female Hormones Affect Insulin
and Exercise 299
Hormonal swings and insulin action 300
Exercise responses with hormonal changes 301
Staying Active During Pregnancy 301
Keeping insulin lower and fitness higher 302
Avoiding excess weight gain by exercising 302
Exercising throughout pregnancy 303
Managing gestational diabetes 304

CHAPTER 18: **Taking Special Considerations for Kids
and Seniors** 305

Getting at the Root of Physical Inactivity of Today's Youth 306
Encouraging Kids to Be Active 307
Examining the effects of exercise on blood glucose 307
Keeping kids safe during activities 307
Nurturing kids' innate love of movement 308
Making movement a family affair 309
Peeling those couch potatoes off the cushions 310
Looking at Aging and Health in Seniors 311
Being aware of bodily changes over time 312
Slowing the effects of time 312
Recognizing whether decline is due to aging or inactivity 313
Being active raises insulin action 313
Avoiding muscle wasting and fat gain 314
Getting Seniors Up and Moving 315
Cardio training and intervals 316
Resistance and core training 316
Balance training 317
Flexibility training 317
Breaking up sedentary time 317
Moving more all day long 318
Working Out for Your Mental Health and Function 318
Assessing How Well You're Aging, Really 320

CHAPTER 19: **Managing Diabetes as an Athlete** 323

Taking Your Activity to the Next Level 323
Bumping up your training intensity 324
Pumping it up until fatigue sets in 324
Knowing why your training state matters 325
Carb Loading Effectively for the Athlete 326

Training Well with Low-Carb Eating 327
  Scrutinizing whether low-carb eating hurts performance 327
  Using the window of opportunity for carbs 328
Troubleshooting Exercise Blood Glucose for Competitive
and Serious Recreational Athletes 328
  Managing hypoglycemia 329
  Handling hyperglycemia 330
  Avoiding early-onset or excessive fatigue 331
  Considering other performance variables 332
  Moving forward when you're still stumped 334

PART 5: THE PART OF TENS 337

CHAPTER 20: **Ten Tips to Boost Your Overall Health** 339
Get Emotionally Fit with Activity 339
Go for the Endorphin Release 340
Enjoy Higher Dopamine Levels 340
Drop Those Cortisol Levels 342
Boost Your Bodily Satisfaction 342
Listen to Your Body 343
Don't Use Poor Health or Age as an Excuse Not to Exercise 344
Tackle Health Problems Early On 344
Plan Ahead for Exercise Success 345
Know It's Never Too Late to Start Being Active 346

CHAPTER 21: **Ten Easy Exercises to Build a Strong
Core without Leaving the House** 347
#1: Abdominal Squeezes 348
#2: Plank or Modified Plank 349
#3: Side Planks 349
#4: Bridging 351
#5: Pelvic Tilt 351
#6: Superhero Pose 352
#7: Knee Push-Ups 353
#8: Suitcase Lift 353
#9: Squats with Knee Squeezes 354
#10: Lunges 355

CHAPTER 22: **Ten Ways to Get Motivated to Exercise
(When You're Not)** 357
Check Your Blood Glucose 358
Start with Easier Activities 358
Pick Activities You Enjoy 358

Spice It Up..359
Have a Plan B..359
Get an Exercise Buddy (or Several)..........................359
Schedule It 360
Set Goals and Reward Yourself............................360
Take Advantage of Opportunities for Spontaneous
Physical Activity 360
Take Small Steps 361

INDEX...363

Introduction

Although ending up with a chronic disease that you're likely to have to deal with for the rest of your life is never pleasant, the thing about diabetes (or prediabetes, for that matter) is that it's at least a manageable condition. You can keep on top of your blood glucose (sugar in blood) and keep it as near normal as possible, regardless of which type you have. In doing so, you greatly lower your chances of having to deal with any additional health complications arising from having diabetes. You can't say that about many chronic health issues.

Diabetes & Keeping Fit For Dummies doesn't necessarily contain any ground-breaking techniques to conquer diabetes once and for all. In fact, it may not contain anything that seems that new to you. What is does offer, though, is everything you need to know to not only lengthen your life with diabetes or prediabetes but also live well in a healthy body with a sharp mind until the end of your life, all from the world's leading expert on the topic of diabetes and exercise.

Living a long life is one thing; living it well is something else completely. Really, what's the point of living long if you can't live well and feel your best every day of your life?

About This Book

Diabetes & Keeping Fit For Dummies tries to give you all the tools you need in your lifestyle toolbox to live long and well with any type of diabetes or prediabetes. It provides an overview of the types of diabetes, what makes you more likely to get one type or another, and why your health can benefit so much from managing it and your diabetes simultaneously. Sometimes that involves using the right medications for your diabetes.

You really need to know the basics about how being active affects your body and your blood glucose, why you want to avoid glucose extremes (and how to do it), and how to set up a fitness program that works for you. And, of course, you need to understand how your food choices impact your health and your ability to be active.

Really, there are no wrong activities for someone who wants to get keep fit with diabetes. The right activities for you basically mean anything you can get yourself to do regularly. But some specific options are recommended more than others when you have diabetes, and this book tells you what you need to know about doing those. You should aim to boost your endurance, pump up your strength, find your balance, flex all your joints, and mix it all up to keep it fun and impactful — not too much to ask.

You keep fit at any age (young, old, or in between) or with any health complication typical with diabetes. If you're overweight, no problem. If you're female and/or an athlete, it's more complicated, but I've got you covered.

You now have no reason to consider *exercise* a four-letter word anymore.

Foolish Assumptions

If you bought this book — or even if you got it as a gift and actually opened it to start reading — I can only assume that you're at least a little bit interested in seeing whether you can get more fit. In writing it, I assume that at least one of the following situations applies to you as a unique individual:

>> You're a complete fitness novice who needs all the help you can get, and you're actually willing to read this book to find out how.

>> You know you should be more physically active, but maybe you're lacking the motivation to get active and stay active.

>> You're up off the couch already, but you want to know more about which activities are best for you.

>> Being active is hard for you given the health issues you're dealing with, and you want some help getting as fit as you can just to be healthier or to lose a few pounds in the process.

>> You're an athletic person already, but you hope to pick up some new trick that will make you a better athlete or allow you to easily try a new activity.

Icons Used in This Book

Throughout this book, I use a number of icons in the margins that are intended to grab your attention and help you get more out of your keeping-fit-with-diabetes journey:

This icon highlights info that helps you better understand a concept or put it into action to save time or frustration. These paragraphs are worth flagging or writing down to help you get fit and stay active. If you do nothing else with this book, read all the time-saving and stress-reducing tips found in each chapter to get moving more.

This icon points out any information that is worth remembering about getting fit with diabetes — even if you remember nothing else (and you may not!).

When you see the Warning icon, take it seriously. These items can truly cause you harm on your fitness journey if you ignore them.

The Technical Stuff icon lets you know that these paragraphs include nonessential details about certain concepts or the research behind what is known about them. You can skip them if you want to (along with the shaded sidebars), but try reading a few of them as you go through the book, especially if you like to know the why and how about stuff.

Beyond the Book

To access the free online Cheat Sheet that accompanies this book, go to dummies.com and search for this book title. This Cheat Sheet contains articles on various issues related to diabetes nutrition and fitness.

Check out more information about being active with diabetes on my website called Diabetes Motion, which you can access online at www.diabetesmotion.com. It's a free resource, and its blogs and other posts can keep you updated on any new stuff coming out in diabetes fitness.

Another of my websites, Diabetes Motion Academy (www.dmacademy.com), is mostly targeted to fitness professionals and health coaches, but it has some free PDFs you can download that show you additional resistance and flexibility exercises that you can try as part of its fitness resources.

Finally, I've shared a wealth of knowledge over the years on my own website and blogs that you can access for some free advice on just about any topic. Find me online at www.shericolberg.com, and feel free to drop me a line with any questions you have.

Where to Go from Here

You don't have to start at the beginning of this book and read through the chapters in order. If you know enough about the type of diabetes or prediabetes you have and just want to dive deeper into the good stuff, skip the first chapter. If you know a lot about diabetes medications already or just don't want to find out anything else, move on to another topic without looking back.

If you're interested in doing a certain type of activity like balance training or cross-training, just jump straight into the chapter that deals with it. The same goes if you have a certain health issue or need help with taking your training up a notch. Even if you're already a pro on a particular topic, though, you may want to skim through it to see whether anything new has popped up.

If you aren't quite sure where you want to go with your fitness and are willing to invest a little time in your long-term health, just start at the beginning of the book and make your way through it in the usual way — one chapter at a time. You may be surprised at how things have changed in the diabetes world in the past few years.

1

Getting Started with Diabetes

IN THIS PART . . .

Get the basics on diabetes, including the different types, diagnosis and treatment, and importance of keeping fit to manage it and your health.

Understand how diet and exercise can affect diabetes and why physical activity can help insulin work better.

Discover the various types of diabetes medications and find out how exercise can affect you if you use insulin.

and insulin

» Defining the types of diabetes
(including prediabetes)

» Identifying diabetes symptoms
and getting a proper diagnosis

» Working with a blood glucose
meter or a continuous monitor

» Recognizing the important links
between fitness and diabetes
management

Chapter **1**

Getting an Overview of Diabetes

One in three Americans currently has diabetes or prediabetes; that's over 100 million people in the United States alone. This isn't a small health issue, and it's not likely to go away anytime soon. But what do you really know about diabetes, other than it involves having extra "sugar" in your blood? How do you know whether you have type 1, type 2, or prediabetes? What's the difference?

In this chapter, you find out what makes someone develop diabetes and the types, along with how each is diagnosed. I also explain why a blood glucose meter can become your new best friend and how to get the most information you can out of it.

Knowing Your Risks for Diabetes

What's your risk for getting diabetes? It has gone up substantially in the past few decades. In fact, anyone born in the United States from the year 2000 forward has a one-in-three chance of developing diabetes during his or her lifetime, and the incidence is closer to 50 percent if you're part of a minority group (like African Americans, Hispanics, or Native Americans).

More than 29 million Americans — close to 10 percent of the population — are estimated to already have diabetes, and this number is growing rapidly. Over a quarter of them don't even know they have it. Add in prediabetes, and the number goes up to over 100 million Americans, or one person out of every three.

WARNING

Everyone knows someone who has diabetes, so why worry about it? Because high blood glucose levels can be deadly. Having poorly managed diabetes can rob years from your life, and the shorter time you do have may be lived in much poorer health. Ignorance isn't bliss; ignoring diabetes and not attempting to prevent or manage its possible health consequences isn't the way to go if you want to live long and well.

Worldwide, this disease causes more than 3.2 million deaths per year, or 6 deaths every minute. Many more deaths are likely related to health problems caused by diabetes that are attributed to some other direct cause, such as a heart attack or a stroke, even though diabetes lead to those events. Unfortunately, poorly managed blood glucose can cause problems with almost every part of your body, including your heart, blood vessels, brain, kidneys, nerves, muscles, and bones. It can even lead to impotence and hearing loss.

Okay, so far this section has been depressing. Here's some good news: Most diabetes-related health problems are preventable. You simply need to get more physically active and follow a more healthful diet. If your health care provider prescribes medications, taking those may also help prevent future health issues. The combination of these improved lifestyle choices helps lower your blood glucose and prevent systemic inflammation that leads to heart disease, nerve damage, and other health complications when not thwarted.

REMEMBER

Well-managed diabetes can be the cause of nothing — that is, no health problems.

Understanding the Culprits: Glucose and Insulin

The human body has to manage its own blood glucose, which it does quite effectively in most people most of the time. You have to have enough glucose in your blood; it's required for your brain and your nerves to function properly. The amount in blood is regulated by a hormone called insulin. The following sections explain how these two components work.

TIP

Think of glucose and insulin as the actor and the director in a performance. The insulin (director) tells the glucose (actor) where to go and what to do to get the best showing out of it. It takes the two coordinating their roles to get the show done.

Glucose is the actor

When people talk about "blood sugar," they mean *blood glucose,* the primary sugar in your bloodstream that fuels the brain, nerves, muscles, and other cells around the body. Having too little in your blood can kill you. Unfortunately, so can having too much, especially over the long haul.

Normally, your body digests the food you eat and breaks it down into more easily absorbed molecules, of which glucose is one. It's a simple sugar that comes mostly from the carbohydrates you eat.

Blood glucose can come from different sources, but you get it mostly from your food and drinks (although your liver makes some, too). Foods rich in carbohydrates (such as grains, milk, fruit and fruit juice, starchy vegetables, most desserts, and sugary drinks) are released as glucose in your bloodstream after your body digests them. Blood glucose levels normally increase slightly after eating, even if you don't have diabetes. Your brain, nervous system, and active muscles use some of that glucose right away, although all cells in the body use glucose at some point. When everything is working right, the body stores away the rest for later.

TECHNICAL
STUFF

When your blood glucose levels are higher (such as after a meal), extra glucose usually gets packed away and stored in the liver and muscles as *glycogen.* When your blood glucose is low, *glucagon* (a hormone made by the pancreas) is released and signals the liver to let out some of its stored glycogen as blood glucose. When you're active, your muscles also use some of the glycogen stored in them as fuel, but the glucose coming from muscle glycogen stores stays in the muscle and doesn't raise your blood glucose. Using up the glycogen in your muscles by exercising gives your body a place to easily store more carbohydrates after you eat the next time, reducing the amount of excess glucose flowing around in your blood, potentially causing inflammation and damage.

Insulin is the director

When your body is working normally, your blood glucose goes up after you eat a meal, and your pancreas senses this increase and releases a hormone called *insulin* to help lower it. Insulin works by binding to its receptors on cells in muscle and fat, the primary places where the body can store glucose for later use.

Two separate, but related, aspects of diabetes are associated with your body's insulin. One is how effectively insulin works. If you have type 2 diabetes or prediabetes, insulin may be abundant, but it doesn't work well to lower blood glucose — that is, you have *insulin resistance.* People with other types of diabetes can become insulin resistant as well. The second is the amount of insulin that is available. Persons with type 1 diabetes make little or no insulin; people with prediabetes and type 2 diabetes have an inadequate amount of insulin produced to meet their needs.

Insulin is a hormone made by the pancreas that, when released into the bloodstream, works to allow blood glucose to enter your cells that are insulin sensitive, primarily muscle, fat, and liver cells. Some of it gets used as a fuel by those cells, but the rest is stored in these tissues for later use. During rest, insulin works to make sure that glucose leaves the blood and goes into the cells, which keeps your blood glucose from going too high or staying that way after eating. Unfortunately, excess blood glucose that can't enter cells for any reason can cause damage to your body over time.

The other aspect is how much insulin the pancreas produces. You can be deficient in insulin, meaning that you simply don't make much. People with various types of diabetes can also have this issue. In that case, they may need to take medications to stimulate the pancreas to produce more, take insulin to supplement their supply, or use other medications that lower blood glucose other ways. In either case, your blood glucose may rise too high at various times, such as after you eat, when you're stressed out, if you're ill, and when you exercise vigorously.

Regardless of whether you have insulin that doesn't work well or too little of it overall, exercise can help your body use insulin more effectively. Weight loss can also help. Being more sensitive to the insulin you do have means that less insulin can lower blood glucose more. In people who have insulin resistance, improving the action of insulin may even reverse the course of their disease.

When overweight people with type 2 diabetes lose just 7 percent of their body weight, their insulin action increases by 57 percent.

Even if you don't have diabetes, you may still be insulin resistant. Being overweight, staying sedentary, and eating a poor diet can all lead to insulin resistance, in which case your body will need more insulin to get the job done. If you're insulin resistant, you can take steps to improve your insulin action that will benefit your overall health.

UNDERSTANDING INSULIN RESISTANCE

Regardless of which type of diabetes you have, you can become resistant to the effects of the hormone insulin, even if you have to pump or inject it instead of making your own. That fact makes insulin resistance relevant to everyone with diabetes of any type or prediabetes.

Think of insulin resistance with a lock and key analogy. In your body, glucose in the blood is trying to get through the door to your muscle and fat cells. To get inside the cells, the glucose must have a key to open the door. Insulin is the key that goes into the lock (or insulin receptors, in this case) to make it open. If you have the key (insulin), but the keyhole on the lock is blocked or the key won't turn when it goes in, then glucose can't enter, and you have insulin resistance — lots of insulin available but not working well. When the keys and the keyholes are functioning well together, the doors open, and glucose enters the cells and lowers the levels in the blood.

Navigating the Types of Diabetes

Diabetes comes in many forms — type 1, type 2, and gestational are the most common forms — as well as being tied to the related condition prediabetes. The following sections give you a glimpse into these conditions.

Taking a look at type 1 diabetes

About 5 to 10 percent of people have type 1 diabetes, which equates to around 1.25 million American children and adults. Prior to having this name, *type 1 diabetes* used to be called *insulin-dependent diabetes*, which is accurate because you have to take insulin if you have this type. But that name got confusing and was dropped because many people with type 2 diabetes use insulin as well.

Early on, type 1 was called *juvenile onset diabetes* because three-quarters of all cases are diagnosed in youth under 18. You can develop type 1 diabetes at any age, though, and most people living with type 1 are adults who inject or pump insulin daily to survive. Because adults also get type 1 diabetes, this term was inaccurate and misunderstood and was, therefore, abandoned decades ago.

Type 1 diabetes results from a relative insulin deficiency, which occurs after the body's own immune system destroys the *beta cells* of the pancreas that make insulin. Although the trigger for this autoimmune response is unclear, it's likely due to a combination of a genetic predisposition and environmental factors. Some causes under investigation include exposure to certain viruses, early introduction of cow's milk or other proteins in the diet of infants, and lack of vitamin D.

How rapidly type 1 diabetes develops is quite variable; it's rapid in some individuals (mainly infants and children) and slow in others (mainly adults). In either case, the symptoms of elevated blood glucose first appear when only about 10 percent of the insulin-making capacity of the pancreas remains.

Talking about type 2 diabetes

About 90 to 95 percent of cases of diabetes are *type 2 diabetes,* which used to be called *non-insulin-dependent diabetes* and *adult onset diabetes.* Most people diagnosed with type 2 are adults, but it has become more common among teenagers with the current obesity epidemic and prevalence of sedentary lifestyles. It's largely related to lifestyle habits that promote insulin resistance and other bodily changes that lead to high blood glucose levels.

Type 2 diabetes primarily results from an inability of insulin to work well enough to lower blood glucose to normal levels, a state of insulin resistance. However, most people with type 2 diabetes suffer from some degree of beta cell burnout, which leads to a diminishing release of insulin over time and rising blood glucose levels. The beta cells in the pancreas that make insulin lose some or all of their ability to produce insulin when exposed to high levels of blood glucose over time.

REMEMBER

If you develop type 2 diabetes, you likely have insulin resistance, paired with insulin secretion that is maximal but insufficient. In other words, your body can't make enough insulin to fully overcome your body's resistance to it.

Many consider type 2 diabetes a less severe condition than type 1, but type 2 is more complex in its origin. With this type, you likely have an underlying genetic susceptibility that, when exposed to a variety of social, behavioral, and/or environmental factors, unleashes a latent tendency for diabetes. In other words, diabetes genes are triggered by combined environmental and lifestyle factors, such as inactivity, poor eating habits, weight gain, exposure to pollutants, vitamin and mineral deficiencies, and more.

Although having a family history of type 2 increases your risk, the recent, unprecedented increase in type 2 diabetes cases suggests that a bigger cause is a combination of factors that increase insulin resistance, such as a sedentary lifestyle and a poor diet. Many people who get this type of diabetes don't have any relatives with it. Having a parent, sibling, or other close relative who has it increases your risk of developing it, though.

TIP

Particularly when you're first diagnosed with type 2 diabetes, you may be able to manage your blood glucose levels effectively or even reverse your diabetes by making lifestyle changes, such as exercising regularly and eating a better diet.

Getting a handle on gestational diabetes

Women can develop *gestational diabetes* during pregnancy if their blood glucose levels rise too high, which is most likely to happen during the second or third trimester. Pregnancy hormones make the mother more insulin resistant — to spare glucose for the developing fetus — but her blood glucose can rise as a result.

Managing blood glucose during pregnancy is important because elevated levels aren't good for the mother or the baby. Unborn babies make their own insulin during the third trimester and can get too large (over 9 pounds) from gaining extra fat when exposed to high levels of glucose, making the birth process difficult for the mother and the child. Babies can also have other health problems if the mother's glucose levels aren't managed well enough.

If you have ever given birth to a baby weighing 9 pounds or more, then you likely had gestational diabetes during your pregnancy (whether diagnosed or not).

You often can manage blood glucose levels during pregnancy with physical activity and dietary changes (particularly limiting carbohydrate intake). Regular exercise is recommended for all women during pregnancy, but it's even more important if you have or are at high risk for developing gestational diabetes. Some women must take diabetes medications that are acceptable during pregnancy to manage their blood glucose levels.

WARNING

Although gestational diabetes usually disappears after the baby is born, it increases the mother's risk for developing type 2 diabetes later in life.

Previewing prediabetes

Prediabetes is basically a relative state of insulin resistance. About 40 percent of adults between 40 and 74 years old who were screened in 2000 were diagnosed with prediabetes. In 2014, 86 million Americans age 20 and older had prediabetes, up from only 79 million in 2011. That is a huge number of people affected by this condition.

Even though blood glucose levels aren't in a diabetic range yet with prediabetes, having prediabetes puts you at high risk for progressing to type 2 diabetes at some point in your lifetime. What's more, you can develop some of the complications usually associated with diabetes, like nerve damage in your feet, heart disease, and stroke, while only having prediabetes.

TIP

You can reverse prediabetes with improvements to your lifestyle. The same changes that help manage type 2 diabetes — regular exercise, a more healthful diet, and fat weight loss — can help eliminate prediabetes and prevent its progression into full-blown diabetes.

Diagnosing Diabetes or Prediabetes

Some people have symptoms of diabetes before they're diagnosed, but many more never have any or realize that any symptoms they're having are related to diabetes. That makes it even more important to get annual checkups — particularly when you're getting older — that measure your fasting blood glucose. Of course, that's only one way to diagnose it, and testing only fasting levels misses some people who experience spikes in their blood glucose after eating although their morning levels are just fine.

Recognizing the symptoms

The more classic symptoms of *hyperglycemia,* or elevated blood glucose levels, include increased thirst, excessive urination, unusual fatigue, blurred vision, unexplained hunger, rapid weight loss, and slow-healing cuts and infections. These symptoms are common in youth who develop type 1 diabetes rapidly. However, diabetes can have subtle symptoms and may go undetected for some time, particularly in adults who develop it slowly.

TIP

If you or a loved one has complained recently about excessive thirst, frequent urination, or excessive hunger, schedule an appointment with your doctor or health care provider to check for diabetes.

REMEMBER

These symptoms aren't always indicative of diabetes. Sometimes elevated glucose levels can occur temporarily due to illness or medication use.

Testing for diabetes and prediabetes

Three main clinical methods are currently approved for diagnosing diabetes or prediabetes: fasting plasma glucose, oral glucose tolerance, and the A1C test (glycated hemoglobin). Any test that appears to indicate that you have either of these conditions should be repeated a second time (on another day) before your diagnosis is officially confirmed.

REMEMBER

Though this test isn't a usual official method, diabetes can sometimes be diagnosed when someone experiences the classic symptoms of hyperglycemia *and* has a random plasma glucose value of 200 mg/dL or higher.

Fasting plasma glucose

This simple blood test measures your blood glucose levels after an overnight fast of at least eight hours. It determines the amount of glucose in plasma, which is the clear part of the blood with all the red blood cells removed.

The fasting value is reported (in the United States) in mg/dL, which is simply a measure of the amount of glucose (in milligrams, or mg) in a set amount of plasma (100 milliliters, which equals 1 deciliter, or dL). Outside of the United States or in research papers, it's reported as mmol/L (millimoles per liter, or sometimes mM). *Note:* To convert from mg/dL to mmol/L, divide the value in mg/dL by 18.

The fasting plasma levels used for diagnosis are

>> **Normal:** 70 to 99 mg/dL (3.9 to 5.5 mmol/L)

>> **Prediabetes:** 100 to 125 mg/dL (5.6 to 6.9 mmol/L)

>> **Diabetes:** 126 mg/dL (7.0 mmol/L) or above

Prediabetes is diagnosed when your fasting glucose levels are elevated above normal (also known as *impaired fasting glucose,* or IFG). Diabetes is diagnosed when your fasting plasma glucose exceeds the prediabetes range.

Being on the lower end of the normal range in the morning is always better, and you should take steps to lower it if it rises over time toward the high end of normal.

Oral glucose tolerance

An alternate testing method is the oral glucose tolerance test (OGTT), which involves drinking 75 grams of glucose and having your blood glucose monitored for two to three hours afterward. This approach tests your body's ability to respond to a large influx of sugar. If your blood glucose goes up or stays up too high for long from this oral sugar load, you're said to have *impaired glucose tolerance* (IGT). This test is used to diagnose diabetes, prediabetes, and gestational diabetes.

Make sure to have your fasting blood glucose levels tested annually, and an A1C test (discussed in the following section) as well if you can swing it.

A1C test (glycated hemoglobin)

A third approved method to diagnose diabetes is to test your A1C (previously called glycated hemoglobin or hemoglobin A1C). The A1C indicates your average blood glucose over the past two or three months. Basically, the higher your blood glucose has been, the more glucose will be "stuck" to the hemoglobin part of red blood cells, and those blood cells live about 120 days.

This simple blood test can also be used to diagnose prediabetes because it averages in post-meal spikes in your blood glucose that a fasting value may not detect. Finding out your risk for developing diabetes is important because complications can occur when your A1C test is still in the normal range (at the high end).

Interpreting your test results

Table 1-1 illustrates how the results of these tests are used to diagnose diabetes and prediabetes.

Your test results can be confusing because you may not get diagnosed with diabetes with one test, but meet the criteria for another. To be considered as having diabetes, you only have to meet the criteria for one test. But then how your diabetes is managed may vary based on which category you met. For instance, if you just have elevated fasting levels but your A1C is okay, your doctor may put you on a medication that will lower your morning blood glucose. If your blood glucose shoots up after meals (as indicated by an oral glucose test), you may need a medication that makes your pancreas release more insulin when you eat but not at other times of day.

Talk to your doctor or health care provider about your diagnosis and the best course of action to follow based on your test results.

TABLE 1-1   **Diagnosis of Diabetes and Prediabetes**

Diabetes Diagnosis	Fasting Plasma Glucose	Oral Glucose Tolerance Test (OGTT)	A1C	Symptoms
Type 1	≥ 126 mg/dL (7.0 mM)	2-hour value: ≥ 200 mg/dL (11.1 mM)	6.5% or higher	Classic symptoms of hyperglycemia or a random plasma glucose ≥ 200 mg/dL (11.1 mM)
Type 2	≥ 126 mg/dL (7.0 mM)	2-hour value: ≥ 200 mg/dL (11.1 mM)	6.5% or higher	Classic symptoms of hyperglycemia or a random plasma glucose ≥ 200 mg/dL (11.1 mM)
Gestational	≥ 92 mg/dL (5.1 mM)	1-hour value: ≥ 180 mg/dL (10.0 mM) or 2-hour value: ≥ 153 mg/dL (8.5 mM)		
Prediabetes	100–125 mg/dL (5.6–6.9 mM)	2-hour value: 140–199 mg/dL (7.8–11.0 mM)	5.7–6.4%	

Getting tested for gestational diabetes

Gestational diabetes is typically tested for and diagnosed between 24 and 28 weeks of pregnancy with an oral glucose tolerance test. Managing it may involve using insulin or other medications, along with diet changes and regular exercise. All pregnant women should be screened for this condition no later than 28 weeks and possibly even earlier if it was diagnosed during previous pregnancies.

FIND OUT YOUR PREDIABETES RISK ONLINE

A quick and easy way to assess your risk for prediabetes is to take an online risk test created by the American Diabetes Association. It asks you a few simple questions about your diet, activity levels, body shape and size, and more and only takes a couple of minutes to do.

Access the Association's prediabetes risk test online at www.doIhaveprediabetes.org.

The good news is that prediabetes is possible to reverse with some simple and easy lifestyle changes like some small changes in your diet and a little more exercise. Find out if you're at risk and start making those lifestyle improvements now, and you may avoid ever getting prediabetes or type 2 diabetes.

Being misdiagnosed with type 2 diabetes

Given the current diagnosis methods for diabetes, determining which kind of diabetes a person has can sometimes be difficult. In addition, diabetes can sometimes have other causes, such as pancreatic cancer or other rare conditions. Having excess body fat used to lead to an almost guaranteed diagnosis of type 2 diabetes, but that is no longer the case because people who develop type 1 are often overweight and can develop an insulin-resistant state related to weight gain, dietary choices, and physical inactivity.

As many as 20 percent of adults who develop type 1 later in life may initially be misdiagnosed with type 2 due to their older age and slower onset. Being misdiagnosed because of your adult age is common, and you may initially respond well to oral diabetes medications (which further confuses the diagnosis). But you're not likely to be as insulin resistant as someone who has type 2 diabetes.

TIP

If you're an extremely athletic adult (age 25 or older) and you were diagnosed with type 2 over the age of 18 while regularly active and at normal or near-normal body weight, you likely have a slow-onset form of type 1 diabetes instead.

REMEMBER

You can get antibody tests done to help make the diagnosis between type 1 and type 2. Knowing which you have can help because starting insulin therapy (rather than diabetes pills) early may help preserve your remaining beta cells for a little longer.

Self-Monitoring Your Blood Glucose

People living successfully with any type of diabetes use their blood glucose meters regularly. Frequent testing allows you to detect patterns and learn your body's unique response to different things — foods, activities, medications, emotional and physical stress, and more. Then you can adjust your medications, insulin, or lifestyle to better manage your blood glucose and prevent future health problems.

You may wake up every day and test, and your blood glucose is somewhat consistent then. But do you know what it's doing the rest of the day? What effect does eating one food have on it compared with another or doing one type of exercise rather than a different one?

TIP

If you don't know the answers to these questions, consider occasionally monitoring at alternate times — such as before and after exercise — even if you don't increase the number of times a day you check overall. Testing your blood glucose at different times rather than just first thing in the morning or before meals can often reveal trends with your blood glucose that you may not notice otherwise.

Here's another reason monitoring is important. Minimizing post-meal glucose spikes may be the key to preventing microvascular (small blood vessel) complications like diabetic eye disease (retinopathy). Testing not only before meals but also one hour and two hours afterward can let you know how meals and different foods are affecting your blood glucose and how much variability you're experiencing.

Regardless of which type of diabetes you have, your blood glucose typically starts to rise in 20 minutes and peaks in one to two hours after eating. It's recommended that you check blood glucose one to two hours after your first bite of a meal. However, blood glucose changes after meals vary widely from person to person and can even differ within one person depending on the food, time of day, and recent exercise.

How much your blood glucose goes up in the two hours after a meal may be just as important in causing diabetes complications as overall glucose control — maybe even more so.

Using a Blood Glucose Meter

Depending on your medications, you may have to make some changes to keep your levels optimal. Regardless of what type of diabetes you have, using injected or pumped insulin requires you to be vigilant to manage diabetes with activity. Even if you don't typically get low blood glucose during exercise, monitoring frequently is still advisable.

Most insulin users agree that glucose monitoring is essential for detecting patterns and making changes, although it still involves a lot of trial and error for each individual by activity. Blood glucose levels can be monitored in various ways at present, including blood glucose meters and continuous glucose monitors.

Using a meter, you can manage the many factors affecting your unique responses by checking your blood glucose levels before, during, and after exercise.

If you use certain oral medications, you may have higher risk for developing *hypoglycemia*, or low blood glucose. Luckily, type 2 exercisers aren't prone to developing diabetic ketoacidosis (DKA) — which can be life-threatening — even when their blood glucose runs high, but knowing your starting level is still important when you have that type of diabetes. Flip to Chapter 4 to find out more about this condition.

Monitoring can be motivational, especially when your blood glucose goes down from an activity and you're hoping to lower it that way.

Tackling types of meters

Many different blood glucose meters are available for self-monitoring. Most give readings in only five seconds and are small enough to carry around in your pocket or small bag. They vary somewhat in accuracy, but using whichever one you have access to is still better than checking infrequently or not at all. Talking to a certified diabetes educator may help you find the meter that is right for you.

You may want to consider these factors when choosing a meter:

>> **Insurance coverage:** Your provider may limit your coverage to certain models or only reimburse for a limited number of test strips per month. Choose a meter that gives you the greatest flexibility when it comes to testing as much as possible.

>> **Cost:** Although costs for the meters themselves have come down tremendously over time, they still vary in price, as do the test strips. Be sure to factor that in when making your selection.

>> **Ease of use and features:** Check out a variety of meters to see which ones are easier for you to use. Do you need one with big numbers on the screen that are easier to read? Do you need one with auditory cues? Is it easy to hold in your hand? Some meters are equipped with large, easy-to-handle buttons and test strips; illuminated screens; and audio, which may be useful for people with impaired vision. Consider these factors when making your choice.

>> **Data storage:** Many meters now track everything so you don't have to write anything down (including time, date, trends, and so on), and others let you input data like whether the reading is before or after a meal or exercise. Most allow you to download all your results to a computer or upload them to a mobile device or app. Consider which of these features would make your life and diabetes management easier.

Examining what affects meter readings

Many things can cause you to get erroneous readings using your blood glucose meter, which can then lead you to make incorrect or inappropriate adjustments to your diabetes regimen. Be careful to avoid these situations if you can. Some meters are rather inaccurate, but you can throw your measured values off further with the following:

>> **Dirty fingers:** Wash your hands before testing.

>> **Cold fingers:** Warm them up before attempting to get a finger stick sample.

>> **Calluses on fingertips:** Choose a less callused spot to prick.

>> **Excessive squeezing of fingers:** You can dilute your blood this way.

>> **Dehydration:** Being dehydrated makes blood glucose seem higher than it is.

Looking ahead to other ways to measure blood glucose

For many years, the race has been on to develop an effective noninvasive monitor that doesn't require actual blood samples, or at least not pricking your fingers or other body part with a lancet, but such devices are still in development (like the Google contact lenses that are supposed to monitor glucose levels in the eye). Such devices will likely be available in the near future and make exercise and daily monitoring even easier. Make sure you only rely on ones that have been approved by the FDA, though, as some fitness vendors have started hawking unapproved ones that may not be accurate enough for making safe and effective diabetes management decisions.

Exploring the pros and cons of continuous glucose monitors

Other glucose monitoring devices called *continuous glucose monitors* (CGMs) have been approved by the FDA for use in the past decade or so. They're still invasive, requiring that you place a small and thin wire filament under your skin. Most of these monitors aren't a complete closed-loop system (yet), meaning that currently you still have to check the blood glucose readings and make regimen adjustments yourself based on those results. One combined insulin pump and CGM sensor system that adjusts basal rates overnight and throughout the day without your input is now approved and on the market, and more with this feature are coming soon. Even with just the readings, however, obtaining a glucose reading every 5 minutes 24 hours a day can be quite useful to people who are trying to learn their patterns and keep blood glucose in tighter, more normal ranges.

REMEMBER

Though it's worn more frequently by people with type 1 diabetes, CGM technology can be used to determine which exercise programs are most beneficial for lowering blood glucose in people with type 2 diabetes.

CGM can provide useful information on glucose fluctuations. Although this technology is advancing, it still is imperfect. These systems currently measure glucose levels in the skin (in interstitial fluids between cells) rather than the blood, a lag between actual and measured blood glucose levels of anywhere from 6 to 12 or more minutes, and the values it displays are also time-delayed from 2.5 to 7.5 minutes.

Thus, its trend arrows (for example, one or two arrows down or up, with more arrows indicating a faster rate of change) aren't perfectly in sync with rapidly changing blood glucose levels that can occur during exercise or after eating a meal. When blood glucose levels are rising, the CGM is likely to display values that are lower than actual blood glucose, and when they're falling, it may display values that are higher than blood glucose actually is. CGM values can also be inaccurate due to other factors, such as improper insertion of the sensors under the skin, irritation of the skin in that area, or improper monitor calibration.

On the helpful side, at least one CGM system now allows cloud sharing of values in real-time, which is especially appealing to parents of children with type 1 diabetes or significant others of adults wearing CGM devices. Wouldn't life be simpler if you always knew in real time that your loved one had a blood glucose level in a safe range?

TECHNICAL STUFF

Some of the newer-generation CGM systems can communicate with insulin pumps and suspend insulin delivery when low blood glucose levels are detected and adjust basal rates based on sensor values. These developments are some of the first steps in creating a viable closed-loop insulin delivery and glucose monitoring system that combines CGM and insulin pumps. Many research groups are using the two technologies together with a central control unit with algorithms to create a system that can balance blood glucose levels in people with type 1 diabetes without much, if any, user input. These so-called artificial pancreas systems are still subject to the many limitations that these technologies currently have, including measurement of interstitial fluid glucose (rather than blood glucose), time lags, and insulin delivery under the skin (rather than directly into the vein that flows from the pancreas to the liver, the *portal vein*). In the near future, other devices like heart rate monitors or accelerometers (movement and activity monitors) may eventually be paired with such systems to make them more effective during exercise.

Discovering Why Being Fit with Diabetes Matters

Without a doubt, being physically active is good for your body, heart, and mind. If you're already an avid exerciser, then you're likely aware of most of the benefits of exercise for your physical health and your diabetes management. If you're just getting serious about engaging in more fitness activities or sports, you have many positive changes to look forward to.

TIP

Exercising regularly is likely the single most important thing you can do to keep your blood glucose in check, prevent or reduce your risk of developing diabetes-related or other health complications, and slow down aging.

Exercise can help you build muscle and lose body fat, suppress your appetite, eat more without gaining fat weight, enhance your mood, reduce stress and anxiety, increase your energy, bolster your immune system, keep your joints and muscles more flexible, and improve the quality of your life — all this and more, especially when you have diabetes.

Getting and staying fit when you have diabetes (or prediabetes) is even more important. For many people, being physically active has made all the difference between managing and living well with diabetes or letting it control them. People who are physically fit live longer, healthier lives. It's not just about living longer, but living well and feeling your best as you age. Having diabetes increases your risk of getting health problems that can reduce your quality of life. You can fight back by keeping fit.

TIP

Confused about which activities you should you be doing or how much is necessary to be as healthy as you can be? You get different (but all good) results from doing a variety of types of daily activity, and that gives you a lot of options.

diabetes

» Raising insulin action with physical activity (and other factors)

» Consulting with your health care provider and establishing training goals

» Considering your chances for cardiovascular disease

» Having a long, full life despite diabetes/prediabetes

Chapter **2**

Managing Health and Diabetes Fitness

G etting fit can benefit your health, whether or not you have diabetes or pre-diabetes. Physical activity makes your insulin work better. More effective insulin action usually results in improved blood glucose.

In this chapter, you get guidance on managing your diabetes and improving your health, along with the keys to making goals that stick and help you get fitter and keep fit for life. You also discover when seeing your doctor before getting started on your new fitness goals may be best — such as before you start working out too hard if you've been a couch potato recently.

Knowing the Importance of Getting Moving

Many people — youth and adults alike — are becoming overweight in large part because they're failing to engage in enough daily physical movement and making unhealthful food choices. Americans have become a society of overweight, sedentary people. Despite knowing the health benefits of exercise, nearly half of all American adults aren't active at all, and 70 percent fail to meet the recommended 30 minutes of exercise a day on most days.

Becoming physically active is more than worth the effort because the more sedentary you stay, the greater your risk of dying prematurely. If that's not convincing enough, think about your daily life. The quality of your life matters even more than just being alive, and staying on the couch increases the chance that you won't feel as good as you can for much of your (shortened) life.

REMEMBER

Feeling well during your lifetime is truly more important than simply living longer, especially if your later years are burdened by health problems and limitations.

For people with diabetes, inactivity is even more rampant. If you have diabetes, you may keep yourself from being active because being active can potentially unbalance your blood glucose, or you may be dealing with another health issue. But you have to ask yourself: Do you really want to spend the last 20 years of your life impaired by even more diabetes-related health complications? You can improve your quality of life with diabetes and prevent most health problems by getting off the couch and keeping fit.

TIP

The time to get your body moving more and your health optimized is now. It's never too late to start reaping the benefits of an active and healthier lifestyle, even if you start by simply standing more each day.

Understanding How Exercise and Food Affect Your Body with Diabetes

Having a basic understanding of what is happening in your body when your glucose levels get high is helpful so you know what you can do about it. Regardless of whether you have prediabetes or diabetes (which I describe in Chapter 1), exercise works to lower insulin resistance and improve your blood glucose management. By combining regular activity with more healthful eating and possibly medications, you can take control of your blood glucose and your overall health.

WHY EXERCISE REALLY IS THE BEST DIABETES MEDICINE

Exercise truly is a magic bullet for optimizing quality of life, and if you have diabetes, the physical and mental health benefits are magnified. From a metabolic standpoint, being fit is always better, no matter what your body weight is. Exercise enhances your body's sensitivity to insulin, usually resulting in better blood glucose levels. Many chronic diseases in addition to type 2 diabetes are associated with reductions in your insulin action (including hypertension and heart disease). Exercise may also enhance your body's ability to produce more insulin — as long as enough functional beta cells remain in your pancreas. (Head to Chapter 1 for more on beta cells.)

Regular exercise also lowers your risk of premature death, heart disease, certain types of cancers (colon, prostate, and breast, to name a few), anxiety and depression, osteoporosis, and severe arthritic symptoms. It even helps you sleep better, which is especially important because sleeping too little (for example, only five hours a night) has been linked with increased incidence of overweight and obesity, not to mention insulin resistance — even in healthy young adults. In fact, if exercise isn't a potential cure for everything that ails you, then I don't know what is. When it comes to diabetes, exercise is powerful medicine, and all the side effects are good ones.

Recognizing why exercise training is critical

In short, exercise bypasses the need for insulin to lower blood glucose, even if you're insulin resistant the rest of the time. That means you have an alternate way to bring glucose levels down without being dependent on your insulin to do it.

During rest, muscles cells depend on insulin to allow blood glucose to enter. Insulin binds to insulin receptors on the surface of individual cells, which starts a series of enzymatic reactions inside the cells that allow glucose to be transported across the cell membrane, thus lowering blood levels.

However, when the muscles are active during exercise, insulin isn't required to start this reaction. The muscle contractions themselves trigger an alternate pathway that gets glucose from the blood into active muscle without using insulin at all.

Your muscles can continue to bring in more glucose — without insulin initially — for a period of time after exercise (typically 2 to 72 hours, depending on the type of activity done). That helps you lower blood glucose naturally and lasts as long as your muscles are replenishing their carbohydrate (glycogen) stores. Several hours after exercise ends, insulin is back to being the main way to lower blood glucose, but its action is higher than it was before you worked out.

REMEMBER

Your insulin action is usually dependent on how long ago you did your last cardio workout. Resistance training also increases insulin action in resting muscles, but that occurs though a different mechanism related to increases in muscle size and mass.

TIP

You can manage your blood glucose better by exercising at least three to four days per week doing any activity. (But to lose weight most effectively, you'll likely need to aim for exercising for 60 minutes six to seven days per week to burn more calories.)

Grasping how food affects your blood glucose

Food and calorie-filled drinks are made up of *macronutrients* (carbohydrate, protein, and fat) that can be converted into usable energy in the body and *micronutrients* (like vitamins and minerals) that help your body break down the macronutrients. These macronutrients supply your body with energy, or calories, although each serves a different primary role:

>> **Carbohydrate** is a major fuel source for the body, especially during physical activity, and the primary supplier of energy for your brain, nerves, and muscles.

>> **Protein** helps build muscle and forms the basis of many hormones, enzymes, and other structures in the body.

>> **Fat** provides an important source of stored energy and adds to the health of your brain, nerves, hair, skin, and nails.

Though each of these nutrients potentially affects your blood glucose in different ways, it's the carbohydrates you eat that have the greatest impact on the amount of glucose in your blood. The body converts carbohydrates into simple sugars — glucose being the primary one — soon after you eat them, usually within five minutes to two hours depending on the type. Only minimal amounts of protein and fat become glucose after digestion, so they don't affect your blood glucose nearly as much.

You should check your blood glucose before and after meals to get a feel for how foods, particularly those containing a lot of carbohydrate (such as potatoes, bread, rice, pasta, fruit, fruit juice, and desserts), affect your blood glucose.

REMEMBER

Your blood glucose is at its highest generally one hour after eating, remains high for up to two hours, and then starts to fall. Check your blood glucose one to two hours after you eat to see how the food you ate affected your levels.

When you eat a higher-fat meal, your digestive process is somewhat slowed down, and your blood glucose may not reach its highest point until four to five hours later. What's more, high-fat foods cause insulin resistance, which, together with slower digestion, may lead to higher blood glucose levels hours after you eat when your muscle, fat, and liver cells aren't using the insulin in your body properly to lower blood glucose. Many of these options are best considered "get you now, get you later" foods because they can raise your blood glucose at both these times if you are a meal-time insulin user.

Uncovering More about Fitness and Aging

Aging by itself causes bodily changes, many of which are independent of disease, even if you remain physically active throughout your lifetime. Diabetes can also cause health complications that are separate from the effects of aging. Sometimes, it's hard to tell whether your health issues are arising from diabetes or normal effects of getting older. For instance, people without diabetes can develop nerve damage (*neuropathy*) in their feet, especially if they're taller.

Questioning whether aging, inactivity, or diabetes is to blame

The changes your body undergoes over time are complex and involve both normal physiological and disease processes. In general, your body experiences very gradual and subtle alterations in how well its different systems like breathing, digestion, and sexual ability function over time.

Human cells apparently can split and reproduce a limited number of times. After your cells slow their rate of turnover, these subtle changes start to accelerate. Unfortunately, such effects are often inseparable from the onset of diseases like heart disease and cancer.

However, much of what people attribute to getting older — such as muscle atrophy or loss of flexibility in joints — results from disuse over time, not just from aging. At one point, researchers believed that greater insulin resistance was practically inevitable with aging due to a natural loss of muscle mass over time. But more recent studies have shown that master athletes are as insulin sensitive as younger individuals who are physically active, and they also have better insulin action than people of any age who are sedentary and either of normal weight or obese. Being sedentary can lead to insulin resistance even if you stay thin, most likely due to dual losses of muscle from aging and inactivity.

REMEMBER

Some health problems *are* directly related to diabetes and elevated blood glucose over time, such as diabetic eye disease. You can prevent or slow the onset of many of these health complications with better blood glucose management, more healthful food choices, and regular physical activity.

TIP

Do what you can to prevent diabetes-related and other health complications by staying active and making better food choices.

Slowing down aging with exercise

TIP

Being regularly active is the most important thing you can do to slow the aging process, manage insulin resistance, and reduce your risk of health problems.

Having diabetes or prediabetes — especially when your insulin resistance is high or your blood glucose is poorly managed — can cause premature aging, accelerated heart disease, and other chronic illnesses. In such cases, regular exercise can keep you looking and feeling younger for longer and even greatly lower your risk of getting any health complications.

Getting in regular workouts has an immediate effect on your overall physical condition by slowing aging and preventing diseases that can shorten your life span or rob you of your vitality as you age. For example, bone density peaks somewhere around 25 years of age, after which time bones may start to lose some stored calcium and other minerals over time — unless you stress the bones with physical movement and stimulate them to retain more minerals. A sedentary lifestyle, conversely, leads to thinning bones, the potential for fractures, and a reduced quality of life.

REMEMBER

You must also routinely use muscles fibers to prevent excess loss of muscle with each passing decade of your life.

Investigating the Impact of Fitness and Other Factors on Insulin Action

Keeping fit is more important to living well than you can possibly know. In fact, it's likely the most critical behavior you can adopt to impact how well your insulin works in your body. Insulin resistance is linked to multiple health problems, including type 2 diabetes, high blood pressure, reduced blood flow, inflammation, heart disease, and many more. A lack of physical activity is linked directly to defects in the action of insulin primarily at the level of your muscle and fat cells.

Looking at what impacts how insulin works

The two main body tissues that are sensitive to the effects of insulin are your muscle cells and *adipose,* or fat, tissue. Obesity is associated with an accumulation of stored fat inside both muscle and adipose cells. Muscle is an important storage site for excess glucose and carbohydrates. But when your muscles get filled with excess fat or carbohydrates, they become less sensitive to insulin, and your pancreas must release more insulin to have the same effect (or if you need insulin, you'll need to take higher doses).

A third tissue also responsive to and affected by insulin is your liver. This organ is responsible for making sure you have enough glucose in your blood at all times. It can both store and release glucose to keep levels constant.

In some people with diabetes, the liver becomes insulin resistant and releases too much glucose, especially overnight when they go for long periods without eating. Gaining a lot of excess fat within your abdomen (called *visceral fat*) and within the liver itself can contribute to an insulin resistance there.

Interestingly, your fat cells usually remain largely responsive to insulin even when your muscle cells become resistant, and much of your excess blood glucose can be converted into storage fat. When the carbohydrates you eat end up spiking your blood glucose, the rise causes the release of more insulin and ultimately more fat storage in fat cells and likely your liver.

REMEMBER

Being active helps reverse insulin resistance in your liver and reduces the amount of metabolically bad, visceral fat stored inside your abdomen.

Revving up your insulin action

Think of your muscles as a glucose tank, a place to store the carbohydrates that you eat and don't need to use right away, as shown in Figure 2-1. When you exercise regularly, you use up glycogen stored in the muscles and have room to put carbohydrates back in after you eat. If the glycogen stores are already full because you've consumed too many carbohydrates or exercised too little, your muscles can't store more carbohydrates after you eat, and you're insulin resistant. This state is reversible with exercise.

TIP

To raise your insulin sensitivity, keep your muscle glucose tank as big as possible (by doing resistance and other training regularly) and partway empty (by being active on a daily basis, or at least every other day).

Physical activity isn't the only factor that can improve your insulin action, however, and most of them you have some control over. Addressing these factors can raise your body's insulin action and consequently reverse prediabetes or improve diabetes management.

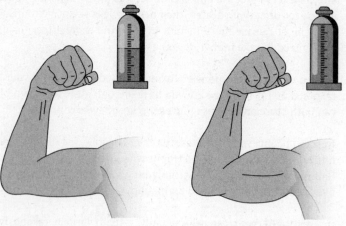

FIGURE 2-1:
The muscle glucose tank.

© John Wiley & Sons, Inc.

REMEMBER

Factors that can boost insulin action in your muscles include the following:

» Regular aerobic, resistance, interval, and other types of exercise

» Tighter blood glucose management

» Increase in overall muscle mass

» Loss of body fat, particularly visceral fat and extra fat stored in the liver

» Intake of more dietary fiber, less manufactured trans fat, and fewer highly refined foods

» Daily consumption of a healthy breakfast

» Lower daily caffeine intake

» Reduced levels of circulating free fatty acids (fat in blood)

» Reduction in mental stressors (depression, anxiety, stress, and so on)

» Better control of physical stressors (illness, infection, exhaustion, and so on)

» Adequate sleep (seven to eight hours a night for most adults)

» Effective treatment of sleep apnea

» Use of insulin-sensitizing medications

>> Reduction in low-level, systemic inflammation

>> Decrease in circulating levels of cortisol

>> Increased testosterone levels in men

TIP

If you're trying to improve your insulin action (or lose weight) and your body releases a large amount of insulin in response to the carbohydrates you eat, you may benefit from eating a food plan that is moderate in carbohydrate. Talk to a registered dietitian or nutritionist about the best plan for you.

Deciding When to Consult with Your Doctor First

How do you know whether you need to see your doctor before you start to exercise? The bottom line is that you probably don't need a checkup before engaging in easy workouts or moderate activities like brisk walking, but having one before you begin more vigorous workouts is a good idea. It also depends on your age, your general health, and your current physical activity level.

If your blood glucose has been in check, you've already been physically active, and you don't have any serious diabetic complications, then exercise away. If you're very active, getting an extra checkup before you replace your current exercise regime with another exercise routine is definitely unnecessary. Having regular visits to your doctor or other health care provider, though, is a good idea for anyone who has diabetes or prediabetes.

If you have a checkup, get your blood pressure, heart rate, and body weight measured, and ask whether you need to do an exercise stress test, which usually involves walking on a treadmill or riding a stationary bike for around ten minutes. *Note:* The American Diabetes Association recommends an exercise stress test only if you're over 40 and have diabetes or if you're over 30 and have had diabetes for 10 or more years, smoke, have high blood pressure, have high cholesterol, or have eye or kidney problems related to diabetes. Above all, this recommendation applies only to people planning to do vigorous training that gets their heart rates up high. If you'll just be doing mild or moderate aerobic activity or resistance training, such extensive (and often expensive) testing may not be necessary.

Your checkup may also include a urinalysis, kidney function testing, serum lipid evaluation, and electrolyte analysis, along with screening for any diabetes-related complications, including heart, nerve, eye, and kidney disease. Though such health problems don't usually keep you from exercising, doing so safely and effectively with them may require special accommodations or precautions.

CURRENTLY SEDENTARY? YOU MAY NEED A CHECKUP

Get a checkup from your doctor or health care provider first if you're sedentary and you

- Are planning on participating in vigorous activities, not just easy or moderate ones

- Are over 40 years old (or over 30, if you have any of the indicators in the remaining bullets)

- Have had diabetes for more than ten years

- Have heart disease, a strong family history of heart disease, or high cholesterol

- Have poor circulation in your feet or legs (or lower leg pain while walking)

- Have diabetic eye disease, kidney disease, numbness, burning, tingling, or loss of sensation in your feet, and/or dizziness when going from sitting to standing

- Haven't consistently managed your blood glucose levels well

- Have any other concerns about exercising, including joint pain, arthritis, or other chronic health problems

REMEMBER

Exercise most days of the week because regular, moderate to vigorous activity can reduce your risk of having a heart attack, even if you've already had one before. Just realize and respect your limitations.

WARNING

If you have any preexisting health complications, you may need to take extra care to prevent problems during exercise. You may also still need to take certain precautions, particularly related to hypoglycemia, hyperglycemia, and dehydration. (Flip to Chapters 6 and 7, respectively, for more on blood glucose management and hydration during exercise.) If you have any concerns, check with your health care provider at your next visit to discuss any measures that may be important for your health when exercising.

Setting Diabetes, Health, and Fitness Goals

Health and training goals for most people revolve around lowering insulin resistance, managing diabetes and blood glucose levels, and losing weight and keeping it off. Regardless of your motivation for keeping fit, your overall health and your diabetes management can both benefit immensely from any physical activity that you do regularly.

REMEMBER

You may be able to completely avoid many health issues associated with long-term diabetes by adopting a healthier lifestyle and using exercise as a daily dose of medicine.

TIP

Whether you're setting goals related to your blood glucose or cholesterol levels or how often you're going to be active, you want goals that aren't too vague, broad, or difficult to reach. Chapter 8 has guidance on how to set up activity goals that are SMART (specific, measurable, attainable, realistic, and time-frame specific).

Diabetes targets and goals

Preventing your blood glucose from getting too low or too high during exercise is critical to exercising safely and effectively, particularly if you use certain diabetes medications or insulin. Whenever you start doing new or different activities, plan on testing your blood glucose to determine how your body reacts, including before and after exercise and even sometimes during a workout.

You should have a target for your blood glucose, both for certain times of day and for average levels over two to three months. Exercise has a short-term effect on your blood glucose (see the earlier section "Recognizing why exercise training is critical"), but it also has a longer lasting benefit: Your insulin (natural or injected) is more effective. With regular exercise, better insulin action helps lower your blood glucose levels, improve your diabetes management, and prevent health complications.

Table 2-1 gives the recommended targets for all your blood glucose numbers. It includes what you should aim for both before and after meals, as well as what a good average glucose (A1C) would be and how that corresponds to the values you see on your blood glucose meter.

TABLE 2-1 **Recommended Blood Glucose and A1C Targets**

Glucose Measure	Goals
Blood glucose (before and after meals) ADA goal – not AACE	70–120 mg/dL (3.9–6.7 mmol/L), before meals
	< 180 mg/dL (10.0 mmol/L), 2 hours after meals
A1C (glycated hemoglobin)	American Diabetes Association goal: < 7.0%
	American Association of Clinical Endocrinologists goal: < 6.5%
Average glucose (from A1C values)	American Diabetes Association goal: < 154 mg/dL (8.6 mmol/L)
	American Association of Clinical Endocrinologists goal: < 140 mg/dL (7.8 mmol/L)

Unlike a finger stick glucose, which represents only one point in time, an A1C value gives you an idea how your blood glucose has been averaging during the past several months, particularly the previous four weeks. Current recommendations suggest you should aim for a value of 7 percent (equivalent to average blood glucose levels of 154 mg/dL) or less. Some groups recommend a goal of less than 6.5 percent (non-diabetes values usually fall in the range of 4.0 to 5.6 percent). The lower your A1C is, the better it generally is for your health. If you have diabetes, you should routinely get your A1C tested every three to six months.

You can convert your A1C value into an equivalent glucose reading (shown in Table 2-2) to make it more meaningful when you see it. This average glucose tells you what your glucose has been in the same values you're used to seeing on your blood glucose meter.

TABLE 2-2   **A1C Converter to Average Glucose Equivalent**

A1C (%)	Average Glucose (mg/dL)	Average Glucose (mmol/L)
5.0	97	5.4
5.5	112	6.2
6.0	126	7.0
6.5	140	7.8
7.0	154	8.6
7.5	169	9.4
8.0	183	10.1
8.5	197	10.9
9.0	212	11.8
9.5	226	12.6
10.0	240	13.4
10.5	255	14.1
11.0	269	14.9
11.5	283	15.7
12.0	298	16.5
13.0	326	18.1
14.0	365	20.3

REMEMBER

Although useful for other reasons, an A1C test is an average and doesn't tell you about your glucose fluctuations — that is, the highest or lowest blood glucose levels that you've had or any variations that occurred with eating and exercise. Having frequent or large swings in blood glucose values is unhealthy, even if your A1C is within range, and you should avoid spikes and lows as much as possible.

Health goals

Many people with diabetes also have elevated levels of blood lipids (fats like triglycerides and cholesterol) that are associated with an increased risk for heart disease and stroke. Having diabetes by itself already increases your risk of having cardiovascular disease.

You likely can reach most of your health goals by adopting a physically active lifestyle and making better food choices. Losing weight usually helps improve blood lipid profiles, although aerobic exercise training without significant weight loss has been shown to improve metabolism, cholesterol levels, fasting glucose, and more in people with type 2 diabetes. Eating more fiber and fewer refined foods can also improve these health variables. You may be able to reduce or eliminate your need for cholesterol-lowering medications like statins.

Fitness goals

People decide to become more physically active for all sorts of reasons. Some are new to exercise and realize that making important lifestyle changes may allow them to manage type 2 diabetes, reverse prediabetes, and avoid diabetes medications early after their diagnosis. Others with type 1 diabetes are suffering from "double diabetes" due to being sedentary and gaining weight, and they may choose to benefit from starting an exercise program.

Many people are already active and want to train for a specific event, such as a 10K race or a half-marathon, and they need to increase their fitness to cross the finish line in style. Others may simply want to try a new sport or activity or get involved in cross-training to raise their level of fitness.

All these reasons for getting more physically active are appropriate. There is no wrong reason for getting and keeping fit when you have diabetes or prediabetes. (In fact, everyone should set some fitness goals — even if they don't have diabetes.) Just make sure your goals are realistic and achievable so that you don't get discouraged.

REMEMBER

Keeping fit should be a lifetime goal, not just a short-term one.

Surveying Cardiovascular Risks That May Limit Exercise

As I note earlier in the chapter, people with diabetes have a higher risk of developing cardiovascular disease. If you have additional risk factors for heart disease, your chances of having a heart attack or stroke during exercise are greater. For that reason alone, you should figure out what your risk factors are. The major cardiovascular risk factors include the following:

>> **Age:** The older you are, the higher your risk becomes simply because your body has had more time to develop plaque in arteries in various parts of your body, including your *coronary* (heart), *carotid* (neck), and other arteries.

>> **Sex:** Although men have a higher risk than women (at least until women go through menopause), having a disease like diabetes can even the playing field.

>> **Family history:** Having a *positive family history* means that you have close male relatives (father, brother, or son) with cardiovascular disease before age 55 or a close female relative (mother, sister, or daughter) with it before age 65.

>> **Elevated blood fats:** Aim for HDL (so-called good cholesterol) levels that are higher than 40 mg/dL in men and 50 mg/dL in women, and LDL (bad cholesterol) levels as low as possible. You can raise your HDL levels with regular exercise and lower LDL with a healthful diet that includes more vegetables, fresh fruit, whole grains, and fish and fewer fatty meats and trans fats.

>> **Cigarette smoking:** Cigarettes cause more cases of heart disease than they do lung cancer. Just cutting back on how much you smoke a day lowers your risk, but stopping completely is the way to go to remove this risk factor.

>> **Hypertension (high blood pressure):** Keeping your blood pressure under control greatly lowers your risk of having a stroke or developing heart disease; you can use exercise, diet, stress management, and medications to achieve this goal.

>> **Physical inactivity:** Simply being sedentary increases your risk for all forms of cardiovascular disease; doing any physical activity is far better than none, and any movement you do reduces your risk, even low-intensity activities.

>> **Poorly controlled diabetes and prediabetes:** Though diabetes by itself is an independent risk factor for cardiovascular problems, well-managed diabetes doesn't have the same bad effect. Change your lifestyle to better control your blood glucose, and you substantially lower your risk as well.

>> **Obesity:** Being obese or overweight increases your risk, especially if you carry your extra body weight in your abdominal region. Obesity increases blood fat levels and inflammation, both of which contribute to the formation of plaque in arteries, so use regular exercise and dietary changes to lose weight or prevent more weight gain.

The more risk factors you have, the greater your chance of developing heart disease, stroke, or peripheral artery disease. You can't really do much about some of these risks (like age or biological sex), but others you can. For example, getting rid of some of the fat inside your belly through exercise usually helps more than just lowering your overall weight with dieting.

Having an elevated degree of a particular risk increases your overall chances, too. For example, if your total cholesterol level is 300 mg/dL, your risk is higher than the risk for someone whose cholesterol runs 245 mg/dL, even though both numbers are in the same high-risk category. Likewise, you can stop — or at least reduce — cigarette smoking and lower your risk, given that the relative risk of stroke in heavy smokers (defined as smoking more than 40 cigarettes a day) is twice that of light smokers (fewer than 10 cigarettes a day).

Living Long and Well with Diabetes or Prediabetes

Despite any horror stories you may have heard about diabetes and its potentially bad effects, you can live long and well with any type of diabetes or prediabetes. You just have to learn all you can about what to do to stay healthy. Most of the advice from long-living people with diabetes about how to live well applies to everyone — not just to those with diabetes.

Get started today on improving your fitness and also follow these tips for optimal health and a long life:

>> Regularly monitor your blood glucose levels.

>> Exercise and stay as physically active as possible on a daily basis.

>> Make more healthful food choices by eating fewer refined foods, focusing on less refined ones naturally rich in antioxidants, vitamins, minerals, and fiber, such as vegetables, whole fruits, and whole grains.

>> Set reasonable goals, particularly ones that focus on good health habits.

>> Get all the information you can about diabetes, how to manage it, and how to avoid short-term and long-term health problems. Share your diabetes knowledge with others; you'll likely learn more in the process.

>> Involve a supportive spouse, family, or friends in managing your health.

>> Maintain a positive attitude about diabetes and life in general.

>> Find a good doctor (preferably an endocrinologist), a diabetes educator, or other health care provider with diabetes knowledge that you trust who can help you better manage your condition.

>> Always take your insulin or other prescribed medications to better manage your blood glucose, along with maintaining your healthy lifestyle (which is equally if not more important).

Chapter **3**

Understanding Diabetes Medications

U sing prescribed medications to treat diabetes — type 2 in particular — never used to be so complicated. You had one main class of drugs (sulfonylureas), along with insulin, but no other options. Now, multiple classes of medications are available that target tissues from your pancreas to your liver, intestines (gut), and kidneys. Which ones are best to use can be hard to sort out.

In this chapter, you uncover information about these options and how they work. The various insulins may need to be adjusted based on your physical activities, and being regularly active may allow you to lower doses of other medications, too. You also find out more about the effects of some other medications that you may be taking and whether exercise impacts them so you can get the most out of your workouts and get as fit as possible.

Knowing How Oral Diabetes Medications Work

If you have type 2 diabetes and use diabetes medications that you take as a pill by mouth, you benefit by understanding how they may or may not lower your blood glucose during activities. When you get more active, you may need lower doses, even of oral medications that don't usually cause low blood glucose with exercise.

If you have type 1 diabetes, most oral medications won't manage your blood glucose (except possibly metformin if you're insulin resistant). However, some people with type 1 diabetes use pills to lose more glucose through urine or other medications to help lower glucose variability and lose weight (but they're using them off label, which means that they're not approved by the FDA for use by people with type 1).

Targeting specific tissues

The number of diabetes medications available for persons with type 2 diabetes has skyrocketed recently, with 12 classes of medications now available that target different tissues in your body. The targets now include the pancreas (increasing insulin release), liver (decreasing blood glucose release), muscles (making them more responsive to insulin), gut (slowing down absorption of carbohydrates), and kidneys (releasing excess glucose in urine).

Among oral medications, only the ones that target the pancreas and cause insulin release have any significant effect on your exercise blood glucose responses.

Metformin works by targeting the liver to reduce blood glucose release overnight and after meals; it also increases insulin action. Sulfonylureas like Amaryl and Glyburide help stimulate your pancreas to make more insulin (if it can). Both Actos and Avandia, drugs in the thiazolidinedione (TZD) class, sensitize fat and muscle cells to insulin. A newer class of drugs (SGLT-2 inhibitors) acts on the kidneys to cause excess blood glucose to be peed out.

Identifying which pills work best to lower glucose

Some people have elevated blood glucose levels in the morning only, while others experience spikes after eating. Your doctor may prescribe medications for you based on which body tissues are the target (see the preceding section) and add other ones to the mix if your blood glucose isn't coming down enough. Here's a breakdown of how each of the following classes of medications works:

>> **Sulfonylureas:** These medications stimulate your pancreas to release most insulin and have been around the longest to treat type 2 diabetes. They include Amaryl, DiaBeta, Diabinese, Glynase, Glucotrol, Micronase, and others.

The newer generation sulfonylureas have fewer bad side effects than the older ones. These medications are generally less expensive than newer types.

If your pancreas loses the capacity to make much insulin, no medication will be able to stimulate your beta cells to make enough to manage your blood glucose.

>> **Biguanides (metformin):** Metformin is the generic name of the only medication in this class. It's one of the most widely prescribed medications for type 2 diabetes and prediabetes (and other insulin-resistant states) and the drug of first choice for these conditions. It doesn't cause hypoglycemia, but it can shut down your liver's release of glucose overnight, making it excellent for preventing morning elevations. It also improves the action of your insulin in both the liver and muscles.

>> **Thiazolidinediones (TZDs):** These medications act as insulin sensitizers to boost insulin action. Two medications in this class, Avandia and Actos, are available. They can increase bone fractures and swelling of the feet and ankles, and you can't take them if you have heart failure. Both may cause you to gain weight.

>> **DPP-4 inhibitors:** DPP-4 inhibitors work with gut hormones, natural enzymes, and your body's own insulin to lower blood glucose. They may help preserve the ability of the beta cells of the pancreas to make insulin.

Incretin hormones, called GLP-1 and GIP, are naturally occurring substances produced in the intestines when you eat, and they help regulate blood glucose by stimulating both the alpha and beta cells of the pancreas. Alpha cells secrete glucagon, which mobilizes glucose when your blood glucose is low (such as overnight or during prolonged activity). These medications boost the incretin response by inhibiting DPP-4, an enzyme that breaks down incretin hormones before they have time to work effectively.

>> **Meglitinides:** Prandin and Starlix are the two drugs in this class, which may work well for you if you eat sporadically. You take a dose when you eat to cause your pancreas to release enough insulin then to reduce blood glucose spikes after meals. They are one of the oral medications sometimes prescribed for women who have gestational diabetes (during pregnancy).

If your blood glucose rises sharply after you eat, you can benefit from these medications, assuming your beta cells can still release enough insulin.

>> **Alpha-glucosidase inhibitors:** These medications control your post-meal spikes by slowing how quickly you digest carbohydrates after eating. You can dose with either Precose or Glyset, the two medications in this class, but only if you don't have slowing of your digestion caused by *gastroparesis* (central nerve damage). This medication is also an option for women who are pregnant and have gestational or type 2 diabetes.

>> **SGLT-2 inhibitors:** This more recent class of medications treats diabetes by making you lose glucose through your urine. Because more glucose appears in the urine, taking these medications raises your risk of yeast infections slightly, especially in women, as well as of urinary tract (bladder) infections and dehydration. These medications have been associated with *ketoacidosis* (elevated levels of ketones in the blood) in both individuals with type 1 and type 2 diabetes even with only moderate elevations in blood glucose.

TECHNICAL STUFF

Around 160 to 180 grams of glucose a day are filtered through the kidneys, but they don't appear in urine because they're reabsorbed back into your bloodstream. When your blood glucose rises above 180 mg/dL, however, some glucose normally ends up in your urine. These SGLT-2 (sodium-glucose co-transporter-2) inhibitors block glucose reabsorption and cause you to lose some glucose and calories in urine and usually lose some weight.

Even if you start out taking only one medication, ending up being prescribed two or more is common. Combination drugs that have two of these drugs in one pill are popular for that reason. For instance, Glucovance and Metaglip combine a sulfonylurea and a biguanide, and Avandamet is a combination of a glitazone and a biguanide. Combinations of some of the newer medications (like DPP-4 and SGLT-2 inhibitors together in Glyxambi, a combination of Tradjenta and Jardiance) are now available. Expect many new combination diabetes pills to be available in the future, reducing the number of pills you may take on a daily basis.

TIP

Table 3-1 provides a handy summary of the various types of oral diabetes medications currently available.

TABLE 3-1   **Oral Diabetes Medications**

Class of Medication	What They're Called	How They Work
Sulfonylureas	Amaryl, DiaBeta, Diabinese, Glynase, Glucotrol, Micronase	Promote insulin release from the beta cells of the pancreas; some increase insulin action
Biguanides	Metformin (generic), Glucophage, Glucophage XR, Riomet, Glumetza	Decrease glucose release from the liver; increase liver and muscle insulin sensitivity
Thiazolidenediones or glitazones	Avandia, Actos	Increase insulin sensitivity in muscles
DPP-4 inhibitors	Januvia, Onglyza, Nesina/ Galvus, Tradjenta	Inhibit DPP-4 that breaks down GLP-1; improve insulin action, lower glucagon

Class of Medication	What They're Called	How They Work
Meglitinides	Prandin, Starlix	Stimulate beta cells to release insulin, but only enough to cover meals
Alpha-glucosidase inhibitors	Precose, Glyset	Work in gut to slow carbohydrate digestion and lower post-meal blood glucose spikes
SGLT-2 inhibitors	Invokana, Farxiga, Jardiance, Steglatro	Prevent kidneys from reabsorbing glucose; lost in urine when above a certain level
Combination therapies	Glucovance, Metaglip, Avandamet, Avandaryl, Duetact, Glyxambi	Combine effects of two medication classes in each pill

Using (Non-Insulin) Injected Medication

You can use other medications besides insulin that are injected and treat type 1 and type 2 diabetes. One class (amylin) replaces a hormone secreted with insulin, and the other (GLP-1 agonists) affects the gut hormones. Table 3-2 summarizes these two classes quickly, and the following sections provide more detail.

TABLE 3-2 **Injected (Non-Insulin) Diabetes Medications**

Class of Medication	What They're Called	How They Work
Amylin	Symlin	Work with insulin to control glucose spikes for three hours after meals
GLP-1 agonists (incretins and incretin mimetics)	Byetta, Victoza, Lyxumia, Bydureon, Trulicity, Ozempic, Eperzan, Adlyxin	Stimulate insulin release; inhibit the liver's release of glucose; delay emptying of stomach

Amylin

If your body makes very little or no insulin, you're missing a hormone called amylin. A replacement form, Symlin (pramlintide), can be injected by people with type 1 diabetes or anyone with type 2 using insulin. Symlin works with insulin after meals to slow the glucose coming into the blood from digested foods. It can help you lose weight by making you feel full sooner, as well as improve your diabetes management and lower the risk of complications.

Symlin has some potential side effects, including severe *hypoglycemia* (low blood glucose, mostly in type 1s), nausea, vomiting, abdominal pain, headache, fatigue, and dizziness. Another drawback is that it can only be injected, not taken by mouth. If you have diabetes-related digestive problems (gastroparesis), you shouldn't use this medication.

GLP-1 agonists

People with type 2 diabetes can also use a class of injected medications known as *glucagon-like peptide-1 agonists*, or GLP-1 agonists. These medications delay digestion and cause you to feel full sooner and possibly lose weight.

TECHNICAL STUFF

GLP-1 agonists replicate a synthetic version of a small protein derived from the venom of the Gila monster (a poisonous lizard found in the southwestern United States and in Mexico). These gut hormones stimulate the release of insulin when you eat. They also protect your pancreatic beta cells from burnout, inhibit the liver's release of glucose (by blocking glucagon), delay the emptying of food from your stomach, and promote early fullness.

Despite occasional side effects such as nausea, vomiting, temporary headaches, and increased risk of blood glucose lows when used with sulfonylureas or insulin, replacement of these natural hormones can treat type 2 diabetes quite effectively. A drawback for many potential users, though, is that some types must be injected daily (Byetta and Victoza), although once-weekly forms (Bydureon, Trulicity, and Ozempic) are available.

Changing Doses for Exercise

The medications you take to manage diabetes or other health conditions can alter your blood glucose responses to being active. If you take certain pills or insulin, you must be vigilant about adjusting how much you take and what you eat to avoid ending up with blood glucose that is too low or too high from exercise.

If you take medications that increase the secretion of insulin, or if you take insulin, you have a greater risk of exercise-induced blood glucose lows. To prevent hypoglycemia, you may have to adjust other medications for regular exercise or lower your insulin doses before and possibly after your workouts. (The earlier sections in this chapter explain the basics of the various classes of diabetes medications.)

Oral medications that may cause exercise lows

Most oral medications are unlikely to cause lows, with a few exceptions. Any pills that cause your pancreas to release insulin increase your risk of hypoglycemia with exercise. For the sulfonylureas, the actual risk varies with how long the medication works. For the meglitinides, the timing of when you take the pill before exercise matters.

Sulfonylureas

Sulfonylureas are one class of medications with definite potential effects on exercise, increasing the risk for hypoglycemia in people with type 2 diabetes. Older-generation sulfonylureas (such as Diabinese, Orinase, Tolinase, and Dymelor) cause insulin to be released from the pancreas and reduce insulin resistance. These typically have a longer duration (up to 72 hours) than the newer ones, creating the greatest potential for lows during and after exercise.

Second-generation sulfonylureas, such as Amaryl, DiaBeta, Micronase, and Glucotrol, don't last as long and carry a lesser risk. DiaBeta and Micronase have a slightly longer duration (24 hours) versus 12 to 16 hours for Amaryl and Glucotrol.

TIP

Keep these guidelines in mind if you use any of these medications:

>> Frequently monitor your blood glucose levels when exercising if you take any sulfonylureas that stay in your body for 24 hours or longer.

>> Choose to take Amaryl and Glucotrol if you want a reduced chance of getting low during or after exercise because their effects don't last as long.

>> Check with your health care provider about lowering your doses of sulfonylureas, particularly if you begin to have lows more frequently.

Meglitinides

Prandin or Starlix only potentially increase your risk of low blood glucose if you take them immediately before prolonged exercise because they increase insulin levels in the blood temporarily when taken with meals.

WARNING

However, if you take Prandin or Starlix before meals after which you plan to exercise, you may need to lower your doses to avoid hypoglycemia.

Medications unlikely to cause lows

Other diabetes medications may affect exercise even less or not at all. The following list and Table 3-3 spell out some of their other possible effects so you can be informed before you get active.

>> **Insulin sensitizers:** Medications that increase insulin sensitivity (Avandia, Actos, and metformin) only affect it when you're resting. They don't cause exercise lows.

>> **Alpha-glucosidase inhibitors:** The slower absorption of carbohydrates Precose and Glyset cause doesn't directly affect exercise blood glucose levels. However, these medications can slightly delay your treatment of a low blood glucose level during workouts.

>> **DPP-4 inhibitors:** During low blood glucose, people taking these medications have a greater release of glucagon, which helps raise glucose levels. They don't cause lows.

>> **SGLT-2 inhibitors:** These medications have no known exercise effects, even though they may lower blood pressure by causing you to pee out extra water when your blood glucose goes high. To be on the safe side, drink plenty of fluids to stay hydrated.

TABLE 3-3   **Oral Diabetes Medications and Risk of Exercise Lows**

Class of Medication	Specific Medications	Risk of Exercise Lows
Sulfonylureas	Diabinese, Glynase, Orinase	High (last > 24 hours)
	DiaBeta, Micronase	Medium-high (24 hours)
	Amaryl, Glucotrol	Medium (12 to 16 hours)
Biguanides	All formulations	Low
Thiazolidenediones	Avandia, Actos	Low
DPP-4 inhibitors	Januvia, Onglyza, Nesina, Tradjenta	Low
Meglitinides	Prandin, Starlix	Moderate (during exercise after meals)
Alpha-glucosidase inhibitors	Precose, Glyset	Low
SGLT-2 inhibitors	Invokana, Farxiga, Jardiance, Steglatro	Low

Injected (non-insulin) medications

None of the non-insulin, injectable medications impact glucose responses to exercise unless you take them with insulin or you have slower digestion from diabetes. Problems may arise if your blood glucose drops for other reasons.

By slowing how quickly carbohydrates are digested, these medications make exercise lows harder to treat. This difficulty can occur with use of either Symlin that you inject for meals or GLP-1 agonists that you inject daily or weekly.

WARNING If you use Symlin and try to treat a low, your body will digest the carbohydrates you take more slowly, making raising your blood glucose quickly more difficult.

WARNING Some individuals with type 2 diabetes find that long bouts of exercise are much more difficult to accomplish when using GLP-1 agonists because they feel more sluggish and less able to do their fitness routines.

Check out Table 3-4 for a handy summary of the risk of exercise lows with injected diabetes medications.

TABLE 3-4   ## Injected Medications and Risk of Exercise Lows

Class of Medication	Examples	Risk of Exercise Lows
Insulin (*bolus:* injected or pumped)	Humalog, NovoLog, Apidra, Fiasp, Regular (R)	High (given within 2–3 hours of last bolus)
Insulin (*basal:* injected, not pumped)	Lantus, Basaglar, Levemir, Toujeo, Tresiba, Novolin N, Humulin N	Moderate (but lower overall doses may be needed when active)
Amylin	Symlin	Low (can make hypoglycemia harder to treat effectively)
GLP-1 agonists	Byetta, Victoza, Lyxumia, Bydureon, Trulicity, Ozempic, Eperzan, Adlyxin	Low

Understanding Insulin Use

All people with type 1 diabetes and many with type 2 must give themselves insulin to manage blood glucose, whether that insulin is injected, pumped, or inhaled. (In the future, a swallowed form may be an option.)

REMEMBER

If your blood glucose is high (greater than 250 mg/dL) at diagnosis, your doctor may start you on insulin right away, regardless of your diabetes type.

Taking insulin allows you to rapidly achieve better blood glucose and may give your beta cells a rest so they can recover at least some of their function. Being put on insulin with type 2 diabetes isn't a sign that you have failed or that your diabetes is worse. In fact, when people with type 2 diabetes are started on insulin early, they're unlikely to need to take it a year later (although they may need it years down the road).

If you have type 2 diabetes, your insulin doses may be decreased or withdrawn if lifestyle changes (improvements in food, diet, stress management, and more) can manage your blood glucose. That period of improved blood glucose when you start using insulin also has a lasting effect in terms of preventing diabetes complications for both types.

Often when adults develop type 1 diabetes, their insulin needs are low for several years and result in a misdiagnosis of type 2. Most individuals with type 1, however, require insulin from diagnosis on, and oral medications don't effectively lower blood glucose.

Basal and bolus insulins and their actions

Insulins have been formulated to act differently. Depending on the type, they lower glucose at different times after you take them (*onset*), reach maximal concentrations in the blood (*peak*) at varying times, and last for shorter or longer times in the body (*duration*).

Most people with type 1 diabetes follow a *basal-bolus regimen*, meaning that they take *basal* (longer-lasting, or background) insulin to cover their needs all day long and *bolus* (shorter-acting) insulin to cover increases in blood glucose from meals and snacks. See Table 3-5 for more about the actions of the various insulins. You can follow this regimen whether you inject or pump insulin. In the case of pumps, they are unique in that they use shorter-acting insulins only but are programmed to deliver doses over time that cover basal insulin needs. People using them have a separate program in the pump to give bolus dose for meals and snacks.

REMEMBER

If you have type 2 diabetes and need to take insulin, your doctor may first put you on only basal insulin, which covers your non–food-related insulin needs and provides stable amounts of insulin during the day.

TABLE 3-5   ## Characteristics of Insulins and Insulin Analogs

Insulin/Insulin Analog	Onset	Peak	Duration
Fiasp	2–15 minutes	0.25–2.0 hours	2–5 hours
Humalog, NovoLog, Apidra, Admelog	10–30 minutes	0.5–3.0 hours	3–5 hours
Regular (R)	30–60 minutes	2–5 hours	5–8 hours
N (NPH)	1–2 hours	2–12 hours	14–24 hours
Lantus, Basaglar, Toujeo	1.5 hours	None	20–24 hours
Levemir	1–3 hours	8–10 hours	Up to 24 hours
Tresiba	30–90 minutes	None	Over 24 hours

Basal insulins

At present, the most widely used basal insulins are Lantus, Basaglar, and Levemir, all of which you can inject once or twice a day. *Note:* For many Lantus/Basaglar users who need small total daily doses of basal insulin, their insulin lasts significantly less than 24 hours, and they may need to take it twice a day.

REMEMBER

Basal insulins don't directly cover the carbohydrates you eat during the day, but they help you start the day with better glucose readings. They also maintain your blood glucose throughout the day by covering your body's insulin needs that remain the same regardless of whether you eat.

An even longer-acting one called Tresiba covers your basal insulin needs for well over 24 hours. In addition, the manufacturers of Lantus recently created a version of basal insulin called Toujeo at three times the strength per volume (especially made for people who take large doses of basal insulin).

Combination basal and bolus insulins (intermediate-acting)

Intermediate-action insulins like Humulin N can cover both basal needs and some meals (like lunch, which is when it peaks if given before breakfast), but they've become less popular than longer-acting basal insulins that better mimic the normal release of insulin. People with type 2 diabetes may also be put on combination insulins, such as 70/30 or 75/25, containing more basal or intermediate insulin (70 or 75 percent) with less of a rapid-acting one (the other 25 or 30 percent) to cover meals. Using premixed insulin may increase the risk of hypoglycemia.

For many with type 2 diabetes, using combination insulins is effective. Premixed formulations may make taking the proper combination of insulin to best cover all your body's daily needs easier, although these options aren't as effective for people who make none of their own insulin (that is, those with type 1 diabetes).

Bolus (mealtime) insulins

The main rapid-acting insulin *analogs* (all synthesized and slightly altered forms of human insulin) you can use are Humalog, NovoLog (or NovoRapid), Admelog, and Apidra. Their differences in onset and peak times are minimal, but all work more rapidly than regular (for example, Humulin R) insulin. Another one, Fiasp, just gained FDA approval and is even more rapid-acting than all of these insulins, with a quicker onset and 50% more insulin delivered during the first hour after you inject it. You can use any of these to cover food at meals or to correct high blood glucose, and usually one is used in insulin pumps.

Insulin delivery methods

You have many options to choose from on how to take insulin, such as syringes (of varying needle length and dosing scales), insulin pens, insulin pumps, or inhaled insulin, with other possibilities likely coming down the pike soon. The following sections outline some of these choices.

Syringes and pens

You can use syringes or choose insulin pens that contain prefilled insulin cartridges. Using insulin pens reduces the chances of giving yourself a dose of the wrong insulin when you use more than one type because each insulin has its own unique injection pen. Giving an exact dose dialed on a pen is also easier than filling a syringe from an insulin vial to the correct amount (which can be particularly difficult if you can't see well).

TIP

If you take insulin, ask your doctor whether an insulin pen would be better for you than syringes. Several pens now have memory functions (recording the last dose and time), and some have half-unit dosing rather than just whole units.

REMEMBER

For all injected insulins, smaller doses are generally absorbed from your skin and available in your bloodstream more rapidly than larger ones, but smaller doses also have a shorter duration.

Insulin pumps

You may take insulin by using a specialized insulin pump, which is usually about the size of a pager or small cellphone (or smaller). *Pumps* use a small catheter or needle under your skin to frequently deliver basal doses of short- or rapid-acting insulin to mimic normal insulin release by the pancreas. You program the pump to give yourself boluses to cover your meals and snacks.

REMEMBER

In other words, pumps provide insulin more like your own pancreas would: in small doses all day long, with bigger doses following eating.

You can closely mimic this same pattern with the newer basal/bolus regimens (for example, Lantus insulin for basal, Humalog for boluses), but insulin pumps make insulin delivery easier and are flexible enough to allow you to change basal rates of insulin delivery at any time or put in a temporary basal rate for exercise or anything else that changes your insulin needs.

REMEMBER

Using an insulin pump requires having an understanding of the impact of your food and doing frequent blood glucose monitoring (just like if you take multiple daily injections). But you only have one needle stick when the infusion set is inserted every three to five days. The insulin is directly infused into the skin through the same catheter, which stays under your skin.

TECHNICAL STUFF

Insulin pumps have been available since the 1980s. You now have several models from which to choose. Most still require tubing to deliver insulin from the pump through the infusion site below the skin, but several tubeless patch pumps are now available. On most pumps, the built-in features routinely include a bolus calculator that helps to determine how much insulin to give for food and correction, along with a dual wave or square wave to change the duration of the bolus delivery itself. The "active insulin" feature for the insulin still available in the system can help prevent stacking (that is, giving doses too close together). By checking blood glucose frequently after a bolus to see when levels stop falling, you can figure out how long it lasts.

Inhaled insulin

One inhaled insulin, Afrezza, is another option for administering rapid-acting insulin for meals. It makes insulin available sooner but doesn't last as long compared to other rapid-acting insulins. One issue with its use is that the possible doses are only four or eight units at a time. Also, it can cause a cough and throat pain or irritation, and smokers or people with asthma or lung problems like emphysema can't use it.

Insulin and exercise interactions

Using insulin creates the most problems when you're being active. Insulin is the only hormone that lowers blood glucose. The body normally decreases insulin release during exercise, but when people inject or pump insulin that is absorbed slowly, lowering insulin levels during activities is harder, and hypoglycemia can result.

WARNING

If you take insulin, exercise can cause dramatic reductions in blood glucose.

Here are critical points that you need to understand about taking insulin and balancing your blood glucose during and after exercise:

>> Insulin and contractions use separate mechanisms to take up glucose from the blood, and they additively increase what's going into muscles.

>> The type of insulin you use and its timing (peak, onset, and duration) can have a large effect on your blood glucose responses.

>> When no more than basal levels of insulin are circulating in your body during exercise, your body's response is more normal.

>> If you exercise when your insulin levels are peaking, you have an increased chance of getting low.

>> If you use basal insulin only, or your last bolus insulin dose has peaked and waned before you start exercising (usually within two to three hours), your risk of developing hypoglycemia will be much lower.

>> Insulin pump users can prevent lows by either disconnecting their pumps or reducing their basal rates during activity.

>> Some pump users decrease their basal rates before and/or after the activity, depending on how long it lasts and on blood glucose responses.

>> Taking twice-daily doses of basal insulin gives you a greater ability to adjust dosing to prevent hypoglycemia before and after exercise.

>> Exercise, as well as hot tub use and vigorous massage, can increase the absorption of insulin and cause hypoglycemia.

Lowering insulin for physical activity

Physical activity is one of the main causes of hypoglycemia when you use insulin. Knowing when and how to adjust your insulin doses can be critically important to managing your blood glucose. How much insulin is in your bloodstream when you exercise determines much of your response.

REMEMBER

Exercising with low levels of insulin in your blood is a much more normal physiological response.

WARNING

If your insulin levels are high during an activity, your muscles will take up even more blood glucose, and you're more likely to end up with low blood glucose for up to 48 hours after you're done exercising.

Being able to adjust your insulin doses takes a higher level of knowledge about how insulins work, experience adjusting doses, and quite a bit of trial and error, no matter how much you know about your own body's responses. If you're unsure about how to adjust insulin doses, consult with your health care provider, particularly if you begin to experience lows related to your activities and are relatively new to being active. Alternatively, you may be able to gauge how to lower pre-exercise insulin doses or increase carbohydrate intake yourself by determining the effects of the activity.

To lower your insulin during exercise, you may need to decrease your insulin doses before meals, as shown in Table 3-6. The general recommendations for insulin adjustments that follow apply to bolus insulins given within two to three hours of when you start to exercise only.

TABLE 3-6   ## Reduction of Mealtime Insulin Taken Before Exercise

Duration	Low Intensity	Moderate Intensity	High Intensity
30 minutes	None	10–20%	10–30%
60 minutes	10–20%	20–40%	30–60%
90 minutes	15–30%	30–55%	45–75%
120 minutes	20–40%	40–70%	60–90%
180 minutes	30–60%	60–90%	75–100%

Adapted from Colberg, S., Diabetic Athlete's Handbook (Human Kinetics, 2009).

Consider these general guidelines related to making insulin adjustments to manage your blood glucose during exercise:

>> These recommendations only give you a starting point for making insulin changes; you need to do some trial and error to find what works for you.

>> If you eat extra for exercise, your insulin adjustments may be less, or you may need to both lower insulin and eat more for longer activities.

>> Reduce your carbohydrate intake at meals before exercise to allow you to take smaller doses of insulin (to keep insulin lower during exercise).

>> Larger insulin doses take longer to fully absorb, so they stick around in your body longer and can cause lows later on.

>> Basal rate reductions on pumps may be more or less than recommended for boluses, and they may be done alone or with reduced boluses.

>> You may need to reduce insulin less when exercising more than three hours after your last dose (injected or pumped) of bolus insulin.

>> For the meal after exercise, you may need to reduce bolus insulin doses (such as cutting back by a unit or two).

>> You may also need to lower doses after exercise (bolus and basal), both in the short run and longer term (if your training is consistent).

>> If your activities are seasonal, you may have to lower your insulin doses during the season and raise them again during the off-season.

>> When doing intense, near-maximal exercise, you may need to increase your bolus insulin rather than lower it.

>> Competitions usually have more of a glucose-raising effect (especially when you're nervous) compared to practices, which usually lower blood glucose.

>> If you use a pump and disconnect it during exercise, check your blood glucose once per hour, reconnect and correct with dosing suggested by the insulin pump (usually at least half of what you missed per hour off the pump).

>> If you use Lantus or Basaglar as your basal insulin and take small doses, you may want to split it into two daily doses. You can then give less to cover the hours during which you'll be exercising or a smaller dose for the 12 hours following prolonged activities.

>> If you're ever in doubt about how to adjust your own insulin, check with your health care provider for recommended changes and further guidance.

TIP

For additional guidance, consult specific activity recommendations in my book *Diabetic Athlete's Handbook* (published by Human Kinetics).

Exercise and insulin needs in athletes

As I note in Chapter 2, regular physical training increases your muscle mass, in effect giving you a larger glucose tank in which to put excess glucose after meals. What you may not know is that trained athletes generally have low levels of circulating insulin for this reason and are extremely insulin sensitive. Insulin action, though, begins to decline after a period with no exercise, in as little as one to two days, even if you're normally active.

REMEMBER

Many athletes report that their total insulin requirements increase after two to three days without regular exercise (such as when they're too busy to exercise or are injured or ill).

Monitoring Effects of Other Medications

Other medications that don't have a direct effect on your blood glucose can still impact your ability to be physically active, while others have no influence at all. The following sections break down some of the categories other medications you may be taking fall into so you can assess your risk.

Non-diabetes medications with exercise effects

You may be taking medications to lower your blood cholesterol, manage blood pressure, or control other cardiovascular problems. Certain medications for each of these health issues can have an impact on exercise.

Statins

Statins are a class of medications you may be taking to lower cholesterol levels or abnormal levels of blood fats to reduce your risk of having heart attack or stroke. Brand names include Altoprev, Crestor, Lescol, Lipitor, Livalo, Mevacor, Pravachol, and Zocor. In individuals who are unwilling or unable to change their diets and lifestyles sufficiently or have genetically high levels of blood fat (lipids), the benefits of statins on lowering cardiovascular risk likely greatly exceed the risks.

Statin use can cause undesirable muscular effects, such as unexplained muscle pain and weakness with physical activity that may be related to these medications' compromising the ability of your muscles to generate energy. The occurrence of muscular conditions like myalgia, mild or severe myositis, and rhabdomyolysis, although relatively rare, is doubled in people with diabetes. Others have reported an increased susceptibility to exercise-induced muscle injury when taking statins, particularly active, older individuals. Other symptoms, such as muscle cramps during or after exercise, nocturnal cramping, and general fatigue, generally resolve when you stop taking them. If you experience any of these symptoms, talk with your doctor about switching to another cholesterol-lowering drug.

WARNING

A major issue related to statins is that their long-term use negatively impacts the organization of collagen and decreases the biomechanical strength of the tendons and ligaments (which connect muscles to bones and stabilize your joints). These changes make them more predisposed to ruptures. In fact, statin users experience more spontaneous ruptures of both their biceps and Achilles tendons.

Talk to your doctor about whether you may be able to manage your cardiovascular risk and lipid levels without taking statins long-term for this reason. The potential impact of other cholesterol medications like Repatha (which is injected) on muscles and joints is presently unknown.

Beta-blockers

Beta-blockers (such as Lopressor, Inderal, Levatol, Corgard, Tenormin, and Zebeta) treat heart disease and hypertension (high blood pressure). These medications lower both your resting and your exercise heart rate. If you're taking one, your heart rate doesn't reach an age-expected value at any intensity of exercise, and your ability to reach greater intensities is likely compromised. Take them as prescribed, but just be aware of how your exercise responses may differ from normal.

WARNING

Beta-blockers also blunt your normal hormonal response to hypoglycemia and exercise and increase your risk of more severe lows.

Diuretics

Diuretics — often known as "water pills" — such as Lasix, Microzide, Enduron, and Lozol that reduce the amount of water in your body lower blood pressure, but they can also lead to dehydration if you lose too much fluid. They aren't likely to affect your blood glucose, although they may interfere with insulin secretion.

WARNING

Using diuretics can cause low blood pressure, dehydration, and dizziness during exercise.

Vasodilators (nitroglycerin)

Taking *vasodilators* like nitroglycerin allows more blood to flow to your heart during exercise. These medications are used to treat chest pain (angina) both at rest and during exercise.

WARNING

Vasodilators can also induce hypotension, or a drop in your blood pressure that may cause you to faint during or following an activity.

Blood thinners

WARNING

Aspirin and other blood thinners (such as Coumadin) have the potential to make you bruise more easily or extensively in response to athletic injuries. They usually don't have any impact on your ability to exercise, though.

Other medications with no exercise effects

If you take ACE inhibitors (for example, Capoten, Accupril, Vasotec, Lotensin, or Zestril) or angiotensin II receptor blockers (ARBs, such as Cozaar, Benicar, and Avapro) to reduce your blood pressure or protect your kidneys from possible damage, you should expect no negative effects during exercise. In fact, using certain ACE inhibitors may lower your risk of a heart attack during exercise if you have heart disease.

Other medications that treat heart disease and high blood pressure (calcium-channel blockers like Procardia, Sular, Cardene, Cardizem, and Norvasc), depression (such as Wellbutrin and Prozac), or chronic pain (Celebrex) have no effect on exercise.

Non-diabetes medications affecting blood glucose

Very few non-diabetes medications have a direct impact on your blood glucose levels. The exception is any type of corticosteroids — like Prednisone or cortisone (pills or injections into inflamed joints) — which make you more insulin resistant and cause blood glucose to rise, sometimes dramatically. Statins also raise the overall risk of developing type 2 diabetes. (Head to the earlier section "Statins" for information on how these drugs affect exercise risk as well.)

2

Mastering Exercise and Nutrition Basics

Find out how exercise gets you fit and keeps your diabetes in check.

Get your blood glucose on an even keel with exercise and dietary changes guaranteed to make your life easier.

Ramp up your diet for better health and eat right for exercise.

Set up your fitness routine and get started on the path to keeping fit and healthy with diabetes or prediabetes.

Chapter **4**

Finding Out How Exercise Works

What exactly happens to your body when you exercise? Your metabolism gets revved up, and you're off and running (maybe not literally). Have you ever wondered how your body fuels itself during these physical endeavors?

Clearly, your body uses a lot of calories that come from somewhere that isn't always obvious, particularly if you're active first thing in the morning before you eat anything. Your body can run like a well-tuned car or like one that needs a tune-up. You want to aim for the former.

In this chapter, I explain how hormones in your body keep your blood glucose from dropping too much when you're active. You also find out why activities don't always affect your blood glucose the way you expect or want them to, and what to do if that happens. You can keep your blood glucose levels in check when you're active, but doing so often takes a bit of planning.

Knowing How Hormones React

Hormones in your body act like traffic lights when managing your blood glucose. When one turns green, another one with an opposite action turns red, and traffic flows one way. Then the lights reverse, and traffic flows in the opposite direction. It's usually a tightly regulated process because of how critical glucose is to the function of your brain and nerves.

Directing the flow of glucose in blood

In the case of your body, the traffic lights are controlled by insulin and a bunch of glucose-raising hormones that work in concert (see Table 4-1). Insulin has a lowering effect on blood glucose, and the rest have the ability to raise it.

TABLE 4-1   **Actions of Glucose-Raising Hormones**

Hormone	Where It Comes From	Effects During Exercise
Glucagon	Pancreas (alpha cells)	Stimulates liver glycogen to break down and new glucose to be formed to raise glucose; affected by balance with insulin in liver circulation
Epinephrine (adrenaline)	Adrenal medulla	Stimulates muscle and some liver glycogen to break down; releases fat into the bloodstream
Norepinephrine	Adrenal medulla, sympathetic nerve endings	Stimulates liver to produce new glucose; greater release during intense exercise raises blood glucose more
Growth hormone	Anterior pituitary	Directly stimulates fat release in blood; suppresses glucose use; stimulates protein storage in muscles
Cortisol	Adrenal cortex	Mobilizes amino acids and glycerol to use to make glucose; releases fat for muscle use rather than blood glucose

At rest, you need insulin to keep your blood glucose from going too high after meals. But when you're fasting overnight or exercising, your liver needs to release more glucose into the blood, and that requires the opposing hormones.

TECHNICAL STUFF

The glucose-raising hormones the body releases during exercise (and fasting) include *epinephrine* (more commonly known as *adrenaline*), *norepinephrine,* and *glucagon.* Specifically, the hormone release comes from the sympathetic arm of your nervous system — that's the one that helps your body to respond to physical or mental stressors with an increased heart rate (pulse). It's the fight-or-flight system that gets you moving quickly. Other hormones that factor in more during longer workouts include *growth hormone* and *cortisol.*

REMEMBER

Insulin is the only hormone that lowers blood glucose, while all the others raise it either directly or indirectly.

The most common response is that your blood glucose goes down when you exercise moderately. This happens because contracting muscles take up blood glucose directly without insulin, although insulin can add to the drop. Exercise responses aren't always predictable, though, and many things can affect how your blood glucose reacts. Sometimes it goes up rather than down when you're active. (See the following section for more on this effect.)

TIP

Working out can be an effective way to lower your blood glucose when it gets higher than you want it to be.

Understanding why your glucose sometimes goes up with exercise

When you do high-intensity or vigorous exercise like sprinting, intervals, heavy resistance training, and competitions, you often experience an immediate rise in your blood glucose, primarily due to the hormones epinephrine and glucagon. Intense exercise causes your body to release more of the hormones that boost how much glucose your liver releases into your blood, all while keeping your muscles from taking up as much by temporarily raising their insulin resistance. Even when you don't have diabetes, insulin increases after (and sometimes during) intense workouts.

Glucose-raising hormones work so well that they can easily exceed your body's immediate need for glucose, especially because you can't sustain working out at high intensity for long. In such cases, you don't have to worry about getting low during exercise because your blood glucose goes up during and for a brief time after these activities.

Your body needs some insulin in your system to keep a check and balance on this exaggerated release of glucose-raising hormones during intense exercise, but not so much that your blood glucose drops excessively. If you make your own insulin, your body releases less (but still some) during exercise, and then it releases more as blood glucose rises to lower it back to normal after you stop.

Staying elevated too long after a workout

Due to the residual effects of these glucose-raising hormones, you may experience some insulin resistance immediately after intense exercise, which can last for a few hours. For instance, after doing near-maximal cycling — like cycling up a hill or working against a hard resistance in a spin class — to exhaustion, adults with type 1 diabetes on insulin pumps have elevated blood glucose levels for two hours afterward. If you take insulin, you'll likely need some extra insulin to bring your blood glucose levels back to normal.

Similarly, in type 2 diabetes, blood glucose can rise in response to a maximal hard cycling workout and stay that way afterward for an hour or two. Eventually, your blood glucose comes down because many people with type 2 diabetes are still making some of their own insulin. Even if you don't make insulin anymore, it usually comes down over time since your body is more sensitive to the effects of any insulin in your body after a workout. Doing an easier cool-down before you stop entirely may bring your glucose down faster.

WARNING

After these hormones wane, your blood glucose can easily drop later while your body is restoring the muscle glycogen that you used during your workout. Beware of later-onset lows after intense exercise if you take insulin.

Engaging Your Exercise Energy Systems

The way your muscles make and use energy depends on how fast you move, how much force your muscles produce, and how long the activity lasts. Your body has three distinct energy systems (Figure 4-1) to supply your muscles with *adenosine triphosphate (ATP)*, a high-energy compound found in all cells that directly fuels muscle contractions. The three systems act on a continuum, meaning that the first one, followed by the second and finally the third, make ATP as your exercise continues longer than two minutes.

REMEMBER

If you exercise even for just a minute, you end up using all three energy systems to varying degrees. Both of your anaerobic energy systems (phosphagens and lactic acid systems) are important at the beginning of any longer-lasting activity before your aerobic metabolism can supply enough ATP. These first two systems are also important whenever you pick up the pace or work harder, such as when you start going uphill or sprint to the finish line.

TECHNICAL STUFF

All three energy systems work by increasing the production of ATP to fuel contractions. When a nerve stimulates your muscle to contract, calcium is released within recruited muscle cells, ATP "energizes" the muscle fibers, and they go into action. Without ATP, your muscles can't contract, and you can't exercise.

Muscle cells contain only small quantities of ATP ready for use when you start — enough to fuel any activity for about a second, at best. If you want to keep going longer, your muscles need to get ATP from another source right away. Although all the systems can make ATP, the rate at which they supply it varies. The fuels used to make the ATP and the amount of time needed to produce it also differ by system.

REMEMBER

Due to how your energy systems work, the type and intensity of the exercise you do can affect your blood glucose responses differently.

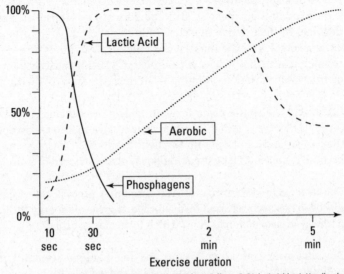

FIGURE 4-1:
Exercise energy systems.

© John Wiley & Sons, Inc. (Adapted from Colberg, S. Diabetic Athlete's Handbook, Human Kinetics, 2009.)

Phosphagens system (short and powerful)

For short activities or power moves, your *phosphagens system* (also called *ATP–CP* or *glycolytic system*) supplies almost all the energy you need. It's called an *anaerobic* system because it doesn't need oxygen to operate. It consists of ATP that is already stored in muscle and *creatine phosphate (CP)* that can be used to rapidly replenish that ATP supply.

The compound CP can't fuel an activity directly, but it can make more ATP that can after you've used up your muscles' initial one-second supply. The energy released from the rapid breakdown of CP then replenishes ATP to fuel your muscles for another five to nine seconds of activity.

Any activity that lasts less than 10 seconds is fueled mainly by phosphagens. Some examples include a power lift, a 40-meter sprint, a pole vault, a long jump, a baseball pitch, or a basketball dunk.

Generally, these types of activities don't lower your blood glucose because glucose isn't used to produce the energy. On the contrary, they can raise your glucose levels because, being short and intense, they can cause your body to release an excess of glucose-raising hormones, and then they end. The extra glucose released stays in your bloodstream.

Lactic acid system (fast, furious, and painful)

You've probably heard of lactic acid already because it gets a bad rap. People blame it for making their muscles stiff and sore after exercise, as well as for the pain they feel in their active muscles. Only the second part is true, though, because lactic acid stays in the muscles for only a few minutes after it's formed, and it certainly isn't what makes you sore later. (That's caused by muscle damage and increased blood flow — swelling — in those areas to fix them.)

Lactic acid is also the name for your body's second energy system, the *lactic acid* (or *rapid glycolysis*) *system*. It supplies the extra fuel for activities that last longer than 10 seconds, but only up to about 2 minutes. This system is also anaerobic because it makes ATP by breaking down glucose stored in muscle as glycogen.

TECHNICAL STUFF

The lactic acid system makes ATP through a process called *glycogenolysis*. After glycogen has been released from storage, it gives off energy through the metabolic pathway of *anaerobic glycolysis*, which forms lactic acid.

REMEMBER

If you've ever started exercising and felt like you wouldn't make it past two minutes, you've experienced the peak of the lactic acid system at work. When you get past two minutes, you usually feel better and are able to continue, but not at the same high intensity. You are switching to rely on the aerobic system, which is good because it can last much longer.

Activities that get most of their fuel from this energy system are less than two minutes in duration at a higher intensity. They include 800-meter runs; 200-meter swimming events; and stop-and-start activities with short, intense activity like basketball, lacrosse, field hockey, and ice hockey.

TECHNICAL STUFF

Due to your muscles' immediate need for more energy as you exercise for longer than 10 seconds, glycolysis proceeds rapidly to provide more ATP. It also makes lots of lactic and other acids that build up in the muscle and blood.

TIP

The best way to clear lactic acid out of your muscles and blood quickly after intense exercise is to do an active recovery at an easy to moderate pace, rather than just stopping movement and sitting down.

Aerobic system (lasts longer)

The other end of the spectrum from the first two energy systems is the aerobic energy system used for endurance activities or ultra-endurance exercise. Sometimes called cardio workouts (short for *cardiovascular*, or involving the heart and the blood vessels), aerobic activities mainly depend on production of energy using oxygen.

WHY IS THE LACTIC ACID SYSTEM SO PAINFUL?

When muscles contain large quantities of lactic acid, the lactic acid drops the pH, causing the associated burn in those muscles and making you feel fatigued. This system can make only 3 ATP from each glucose molecule coming from muscle glycogen, which is a relatively small amount compared with the 37 to 39 ATP that the aerobic energy systems can produce. Consequently, the lactic acid system wouldn't be a good way to supply energy for long, even if it could (but it can't).

When you're resting, your muscle cells use the same pathway (glycolysis) to make ATP. But because you're using ATP slowly, the glycogen is processed using oxygen, more energy is released, and little lactic acid builds up.

REMEMBER

The aerobic energy system provides almost all the fuel for any activity you do that lasts longer than two minutes continuously — at least after the first two minutes.

Your muscles require a steady supply of ATP during sustained activities like walking, running, swimming, cycling, rowing, and cross-country skiing, which you usually do for a longer period. Extreme examples of prolonged aerobic activities include running a marathon, doing a triathlon, or participating in successive full days of long-distance cycling or backpacking. This system uses a mix of carbohydrate and fat to make ATP — more fat during rest and greater carbohydrate use during exercise. Your muscles can use some protein as fuel, but it usually contributes less than 5 percent of the total energy. Your body may use slightly more protein (up to 15 percent) during extremely prolonged endurance activities like running a marathon.

REMEMBER

Most protein in your body is part of structures like muscles, hormones, and enzymes and is your body's last choice for exercise fuel.

At rest, your diet and how recently you last exercised affect the mix of fuels your body uses, but most people use about 60 percent fat and 40 percent carbohydrate. If you're exercising with hyperglycemia, your body may use more blood glucose than normal, regardless of your type of diabetes.

TECHNICAL STUFF

Your body rapidly begins to use more carbohydrate as soon as you start to exercise, and carbohydrate contributes even more to making energy during harder-intensity exercise. High-intensity or hard activities use almost 100 percent carbohydrate. Muscle glycogen provides more — usually close to 80 percent — than blood glucose, unless you're already glycogen depleted from a long workout or from following a low-carbohydrate diet. The actual aerobic fuels your body uses during the activity depend on your training status, your diet before and during the activity, the intensity and duration of the activity, and insulin levels in your blood. More glucose comes from the liver's making it from scratch (a process called *gluconeogenesis*), particularly when you have diabetes and aren't managing your blood glucose that well overall.

Circulating hormones like adrenaline get the fat out of your fat cells (called *adipocytes*), and those fats go to your working muscles as fatty acids the muscles can use for fuel during less-intense or longer-duration activities. Your body can use more fat during mild and moderate activities, along with some carbohydrate. The fats stored in the muscles themselves (*intramuscular triglycerides*) are more important to fuel helping you recover from exercise or during very prolonged workouts (lasting more than two to three hours).

Using Carbohydrate and Fat as Fuels

Glucose, the body's main form of energy during exercise, is in the blood, muscles, and liver. All carbohydrate can be converted into glucose. Some of it gets used right away, but more is usually stored in your liver and muscles as glycogen after you eat.

During the first few minutes of exercise, your muscles utilize the glucose stored there almost exclusively, releasing lactic acid as a byproduct. As you continue to exercise, your body releases stress hormones, adrenaline, and other hormones that signal to your liver that your body needs more glucose, and your liver releases the glucose you need.

After 20 minutes or so of doing any activity, your body begins to use slightly more stored fat for energy. How much depends on things like how hard you're working (more intense exercise uses more carbohydrates), how long you exercise (longer workouts increase fat use), how frequently you exercise (because fully restoring extra carbohydrates in your body takes a while), and your usual diet.

REMEMBER

Fat essentially "burns" in a carbohydrate flame, so you can't use fat effectively as an alternative fuel after you've depleted your glycogen stores.

Carbohydrate: A high-octane fuel

Doing moderate or vigorous exercise always requires that you have some carbohydrates available, or you'll be too fatigued to do anything but walk or stop to rest. The body prefers to use carbohydrate because it's more fuel efficient. It's like using a high-octane gas and getting more mileage for the same amount of gas — only in the case of the body, carbohydrates release more energy with less oxygen needed compared to fat.

TIP

If you take in extra carbohydrate during prolonged exercise, your body will use up to about 70 or 80 grams per hour, depending on how hard you're working and how much muscle glycogen you have used up.

Forget the "fat-burning range"

You're always burning calories during exercise, and whether they come from glucose or fat doesn't matter in terms of expending a certain number of calories or losing weight, despite your cardio training machine or cardio tracking app telling you that you're in a "fat-burning range" or a "cardio-training range." (You use more carbohydrate than anything in either range.)

The more calories you burn (from either source), the more weight you can potentially lose. The so-called training range you're in matters only to your duration — you'll be able to do easier exercise for longer — and to its effect on your blood glucose levels, which lower more with easier activities.

Predicting Your Usual Glucose Response

Doing any physical movement increases your body's use of blood glucose, which can cause you to develop hypoglycemia more readily during or after your workout while you're working out. Most of the changes in your blood glucose depend on how much insulin is in your bloodstream when you're active, along with how well that insulin is working when you're resting. For example, if your insulin levels are high during an activity, your muscles take up more blood glucose, and you may end up with low blood glucose. You can even end up low for up to 48 hours after you exercise.

On the other hand, exercising when your blood glucose is too high — especially with ketones from having too little insulin in your body — can cause your blood glucose to go even higher. Exercising under those conditions can put you into a serious state of ketoacidosis (*DKA, or diabetic ketoacidosis*) caused by the combination of too much blood glucose and not enough insulin. Certain types of exercise, such as intense resistance workouts, can also raise your blood glucose, regardless of whether you have diabetes.

WARNING

DKA is a result of the liver producing ketones which makes your blood too acidic and almost always is caused by not having enough insulin in your body. It can be life threatening and land you in the hospital.

Many other factors can impact your usual responses to physical activity. After you learn to anticipate their effects and manage as many as you can, a somewhat predictable pattern emerges over time to help you better predict your blood glucose responses to similar exercise. The type of activity you do can also affect your blood glucose responses, along with how hard, how long, and how often you're active.

WARNING

Though almost anyone with diabetes can exercise safely, if you take insulin (via injections or pump), you have to be more vigilant about managing your food intake and insulin doses to avoid ending up with blood glucose levels that are too low or too high before, during, and after exercise. If you take other medications that increase your natural release of insulin, you also have to be more proactive to prevent lows.

REMEMBER

Having to deal with so many variables that can potentially affect your blood glucose during exercise can be frustrating. But being active to enhance your overall health and well-being is still a better choice.

Factoring in Exercise Variables

A number of different factors impact how your blood glucose responds to any activity you do. In this section, you find out more about what those are and the response you can expect.

Type (which exercises)

What type of activity you do is your choice because almost any movement can benefit your health, including cardio training, resistance work, intervals, and cross-training. In adults with type 2 diabetes, a single bout of cardio or resistance training has similar glycemic benefits.

Choosing activities that help you gain or maintain your muscle mass to better manage your diabetes and your overall health as you age is always a good idea. Muscles are the main place you can store the extra carbohydrates you eat and, the bigger your muscle tank, the more carbohydrates you can store there (which helps keep blood glucose levels down). Plus, regular exercise keeps the tank at least partway empty most of the time.

TIP

Pick activities to gain more muscle or at least keep the muscle you have.

Picking an activity (any activity)

Not surprisingly, people like to do a lot of different types of activities; one type certainly doesn't fit all. In the Big Blue Test (BBT) conducted online a few years back, almost half of people with diabetes walked, while others engaged in running or jogging (12 percent), cycling (9 percent), using conditioning machines

(6 percent), dancing (6 percent), or other activities (19 percent). Choosing between doing cardio training or resistance workouts may be less important than simply choosing to do anything.

The type of activity you choose isn't nearly as critical as simply getting moving is. Pick what you enjoy doing most so you're more likely to keep at it for many years to come.

Managing your blood glucose, regardless

No matter what you do, be aware of your blood glucose numbers and be cautious. If your blood glucose is too high or low, or you're not feeling well, you shouldn't exercise. Also, if your blood glucose goes up, don't take a correction dose of insulin (if you use it) unless your blood glucose is still high one to two hours later. In that case, consider taking a third to a half dose of your usual correction dose so you don't get low later.

If your blood glucose is below your target when you finish being active, have an appropriate snack and/or lower your post-exercise insulin dosing.

Intensity (how hard)

How hard you work out should reflect your training and fitness goals, such as whether you want to get fitter, perform better, or just burn some calories

Considering factors that determine your desired intensity

Your intensity range should be based on how fit you already are, how long you've had diabetes, whether you have any health issues, and your personal goals. For example, to improve your aerobic or muscular fitness the most, pick exercise that's either moderate or vigorous in intensity, not just easy activities.

The biggest impact on blood glucose is likely the intensity of your activity. For example, 75 percent of exercisers have their glucose levels drop when they're active, about 9 percent stay the same, and 15 percent have an increase rather than a decrease.

In general, doing exercise at a low intensity (less than 40 percent heart rate reserve, or HRR) has a lesser glucose-lowering effect than moderate-intensity exercise — unless you do the exercise long enough. How much glucose you use during moderate workouts depends on both how long you work out and how hard you do it. For vigorous exercise (60 percent HRR and higher), you may end up with temporary increases in your blood glucose. (Check out the later section "Heart rate reserve" for details on this measurement.)

Doing any higher-intensity exercise (like interval training) may raise your blood glucose, at least temporarily. In this case, your blood glucose is likely to drop over the next few hours — even more so than if you'd done a similar amount of an easier exercise.

Adding in faster intervals during any moderate activity can keep glucose more stable during the activity.

Doing easy activities can help lower blood glucose over the course of the day for most people. If you're active longer, even just doing an easy activity like walking or standing, your body uses more blood glucose, and your blood levels can decrease over time. How much glucose you use depends on how fit you are doing that activity. Being fitter increases fat use (over glucose) in most cases.

Monitoring your exercise intensity

You have options on how to follow how hard you're working out, if you choose to do that. They're as easy as seeing how well you can talk to thinking about how hard it feels to actually measuring something that reflects your intensity.

TALK TEST

A good way to determine whether to speed up or slow down is by using the *talk test*. Exercising moderately — meaning that you can still carry on a conversation during your activity — is optimal. You're working hard enough, but not so hard that you have to stop early.

If you can sing or whistle while doing the activity, however, the speed or intensity may be too low to get you fit, and you may want to work a little harder. If you're short of breath or winded and can't talk, you're exercising vigorously and may need to slow down (especially when just starting out).

RATING OF PERCEIVED EXERTION

Another measure of intensity is *perceived exertion*, which is how hard you feel you're working. You should base it on your own perception of your heartbeats, breathing rate, sweating, and feelings of fatigue. Although it's a subjective measure, your exertion rating is a reasonable estimate of your actual heart rate (pulse) during activities.

A subjective rating of your workout feeling "somewhat hard" to "hard" means you're working at a moderate to vigorous level.

HEART RATE RESERVE

A third method to monitor exercise intensity uses a target heart rate during your workouts. Having a target allows you to use the latest apps or monitoring devices to get the most out of your activities, especially if your find that having a target is motivating.

TECHNICAL STUFF

The American College of Sports Medicine (ACSM) recommends an exercise intensity of 40 to 89 percent of heart rate reserve. (This range also corresponds to 55 to 90 percent of maximum heart rate.) The recommended intensity range of 40 to 89 percent is broad because unfit people can get fitter doing lower intensities while more fit ones may have to work harder to get similar gains. Using this heart rate method, *moderate* exercise is in the range of 40 to 59 percent HRR, while *vigorous* is 60 to 89 percent HRR. Someone who's out of shape may start at a target as low as 30 to 39 percent HRR and work up to more moderate levels slowly.

What's your *heart rate reserve?* Basically, your reserve is just the total amount you can raise your pulse, or the difference between your heart rate at rest and how high it can go.

Figuring out your target heart rate by using this method is better than using a percentage of your maximal heart rate, and it isn't as complicated as it seems at first. To use this method, you need to know what your maximum heart rate (MHR) is. It's best if you have that measured during a maximal exercise test, but you can also estimate it quite easily. You also need to know your true resting heart rate (RHR). This measurement is your pulse rate right after you wake up and before you've gotten out of bed in the morning.

Here are the relevant equations to figure out your exercise intensity target:

Heart rate reserve (HRR) = Maximum heart rate – resting heart rate

Percent HRR = HRR × desired intensity (percentage as decimal)

Target heart rate = [HRR × target intensity] + resting HR

Estimated maximum heart rate = 220 – Age, or = 208 – (0.7 × Age)

REMEMBER

Your calculated exercise heart rate is simply how much you must raise your heart rate above your resting pulse to meet your target.

Following is a sample calculation of 40–89 percent of heart rate reserve for a 48-year-old woman.

Resting HR (RHR): 72 beats per minute (bpm)

Maximum HR (MHR): 172 bpm (estimated as 220 – age)

$$\textbf{Target heart rate} = \left[\left(\text{MRR} - \text{RHR}\right) \times \text{desired intensity}\right] + \text{resting heart rate}$$

$$\textbf{Lower end of target range}\left(40 \text{ percent, "moderate"}\right) = \left[\left(172 - 72\right) \times 0.40\right] + 72$$
$$= \left[100 \times 0.40\right] + 72$$
$$= 40 + 72$$
$$= \textbf{112 bpm}$$

$$\textbf{Higher end of target range}\left(89 \text{ percent, "vigorous"}\right) = \left[\left(172 - 72\right) \times 0.89\right] + 72$$
$$= \left[100 \times 0.89\right] + 72$$
$$= 89 + 72$$
$$= \textbf{161 bpm}$$

$$\textbf{Target HR range}\left(40 - 89 \text{ percent HRR}\right) = \textbf{112 to 161 beats per minute}$$

This method may also overestimate the maximum HR of some with diabetes, particularly people with *autonomic neuropathy* (central nerve damage). If you have *cardiac autonomic neuropathy*, you need to get your maximum heart rate measured directly, not estimated, for it to be accurate. You may just want to use subjective measures of how hard you feel like you're working instead because this complication will likely blunt your maximum heart rate.

Duration (how long)

To burn an equivalent number of calories and to manage your blood glucose, you have to do lower-intensity exercise for longer than you would one at a higher intensity. The standard recommendation is 30 minutes of moderate-intensity work most days of the week, but doing most activities for longer lowers your blood glucose more. The effect is more similar if, and only if, you use up about the same number of calories doing an activity at any intensity.

Here are some key points about your blood glucose and how long you exercise:

>> When you work out longer, you usually have larger drops in blood glucose during mild and moderate exercise.

>> Doing any exercise for longer tends to drop blood glucose more, but really long activities have effects that can last a day or two.

>> Your glucose responses also depend on whether you're already trained for a specific activity (and use more fat as fuel).

>> Blood glucose responses to vigorous activity are more variable, but it depends on how long you do such activity.

>> Your responses may also vary if you haven't eaten for a while or exercise first thing in the morning, regardless of how long or hard your exercise is.

>> How long each of your workouts lasts may not be as critical as the total duration in a day when it comes to managing blood glucose.

TIP

If desired, you can break your physical activity down into a minimum of 10-minute sessions spread throughout the day. For example, if you have type 2 diabetes, doing moderate-to-high-intensity training for only 10 minutes three times per day may work better with your blood glucose than doing one continuous 30-minute workout. Very unfit people may need to exercise in multiple sessions of short duration (5 to 10 minutes), as well as begin at low intensities, include brief rest intervals, and progress slowly to harder activities.

TIP

When you can work out for 10 to 15 minutes at a time, work up to doing 30 or more minutes. The recommendation for weight loss is closer to 60 minutes a day.

Frequency (how often)

Being active every day is generally better for your blood glucose. The effects of aerobic exercise last 2 to 72 hours, but usually on the shorter end of that range. That means your insulin action usually starts to go down when you go more than two days without being active, and your blood glucose can creep up. Being active daily is best for improving insulin action and more than once during each day can also be helpful.

TIP

Aim to be active daily (although the activity can vary), but do some exercise every other day at a minimum. Shorter but more frequent activity each day also works well and may be easier to fit in.

As long as you do the same total amount of activity, whatever you're doing likely has the same blood glucose benefits whether you do it daily or every other day, at least if you have type 2 diabetes. That's like doing either 30 minutes a day or a full hour every other day. Not surprisingly, doing more total exercise overall (through various combinations of exercise duration, intensity, and frequency) can improve your blood glucose and insulin action even more. Exercising with type 1 diabetes can result in more variable blood glucose levels unless you balance out your food and insulin doses.

Timing (when you work out)

The time of day you exercise also affects how your blood glucose responds. Your body is temporarily more insulin resistant first thing in the morning when you have higher levels of cortisol and other hormones that help your liver keep your blood glucose stable overnight. Exercising before breakfast may not have the glucose-lowering effect that you expect.

REMEMBER

Your insulin levels are generally lower first thing in the morning and cortisol levels higher. For that reason, doing exercise before breakfast often causes blood glucose to rise, regardless of its intensity.

For instance, in men treated with oral type 2 diabetes medications, doing one hour of moderate cycling barely changed their blood glucose when they exercised before breakfast. But it dropped dramatically (down to normal) when they waited two hours after breakfast to exercise.

Eat something (and take your diabetes medications) before exercising in the early morning if you want to lower your blood glucose at that time of day.

On the other hand, if you tend to drop too low during activities, exercising in the early morning may work to prevent low blood glucose. Moderate walking and similar exercises after dinner also help prevent spikes in blood glucose then, more so than doing the same exercise before dinner.

If you often develop hypoglycemia during exercise, you may prefer to exercise in the morning before taking any insulin or eating breakfast, or to do it when your insulin levels are lower, such as three to four hours after your last meal or dose of meal-time insulin.

The largest drops in blood glucose often occur when you exercise longer (at least 30 minutes) and begin working out within one to two hours after eating, which is when insulin levels are at their highest. Knowing when your injected or pumped insulin (or even the insulin your own pancreas releases) is peaking and taking your doses into account can help you predict such changes.

If your doses are too high, insulin may make your blood glucose go too low during exercise. If you exercise shortly after eating breakfast and taking insulin, your insulin dose will affect your levels of circulating insulin. At least in one study, exercisers with type 1 diabetes who did 60 minutes of moderate cycling starting 90 minutes after taking their regular dose with an insulin pump and eating breakfast had to lower their rapid-acting insulin meal boluses by 50 percent and reduce basal insulin to nothing during the activity. If they did the same exercise in the afternoon, they needed to reduce their meal bolus insulin by even more. Any changes you may need to make to your insulin need to be unique to you, though, and could be more or less than the ones from that study.

If you don't like early morning exercise to raise your blood glucose, simply eat a small snack beforehand to make your body release a little bit of insulin (if you can) or give a reduced dose to cover the food if you take insulin.

If you take insulin, you may need to reduce your rapid-acting insulin doses by one to two units at dinner if you plan to exercise later in the evening, to avoid nocturnal lows, or you may need a bedtime snack.

If you exercise for long enough in the morning before eating, you can develop hypoglycemia. Doing longer early morning exercise without eating anything beforehand isn't a good idea for that reason. In many people with diabetes, their carbohydrate stores in their liver are lower than normal, leading them to rely more on making new glucose to keep blood glucose constant, which doesn't always work well during activities that last a long time.

If you exercise in the evening, one benefit is that when you wake up, your fasting blood glucose may be lower because of the residual insulin sensitivity that came from exercising before bedtime. Evening exercise can also lead to a higher risk of hypoglycemia while you're asleep, though, and you may need to adjust your food intake or insulin doses to compensate for that decrease.

Diabetes aside, the best time to exercise is whenever you can make the time.

Training effects (how fit you are)

After you train doing the same activity for several weeks, your blood glucose doesn't drop as much as it did when you first started because training increases your body's ability to use fat. Using more fat decreases how much muscle glycogen and blood glucose you use doing the same exercise after your muscles have adapted. This training effect is evident when you have diabetes because you find need to take in fewer carbohydrates for the same activity after several weeks or to lower your insulin less (if you take any).

Some of these training adaptations occur because of a lesser release of glucose-raising hormones when you're exercising at a moderate or low intensity. People without diabetes experience the same training effect, but it may be harder for them to see it because their blood glucose levels hardly fluctuate. Insulin release usually goes down during exercise (if you make some or all your own), but being trained causes it to go down less.

After training, your body uses less glucose and slightly more fat when you do the same activity, leading to less of a drop in blood glucose and fewer lows.

This change in fuel use explains why you may need more carbohydrate to keep your blood glucose stable when you first start an activity but less after doing it for several weeks. But if you work out harder to reach the same relative intensity (for example, if reaching 65 percent of HRR after training requires you to do a harder workload than at the start), your blood glucose use during the activity will likely be nearly as high as before.

If running 9-minute miles at the start of a workout program is the same *relative* workout intensity for you as running 8-minute miles after training, your glucose and fat use during the activity nearly stay the same. If you continue to run 9-minute miles after training when you could now run faster (that is, you maintain the same *absolute* intensity), your fat use increases and glucose use decreases for the same pace after training.

These training effects are sport-specific, which means that if you've been walking and then decide to try a new activity like swimming, your blood glucose will probably drop more during swimming until you're trained at that.

Accounting for Other Factors

Just when thought you had it all figured out, you need to take some other possible factors into account. Here are the other things that can change your blood glucose responses that you need to consider.

Environment

Whether it's hot, humid, or cold outside when you exercise or you're on top of a mountain (at high altitude), environmental extremes can affect how your blood glucose responds. Usually any environmental extreme causes your body to use more carbohydrates (and blood glucose), although being at very high altitude (over 15,000 feet) can make you insulin resistant, particularly if you develop acute mountain sickness.

TIP

Expect the environment to change your usual responses somewhat and check your blood glucose to adjust your food and medications.

Insulin regimen changes

A normal response to being active is that insulin levels in the body decrease during the activity. If you have to inject or pump insulin, lowering the level of insulin in your blood during exercise isn't as easy.

Because muscle contractions allow your muscles to take up glucose without insulin, too much insulin along with the effects of muscle activity can equal a rapid decrease in blood glucose levels. The effects of the two are additive.

REMEMBER

If you can't lower your insulin, you have to eat more carbohydrates while you're active to try to keep blood glucose from dropping too much.

Of course, any changes you need are dependent on your starting blood glucose and how hard and how long you choose to work out at any given time. Starting out at higher intensity requires fewer changes, as do shorter activities.

Bodily concerns

Many other factors can influence your blood glucose responses to any given workout. If you're sick or have an infection, your blood glucose may go up. If you're mentally stressed out or upset, dehydrated, or in the second half of your menstrual cycle (women only), it may also go up.

If you're in the first half of your menstrual cycle, have been following a low-carbohydrate diet, or have worked out recently, it may go down instead. Trying to anticipate the effects of each of these factors at any given time can be overwhelming.

TIP

Use your blood glucose meter and test frequently to stay on top of everything, and adjust your diet and medications as you go. Using a continuous glucose monitor can also be helpful to see blood glucose changes during and following your activities.

TAKE A DAY (OR TWO) OFF WHEN YOU'RE SICK

Getting a cold or the flu isn't enjoyable for anyone, and it can wreak havoc with your normal exercise routine and your insulin action. You may be wondering whether you should still try to exercise to combat this effect. It really depends on how sick you are and what stage of the illness you're in.

When you're first starting to get a cold or other illness, working out may cause it to get worse faster. Harder exercise depresses your immune system for several hours afterward and may leave you less able to fight off the virus causing the illness.

When you're fully sick, you may feel weak or too tired to exercise. On those days, abstain from working out, but try to keep up your daily movement as best you can. When the worst of the illness is past, start back slowly doing your exercise, but keep the intensity and the duration lower until you feel more like your normal self.

For more severe illnesses like the flu, the recommendation is that you take one day of rest afterward for every day that you were fully sick (that is, sick enough to stay in bed all day). Again, during that time, still try to get in some movement every day, even if it's just walking and standing. Exercising moderately generally improves your immune function and is likely to keep you from getting colds and other illnesses as easily.

Hypoglycemia-associated autonomic failure (HAAF)

People with type 1 diabetes have a higher risk of getting low during exercise when they have *hypoglycemia-associated autonomic failure (HAAF)*, a poorly understood phenomenon. In a series of studies over the years, researchers have found that when individuals who use insulin do exercise, their bodies don't release as many of their glucose-raising hormones as usual the next time that they exercise or develop hypoglycemia (the same day or even the next day). The same thing happens when you've had a bad low blood glucose (that is, one that is below 65 mg/dL, lasts a long time, or someone else has to help you treat) in the prior 24 hours and you exercise.

What experiencing HAAF means is that when you're doing successive days of exercise, you may need to lower insulin further or eat more to prevent hypoglycemia. And the same applies if you ever have a bad bout of hypoglycemia within a day or two before you work out. Thankfully, mild hypoglycemia doesn't have the same lasting effects and usually doesn't cause HAAF to occur.

Chapter 5

Avoiding Exercise Glucose Extremes

There's nothing worse than being in the middle of your workout and realizing that you aren't going to be able to finish it because your blood glucose is out of whack — either too low or too high to continue. You can't always keep this from happening to you, but you can use some tricks to avoid blood glucose extremes most of the time when you're physically active.

In this chapter, I show you what blood glucose numbers to shoot for and how to prevent the highs and the lows. Knowing the symptoms of lows is important, and you have to modify what you're eating or doing to treat and prevent low blood glucose during and following workouts. Running too high can be just as bad, so I also explain how to bring those extremes back into balance to keep on top of your game.

Exercising with an Ideal Blood Glucose

Though good for your health, exercising can create its own set of challenges when you have diabetes. Keeping blood glucose levels in a normal range is a constant balancing act. Adding exercise into the mix as one more variable to figure out can feel overwhelming at times. The more you understand about what makes your blood glucose levels go down (or sometimes up) during exercise, the easier managing it becomes, and the more confident you can be about doing activities and staying in control of your diabetes.

TIP

Most individuals try to keep their blood glucose levels between 80 and 180 mg/dL (4.4 to 10 mmol/L) to perform optimally and feel their best during exercise. Aim to start and stay in this range during your workouts.

Exercising with levels lower than 80 mg/dL can result in low blood glucose (hypoglycemia) and make you stop early, while starting out or exercising with high blood glucose (hyperglycemia) can make you feel sluggish and less motivated to continue. Though hyperglycemia is technically any blood glucose above normal, in this case I'm talking about numbers higher than around 180 mg/dL. You won't have your best workout or perform well when your blood glucose is at either of those extremes.

Check your blood glucose before you start a workout. If your blood glucose is below 70 mg/dL, you should consider raising it slightly or delaying the start of your exercise until it rises a bit higher (either after you take in some carbohydrates or on its own). The only exception is if you're going to be doing high-intensity training or a competition that is likely to raise your blood glucose levels by itself.

WARNING

If you've already had an episode of hypoglycemia in the prior 24 hours, your body's hormonal response to exercise may be blunted, which increases your risk of having another low blood glucose during or after exercise. Have glucose ready and available during exercise sessions. Also consider lowering your pre-exercise insulin dose, if possible, and setting a starting target of 120–180 mg/dL if you take insulin.

Identifying Hypoglycemia (Lows)

Hypoglycemia is usually defined as a blood glucose lower than 70 mg/dL, and it requires immediate treatment when you experience symptoms or check your blood glucose and find it low.

Hypoglycemia is likely the single biggest barrier to being active with diabetes, so being able to recognize it is the first step toward overcoming that obstacle. The following sections delve into the causes and symptoms of this condition; I discuss how to treat and prevent it later in the chapter.

Exploring what causes low blood glucose

Many things can increase your risk for a low. Some common contributors to low blood glucose are

>> Recent vigorous, prolonged, or unusual physical activity

>> Rapid drop in blood glucose

>> Reduced food or inadequate carbohydrate intake during exercise

>> Excessive insulin doses (basal or bolus amounts)

>> Consuming alcoholic drinks in the previous 12 hours

>> Prior hypoglycemic episode in the past 24 to 48 hours

>> Emotional stress or depression

>> Hormonal changes with start of menstrual cycle (women only)

REMEMBER

If you're managing your diabetes with diet and exercise alone, your risk of developing low blood glucose during exercise is minimal.

Although mild or brisk walking generally allows your body to use some fat as a fuel, you can use up a significant amount of blood glucose if you walk even a short distance in some cases. But it's even more likely if you take long walks. Prolonged exercise causes your muscles to use more stored carbohydrates (*muscle glycogen*), and when these become depleted, you have an increased risk of getting low, although the chances are still minimal unless you take supplemental insulin.

If you're running low on muscle or liver glycogen for any reason or your insulin levels are too high, your muscles will use more blood glucose than normal. In that case, you'll likely have to take in some extra carbohydrate.

During high-intensity, prolonged aerobic activities like running, your body relies almost exclusively on carbohydrate as a fuel, depleting muscle glycogen and glucose in your bloodstream if you exercise for longer than two hours. You'll likely also need to snack during long activities for that reason.

TIP

If your blood glucose drops during extended activities, eat an extra 15 grams of carbohydrates during the activity. It may also help to eat some within 30 minutes to 2 hours of when you finish this type of workout.

Recognizing the symptoms of lows

Though numerous symptoms of hypoglycemia exist, they may differ from one activity or situation to another, vary by time of day, and change over time — even in the same person. Also, how low your blood glucose goes before it causes symptoms can change.

REMEMBER

If your blood glucose has been running on the high side, sometimes you'll get symptoms while your blood glucose is still normal if it drops rapidly, without ever getting as low as 70 mg/dL. If you're in tight control normally, your symptoms may not start until you get to 55 mg/dL, or even lower.

What does a typical low feel like?

Typical symptoms of hypoglycemia (Figure 5-1) include shakiness, hand trembling, tingling of your hands or tongue, sweating, mental confusion, irritability, poor physical coordination (that is, clumsiness), and vision changes. Your usual symptoms can vary with your training state, diet, environmental conditions, and more, which is why knowing all the possible symptoms is helpful. Plus, knowing the symptoms means you can treat a low quickly.

Look for signs of any of these typical symptoms of hypoglycemia:

>> Cold or clammy skin

>> Dizziness or lightheadedness

>> Double or blurred vision

>> Elevated pulse rate (beyond exercise-induced increases)

>> Headache

>> Inability to do basic math

>> Insomnia

>> Irritability

>> Mental confusion

>> Nausea

>> Nightmares

>> Poor physical coordination

>> Rapid-onset fatigue (sudden, unusual, or unexpected tiredness)

>> Shakiness in your hands

» Sweating

» Tingling of hands or tongue

» Visual spots

» Weakness

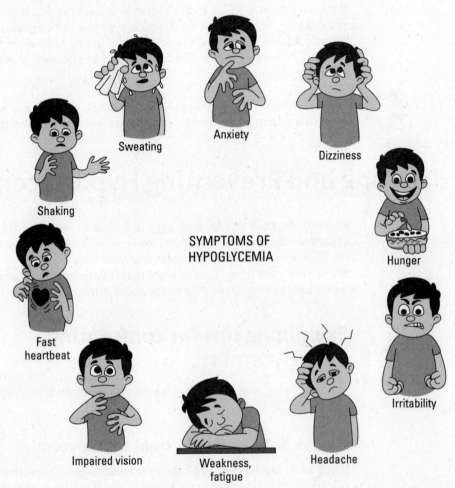

SYMPTOMS OF HYPOGLYCEMIA

Shaking

Sweating

Anxiety

Dizziness

Hunger

Fast heartbeat

Irritability

Impaired vision

Weakness, fatigue

Headache

FIGURE 5-1:
Typical symptoms
of hypoglycemia.

© *John Wiley & Sons, Inc.*

How can you tell if you're low?

You can't always easily tell right away if your blood glucose is too high or low
when you start feeling funny, especially during exercise. When your blood glucose
is changing rapidly, you often can't tell which direction it's going.

In those cases, use your blood glucose meter to check. You can wait until your symptoms progress, but the full-blown symptoms of a low are never fun; checking with a meter if you can may allow you to treat symptoms sooner and avoid feeling worse. Using a continuous glucose monitor may be helpful as well in identifying a trend toward low blood glucose.

If you've ever experienced hypoglycemia, you may be familiar with the effect that it can have on your ability to think straight and act normal. If you ever find yourself thinking, "I know what 2 + 2 equals, but I just can't figure it out right now," you're probably low. If you try for several minutes to program your clock radio with the TV remote, you're also likely experiencing a lack of glucose needed for normal brain function.

Feeling shaky, extremely fatigued all of a sudden, or weak may be symptoms of a low that's affecting your whole body and not just how well you think.

Treating and Preventing Hypoglycemia

Knowing the best way to treat lows is critical to lessening the symptoms you experience. You want to raise your blood glucose back to normal as quickly as you can. If you've never had a low, just ask anyone who has been through one; they'll tell you the same thing. Keep in mind that the amount of carbohydrate needed to treat a low can vary, depending on the reason why you're too low in the first place.

Examining tips for confronting hypoglycemia

In the following sections, I give you some handy suggestions so you can nip hypoglycemia in the bud.

Always be prepared to treat hypoglycemia

If you're an insulin user and have ever been caught somewhere without having anything with you to treat hypoglycemia, you're not likely to forget to bring supplies along the next time. Carry some glucose or other carbohydrates with you whenever you're exercising, even if you're just out walking the dog.

Even if you've never experienced a low before, keep supplies on hand to treat it just in case. You'd hate to be unprepared for your first time.

Check your blood glucose

Keep a blood glucose meter handy to check your blood glucose regularly. Check immediately after exercise and then every 30 to 60 minutes for a couple of hours to determine what kind of lasting effect the exercise is having. If you experience symptoms and have your blood glucose meter handy, confirm that you're having a low. If you don't have a meter, go ahead and treat for hypoglycemia anyway (by eating rapidly absorbed carbohydrates) to be on the safe side.

Treat lows with carbohydrate

Any carbohydrate you take in during and after exercise to prevent or treat hypoglycemia should have a higher glycemic index (GI) value for rapid absorption. That means that the carbohydrate gets into your system quickly. In most circumstances, don't eat things that also have a high fat content — such as chocolate candy, donuts, or potato chips — because the fat in those foods slows down how quickly your body digests the carbohydrates. (Refer to the following section for more on picking the right foods for treating hypoglycemia.)

TIP

Treat low blood glucose immediately with small amounts (4 to 15 grams) of high-GI carbohydrates, wait 5 to 10 minutes for them to take effect, and then recheck your glucose levels or monitor your symptoms. Consume the same amount of carbohydrate again only if your hypoglycemic symptoms haven't started to resolve by then.

Your whole body usually only has about 5 grams of glucose total in your bloodstream, so avoid eating too much, or you'll likely end up with elevated glucose levels later. Unless the insulin levels in your body are high, you may only need anywhere from 4 to 15 grams of glucose to raise your blood glucose to normal.

Choose the carbohydrates that work the fastest

The fastest treatments contain straight glucose (also called *dextrose*). You can find straight glucose in glucose tablets, glucose gels, Gu, most sports drinks, candies like Smarties and SweeTARTS, and more.

Glucose tablets, gels, or liquids have a couple of benefits for treating lows because glucose is the sugar that is normally in the blood, and it gets there most rapidly after you eat or drink it. These products also come in measured amounts — usually 4 grams per tablet or 15 grams per gel or liquid container — making it easy to consume only a specific amount. With trial and error, you can determine how much each tablet, gel, or liquid is likely to raise your blood glucose.

TIP

Using glucose tablets — with 4 grams of glucose per tablet — is an effective way to treat and prevent lows without overshooting on carbohydrates (and ending up high) or calories (which can make you gain weight; see the sidebar "Treating lows without gaining extra fat weight" in this chapter).

You may not always have glucose handy to treat hypoglycemia, though, and you can use other foods and drinks as well. Always carry treatments with you in case of emergency:

>> One to two rolls of Smarties (6 grams each)

>> One to two pieces of hard or sugary candy (but not chocolate)

>> Four ounces of regular soda

>> Eight ounces of juice diluted to be half water (to speed up digestion)

>> Eight ounces of sports drink (6 to 9 grams of carbohydrate)

>> Eight ounces of skim milk

>> Two to three graham crackers or six saltine crackers

The white sugar (sucrose) in regular sodas and candy also works as a treatment because it's half glucose. You can also use skim milk, hard candies, bagels, bread, crackers, cornflakes, and white potatoes.

TIP

Avoid fruit juice as your first choice to treat lows because its primary sugar (fructose) has a relatively low rate of being converted into glucose, and the body absorbs it more slowly. Although juice has traditionally been used for treatment, it may lead to overtreatment of lows while you're waiting for its effects to kick in. Some juices have added glucose, though, and don't contain just fructose, so they may work faster.

Never treat hypoglycemia with low-GI carbohydrates (such as legumes) because the body doesn't absorb them rapidly enough to treat lows quickly. In the preceding section, I note that you shouldn't use chocolate and other high-fat sugary foods to treat hypoglycemia because of their slow absorption rate, and that's generally true. However, how much and what you treat hypoglycemia with may vary by the situation. If you're likely to keep dropping from the insulin in your system or for another reason, you may need to consume additional food or drinks with greater staying power — that is, with some fat or protein to go with the carbohydrate, like peanut butter crackers or energy bars.

Milk is a good treatment option because it contains 7 to 8 grams of protein, along with some fat depending on the type. For prevention of lows that come on later after exercise, whole milk is much more effective than skim milk or even sports drinks, likely because of the extra fat in the whole variety that takes longer to fully digest and impact your blood glucose.

TIP

Chocolate milk is a balanced and effective recovery drink for prevention of lows and recovery from exercise. If you can't drink milk, try soymilk or other options with a mostly equal mix of carbohydrate, protein, and fat.

Keep glucagon on hand for bad lows

Having a glucagon kit on hand may also be beneficial if you experience a bad low that lasts a long time or that you're unable to treat yourself. Of course, your family and friends will need to learn how to use it on you. Glucagon could previously only be given as an injection, but a nasal glucagon spray is in the works. Other companies are working on making more stable formulations to be given as mini-doses with a glucagon pen (similar to the idea of using an insulin pen) to raise blood glucose without taking in glucose or food.

Preventing exercise lows if you use insulin

Few situations are more frustrating than having to stop in the middle of a workout to treat a low blood glucose and not being able to finish working out. What if you're out dancing and you have to stop due to a low? You want to avoid having to stop exercising no matter what fun activity you're doing.

Insulin users must change up their diabetes regimens — possibly including making food changes, modifying insulin doses, and picking different activities — to prevent getting low. You can learn your body's reactions and start to predict what will cause you to drop, which allows you to prevent it.

Some general strategies to prevent hypoglycemia are

>> Learn your body's reaction to specific foods, activities, and stressors by checking your blood glucose often to find your patterns and trends.

>> Test your blood glucose more often when you do new activities, travel, or change up your usual routines.

>> Check more often if you had a bad low or exercised hard in the 24 hours prior to your latest workout.

>> For several hours after a workout, check your blood glucose every hour or so to catch and prevent lows later.

>> Keep in mind that lows can happen not only during or right after exercise but also 6 to 12 hours and even up to 48 hours later.

Carbohydrate and food changes include the following:

>> Consume more carbohydrates or lower your insulin more when doing new or unusual activities, both during them and afterward.

>> Eat extra carbohydrates and possibly other foods before, during, and after exercise.

>> Choose foods that require smaller insulin doses to cover them when you plan on exercising afterward (that is, eat fewer carbohydrates then).

>> Eat at least 15 grams of carbohydrate, along with a little protein and fat, within 30 minutes to 2 hours after exercise to prevent lows.

Insulin dosing changes are also possible:

>> Reduce your insulin doses prior to and during exercise to keep levels low like they'd be in someone without diabetes.

>> Avoid exercise for one to two hours after you give any mealtime insulin, unless you take less insulin or eat more carbohydrates to compensate.

>> If you take insulin for meals and snacks, learn how much you need for a certain intake of carbohydrate to avoid taking too much.

>> If you take any insulin for food you eat within two hours after exercise, lower the dose from your usual amount for that food.

>> If taking more rapid-acting insulin within two hours of your last dose, take a reduced second dose to avoid insulin "stacking."

>> Never skip meals or food for which you've already taken insulin or oral medications that cause insulin to be released.

Suggestions related to the timing, type, or frequency of exercise include these:

>> If you exercise first thing in the morning when you're more insulin resistant, you are less likely to experience a low, and your blood glucose may go up rather than down.

>> When doing both cardio and resistance training, do cardio first if starting with a higher blood glucose, or do resistance work first if it's lower.

>> If you start to feel low, sprint as hard as you can for 10 to 30 seconds to cause a greater release of adrenaline and other hormones to raise glucose. (Flip to the later section "Effects of sprinting" for more on this topic.)

>> Multiple days of exercise training increase the risk of a low, so plan on lower insulin doses on subsequent days and on eating more to prevent a low.

Avoiding lows all the time

You can take some actions to avoid ever getting low. If you hate getting lows or want to minimize how often you get them, follow the advice in this section.

REMEMBER

Most people don't feel nearly as bad when their blood glucose is a little (or even a lot) high compared to being too low, and you may be tempted to run yours on the high side to prevent lows. However, trying to keep your blood glucose normal is much better for your long-term health.

Prevent hypoglycemia after exercise

As I mention earlier in the chapter, after-exercise lows can occur both because your muscle carbohydrates (*glycogen*) are low and being replenished (during which time your insulin action is higher) and because your response of glucose-raising hormones after you've recently exercised may be diminished.

WARNING

If you use insulin or take oral medications that cause insulin release, you need to be on the offensive to prevent getting low in the hours after exercise.

The period in the first 30 minutes to 2 hours after exercise is the critical time when your muscles can take up glucose without much need for insulin. If you can start to restore your muscle glycogen right after exercise at the fastest rate by taking in adequate carbohydrates during this window of opportunity, you're less likely to get as low later. Eating a low-carbohydrate diet during this time not only slows down the rate of glycogen that is being replaced but also sets you up for delayed hypoglycemia if you use insulin.

TIP

If you don't use insulin, eating fewer carbohydrates during the first 30 minutes to 2 hours after exercise may keep your insulin action high for longer.

You may have more than one time following a workout when your body rapidly depletes your blood glucose. One study showed a biphasic increase in carbohydrate requirements — meaning that you can get low at two different times, both right after exercise and again from 7 to 11 hours afterward. Although this effect may not happen in everyone, you should still be on the alert for this second wave of potential hypoglycemia after exercise so you can prevent it.

REMEMBER

Although carbohydrate is most important to replace in the short run, for longer prevention of lows without first causing short-term hyperglycemia, extra protein and fat intake will also help because they have more staying power.

Regularly restore muscle glycogen to lower risk

If you do exercise training on a regular basis, you need to take in enough carbohydrate every day to restore your muscle and liver glycogen between workouts. When you have diabetes, you must manage your blood glucose before and after exercise so that you can put carbohydrate back into those storage places normally.

REMEMBER

To restore glycogen effectively, you need adequate insulin, especially more than an hour after exercise when glucose uptake is more dependent on insulin.

Taking in some carbohydrate immediately after you finish a workout or race will speed up your initial glycogen replacement and help lower your risk of developing low blood glucose later, and your body won't need much insulin then to accomplish that. Adequate carbohydrate intake also helps ensure that your glycogen stores are maximally loaded by the time your next workout rolls around.

REMEMBER

Full muscle glycogen replacement after exercise can take 24 to 48 hours, so that is when your blood glucose needs to stay as close to normal as possible.

TIP

If you eat a low-carbohydrate diet, fully restoring your glycogen takes longer. For that reason, you may want to take in at least 130 grams of carbohydrate per day in your diet on days you exercise. Also, make sure you take enough insulin (if you use it) to get those carbohydrates properly stored in your muscles and liver.

Consider loading with carbohydrates

If you're going to run a half-marathon or a marathon, you need to carbohydrate load to make sure your glycogen stores are full at the start of the race. Keep these points in mind for effective carbohydrate loading when you have diabetes or prediabetes:

» You don't need to spend a week, or even as long as three days, overconsuming carbohydrate to load up your muscle glycogen. Even a single day with a higher carbohydrate intake and rest or tapering can effectively maximize carbohydrate stores in muscles.

» Eating as much carbohydrate as the typical glycogen-loading scenarios recommend may be counterproductive for most people with diabetes. Your carbohydrate intake doesn't need to exceed 50 percent of your calories on the day that you load, assuming you eat enough calories to keep your weight stable with all your exercise training.

>> For carbohydrate loading to be effective with diabetes, your muscles must be able to take up enough glucose.

>> Make sure you have sufficient insulin when you take in carbohydrate to prevent hyperglycemia and promote muscle glucose uptake.

>> Consuming higher-fiber carbohydrate sources will prevent an excessive rise in your blood glucose and still be effective for loading, but it may cause bloating and discomfort if consumed too close to your activity.

>> To optimize your liver glycogen stores, keeping your blood glucose at closer to normal is the most effective strategy.

TIP

To maximize your glycogen stores, combine rest, a carbohydrate-rich diet, and good blood glucose management for a single day.

Beware of hypoglycemia unawareness

Some people develop *hypoglycemia unawareness,* which means they either don't have or fail to recognize the usual symptoms of getting low. This condition appears to be more common if you keep your blood glucose in a tight normal range or you have frequent lows already.

WARNING

Most people who have had type 1 diabetes for longer than 10 years have a blunted release of glucose-raising hormones (for example, glucagon and adrenaline) when they get low from having too much insulin in their bodies.

If you ever get a bad low without being aware of it, you may have this condition, which is estimated to affect up to 20 percent of insulin users. Although it's less common in people with type 2 diabetes, those who have both hypoglycemia unawareness and type 2 diabetes have a greater likelihood of experiencing a severe low and a decline in thinking ability.

Why does this condition happen? Normally, when your blood glucose starts to get too low, you experience symptoms such as sweating, shaking, weakness, and vision changes, due to the release of adrenaline and the other glucose-raising hormones. If you're unaware, though, you may have milder or missing symptoms due to a blunted release of these hormones in response to dropping blood glucose levels. (Check out the earlier section "What does a typical low feel like?" for a fuller list of hypoglycemia symptoms.)

Because low blood glucose affects your ability to think and reason, you may even test your blood glucose when you're low and not realize that the numbers you're seeing mean you need to eat. Some people resist help treating it from others or run away from paramedics who are trying to help them. In other words, the low prevents you from thinking straight and doing things to raise your blood glucose. Given that the nerves use blood glucose as a fuel, this effect isn't entirely surprising — but it certainly is alarming.

WARNING

Though you can easily treat mild hypoglycemia with carbohydrate intake, if your blood glucose drops too low without symptoms or enough time to react and treat it, you may be become unresponsive or unconscious.

If you're experiencing hypoglycemia unawareness, consider trying one of these options:

>> Prevent all hypoglycemia for two to three weeks straight to regain some level of awareness. Set a target blood glucose of 150 mg/dL during that time.

>> Wear a continuous glucose monitoring (CGM) device to alert you to decreases in your blood glucose before they get to a critically low point.

Find out more about HAAF

Many insulin users also experience a condition known as *hypoglycemia-associate autonomic failure* (HAAF), but it's most likely to happen if you have type 1 diabetes and not so much for anyone with type 2. This condition involves an abnormal hormonal response to either exercise or hypoglycemia, but it is most likely to occur when you've exercised within the past 24 hours or you had a bad low during that time frame.

WARNING

If you've had a bad low in the prior 24 hours or exercised during that time, you may be more prone to developing hypoglycemia the next time you exercise.

Because having diabetes for longer than 10 years often results in a blunted release of glucose-raising hormones when you get low, your body may release less of these hormones than it used to, and your blood glucose may stay or go lower than before. However, women's hormonal responses appear to be better preserved during exercise after either prior exercise or a low compared with men's, making the fairer sex better able to respond to exercise-induced lows.

How low you go and how long you stay low also affect whether you experience HAAF during your next hypoglycemia event. For example, short duration hypoglycemia has less of a lasting effect on your ability to respond the next time compared to longer lows, so detecting and treating hypoglycemia early can help prevent this condition.

In one study, participants underwent different levels of induced hypoglycemia for two hours: 70 mg/dL, 60 mg/dL, and 50 mg/dL. When their glucose levels had been normal the previous day, they had perfect hormonal responses to exercise the next day, but any hypoglycemia, even just down to 70 mg/dL, blunted their glucose-raising hormonal responses during their next workout. And the lower it had gone, the worse those next-workout responses were.

You're more likely to develop bad lows within 24 to 48 hours after a day when you exercised more than usual or with greater intensity (such as changing a training schedule or doing a competition). This effect appears to occur rapidly — within a couple of hours — and can increase your risk of getting low for the rest of the day after a workout and the next day.

Using exercise to prevent and treat lows

You may be able to prevent, treat, or reverse your impending hypoglycemia during exercise by some novel means. One way is by doing short sprints, while another is to alter the order of exercises you're doing.

Effects of sprinting

Doing a 10-second sprint either before or immediately after a moderate-intensity workout keeps your blood glucose more stable for at least two hours afterward. This technique works anytime during exercise, but it doesn't reduce the amount of carbohydrate needed to prevent lows during the eight hours following such a sprint.

Sprinting to raise your blood glucose to prevent a low doesn't work if you have a lot of insulin in your bloodstream or experience a blunted hormonal response to activity. The good news is that having a prior low won't affect your release of glucose-raising hormones when you do a short sprint.

You can also keep blood glucose higher during exercise by interspersing four-second sprints into an easier workout every two minutes or so (sort of like doing interval training of sorts). These effects are due to a greater glucose release by the liver during intense exercise and less glucose uptake by muscles during exercise and recovery.

Sprints work best when you have a limited amount of insulin in your system and may not prevent hypoglycemia when you have a lot of insulin on board. When the short-term hormonal effects wear off, however, you can develop hypoglycemia later because doing sprints uses up more muscle glycogen.

Variation in the order of training

Another strategy to manage or prevent lows during activities is to change the order of exercises you do, when your choices are either aerobic or resistance training. Blood glucose levels tend to fall more during moderate aerobic exercise and less afterward compared to resistance workouts, which causes less of a decline during the activity and more overnight.

Aerobic and resistance activities done during the same workout can be ordered strategically to better manage your blood glucose:

>> If you start out on the low side, do resistance training first, followed by aerobic work, to keep glucose higher throughout the first half of your workout.

>> If starting out on the high side with your blood glucose, begin with aerobic training first (assuming it's moderate) to lower blood glucose levels and follow it up with resistance work, during which it will stay more stable.

Dealing with exercise spontaneity

Say someone asks you to go play tennis on the spur of the moment, but you just took some insulin to cover a meal. You now are stuck trying to compensate for this activity entirely with carbohydrate intake (unless you wear a pump and can lower your basal insulin delivery).

TIP

To counter the extra insulin quickly before you start your activity, take in a food or drink with straight glucose.

Items with sucrose (white sugar), such as regular sodas and candy, contain half glucose (half fructose) and are your second choice. Fruit or juice (with fruit sugar) can help prevent lows later because it's absorbed more slowly, but it's not optimal as your first line of defense.

If your activity starts within two hours of the last dose of rapid-acting insulin you took, you may need to take some glucose every 10 to 15 minutes or consume some other types of carbohydrates to cover your insulin (depending on how much insulin you took, the exercise intensity and duration, and so on). You may also need to take in foods or drinks with a balance of carbohydrate, protein, and fat, depending on how long you're active.

REMEMBER

You may need a more balanced food like an energy bar, peanut butter crackers, whole milk, or a mini-meal to prevent lows during and after spontaneous activity.

TREATING LOWS WITHOUT GAINING EXTRA FAT WEIGHT

One issue related to treating lows is that the treatments you use all contain calories. Although hypoglycemia is a medical condition that absolutely requires treatment, having to eat more to treat a low means that you still may be taking in extra calories that can be stored as body fat.

Not surprisingly, some heavily training athletes with type 1 diabetes end up gaining fat weight rather than getting leaner from all their workouts. In almost all cases, this occurs because they're chasing a lot of lows with extra (but necessary to restore blood glucose) calories that end up being packed away into their fat cells.

The best way to treat lows without gaining (much or any) extra body fat is to treat them precisely to avoid taking in too many calories. Don't just grab the nearest candy bar and eat the whole thing. Keep in mind that the body only has 5 grams of glucose total in the blood, and it may not take much more than that (one glucose tablet) to get it back into a normal range. Consider the cause of the low (too much insulin? too much exercise? something else?) and whether you're likely to keep dropping more later.

A key strategy is to kick-start the rise in your blood glucose back to normal with a rapid-acting carbohydrate like glucose (4 to 15 grams to start). Only take in additional glucose or other types of balanced foods if your low doesn't resolve itself within 10 to 15 minutes or if you anticipate needing protein or fat in your system to prevent later lows, such as after a long workout or if you took too much insulin.

Don't overtreat your lows, or you'll end up with rebound hyperglycemia. Taking more insulin later to bring your blood glucose back down from excessive treatment of a low can cause another low later — and more calorie intake and potential weight gain. You get the picture.

Managing Hyperglycemia (Highs) and Exercise

Should you exercise with elevated blood glucose (*hyperglycemia*)? It depends on how high it is, how long it has been elevated, and whether you've developed *ketones* (a byproduct of fat metabolism) in your blood and urine.

When to wait to exercise

A long-standing exercise guideline stated that you should postpone exercising if your blood glucose levels are more than 250 mg/dL and you have moderate or higher amounts of ketones. They can be measured in urine or blood.

TECHNICAL STUFF

Ketones are byproducts of your body's attempt to use fat as a fuel when glucose isn't getting into your cells. They can build up in your blood and spill over into your urine when levels get too high. Going on a low-calorie diet or even one that's just low in carbohydrate can cause ketones to build up as well, but you usually don't have high blood glucose at the same time. Although your brain and your nerves normally use glucose as a fuel, they're able to adapt to using ketones as an alternate fuel when you go for long periods without eating or do extended exercise.

You can also build up ketones when you're sick, have an infection, or have high blood glucose for too long. In any of those cases, don't exercise until you get your blood glucose lower. When you have ketones and elevated blood glucose, doing any exercise can cause your blood glucose to increase even more and may cause *diabetic ketoacidosis* (DKA), which is potentially life-threatening.

Some people with diabetes have never experienced DKA or just never check their urine (or blood) for ketones because their glucose is never that high for long. Most of the time, exercising reduces their blood glucose levels, or a small dose of rapid-acting insulin before an activity brings them right back down to normal.

REMEMBER

If you have insulin in your body or only have high blood glucose because you miscalculated with your last insulin dose, then extended aerobic exercise is likely to lower your blood glucose, regardless of its intensity.

A fairly common practice of the athlete with diabetes is to administer 0.5 to 2 units of rapid-acting insulin before exercise and wait 10 to 15 minutes before beginning. The main danger of doing so is that you may overestimate your insulin needs, so err on the side of caution if you try this correction technique. Underestimating how much insulin you need is far better than ending up with a crashing low blood glucose from taking too much before your workout.

When blood glucose is high, but exercise is okay

If your glucose levels are more than 300 mg/dL without any ketones, then you should simply use caution when exercising. People with type 2 diabetes are much less prone to developing DKA because they still make some of their own insulin, and ketosis is generally the result of a relative lack of insulin in the body. However, you can still be dehydrated from running too high, and you should only exercise with elevated blood glucose if you feel well.

Your body will likely respond normally to exercise with some insulin circulating in your bloodstream, which should bring glucose down during the activity, assuming your workout isn't too intense. Use your blood glucose meter to test your response. Particularly after eating a meal when you take insulin, or your body releases some naturally in response to food intake, your blood glucose levels are more likely to come down naturally during exercise.

WARNING

You likely shouldn't exercise if your blood glucose is above 250 mg/dL and you have moderate or higher levels of ketones because your glucose can go up even more in that case.

Reduce highs after exercise

If your blood glucose is too high after you stop exercising, you have several options about what to do. You can pick one (or more) of these to try:

1. **Do an easy aerobic exercise (such as walking) as a cool-down for 10 to 15 minutes to use up some of the excess glucose.**

2. **Just wait it out to see whether your blood glucose comes down on its own in the next couple of hours due to the increased insulin action caused by your workout.**

3. **Take some insulin (albeit a smaller dose than normal) if you use it; this is probably the best option if you also have high levels of ketones.**

Chapter **6**

Eating Better for Health

Some people literally go days, months, or years without exercising, but everyone has to eat on a (nearly) daily basis to stay alive and healthy, with or without diabetes. What you decide to chow down on matters to your long-term health and your blood glucose. Diabetes makes your food choices even more important.

In this chapter, I explain why your meal plan is so vital to keeping fit and how to get the most out of your body every day by making healthful choices — easily. You have a lot of tasty options that can benefit your body, both today and down the road, even if you don't know it yet.

REMEMBER

No matter what you eat, limiting your portions to amounts that allow you to manage both your blood glucose and your body weight and being active help keep you fitter and more healthy.

Knowing Which Foods Make a Body Healthy

Have you ever chosen the salad for your main meal when you eat out only to find out that it had as many calories as that burger you would've preferred? Not everything you may consider healthful is, and many foods are more nutritious than you realize. Eating right in today's world of confusing messages is tough for everyone — even those supposedly "in the know" about healthful eating.

Here's what's for certain: Eating foods as close to their natural state as possible is almost always best for your health. Processing foods (as when whole wheat is made into white flour, bleached or unbleached) strips numerous nutrients out of food, and only a select few are added back in. The result is that processed foods are far less nutritious than foods in a more natural state. Nutrients in foods work best the way they grew, and often the synergy of the nutrients in food is as vital as the individual nutrients themselves, so just taking supplements is seldom as effective either.

Natural fruits and vegetables are full of vitamins and minerals, and they are particularly rich in compounds called *phytonutrients* (or *phytochemicals*), which are found in plants and have disease-fighting and health-promoting powers; some examples are capsaicin, lycopene, lutein, quercetin, saponins, and terpenes. Most can't be bought in supplement form, and you wouldn't want to consume them without the benefits of the bioactive substances in whole foods anyway. Certain foods containing phytonutrients are considered so powerful for health that they may one day be one of the primary ways we prevent and manage diseases.

Choosing foods that lower inflammation

You've likely heard a lot already about anti-inflammatory diets. They're supposed to be good for your health because low-level, systemic inflammation in your body can lead to plaque clogging up your arteries and insulin that doesn't work well enough to lower your blood glucose.

An inflammatory diet is one laden with highly processed foods (many of which are "white" foods made with white flour and sugar), such as fries, pizza, and other fast foods that many Americans eat daily. This type of diet can cause your blood glucose levels to spike sky high after meals, even if you don't have diabetes or prediabetes. Blood glucose spikes are bad for your health because they cause oxidative stress, which can lead to inflammation, insulin resistance, and so on. You get the picture.

Most of these processed foods are higher in calories and lower in nutrients like essential vitamins and minerals that make your body work well. Processing and refining foods too much takes out the good stuff (good for your body, anyway). To help keep inflammation at bay, avoid highly processed foods and sugar-rich drinks.

Because many complications from diabetes are likely related to unchecked oxidative stress in various tissues and organs, eating foods containing more antioxidant power that lower inflammation certainly can't hurt. Focus on eating minimally processed, high-fiber, plant-based foods — that is, most fruits and vegetables, whole grains, legumes, nuts and seeds, and lean protein sources (like egg whites and whey protein). Other things have been shown to reduce inflammation, such as balsamic vinegar, fish oil, tea, cocoa, and cinnamon, but the research on those is less strong.

Particularly potent fruits to include are blueberries, strawberries, raspberries, oranges, mangoes, grapefruit (particularly pink), kiwi, avocados, concord grapes, cherries, and plums. Also eat more tomatoes, broccoli, red bell peppers, sweet potatoes, carrots, winter squash, kale, spinach, purple cabbage, and eggplant. These are the fruits and vegetables highest in vitamins A and C, folate, iron, copper, calcium, and fiber as well.

COLORIZE YOUR DIET (NATURALLY)

Many people have been brought up in today's world eating an abundance of "white," colorless foods, including white bread, white rice, sugar, and iceberg lettuce. For optimal health from intake of phytonutrients, try to choose to eat a bigger variety of plant-based foods from all of the four color groups daily: red, orange-yellow, green, and blue-purple.

The phytonutrients in each color group vary with the pigment. For example, red foods like tomatoes contain lycopene, which may prevent prostate cancer in men. The carotenoids in yellow-orange foods may reduce heart disease risk, and green foods like broccoli contain *sulforaphane*, a cancer fighter. Finally, blueberries, in the blue-purple color group, contain nearly 100 different phytonutrients including polyphenols, making them a top-ranked food in terms of antioxidants and disease-fighting power.

In general, darker-colored foods have more phytonutrients. Most of these compounds are found in the dark outer coatings that contain the antioxidants plants use to protect themselves from oxidative damage by the sun's ultraviolet rays. Legumes illustrate this concept well: Black beans are highest in antioxidants (flavonoids), followed in decreasing amounts by the red, brown, yellow, and white varieties. Red and purple grapes also contain more of these compounds than green ones.

From a diabetes standpoint, eating more naturally colored food is good as well. For instance, one study showed that tart cherries may be able to increase insulin production in pancreatic beta cells by 50 percent due to their *anthocyanin,* a phytonutrient that contributes to their bright red color. While further research is needed to verify this finding, it is clear that anthocyanin (and many other phytonutrients) are potentially good for your health in many ways. This particular phytonutrient can also be found in other bright red, blue, and purple produce — such as red grapes, strawberries, and blueberries — as well as in wine, cider, and tea.

Dark chocolate and cocoa, red wine, green and black tea, and coffee also have large amounts of disease-fighting antioxidants. Don't consume too much dark chocolate and wine, though, to avoid taking in too many calories. Also limit your coffee intake to moderate amounts because caffeine itself can decrease how well your body's insulin works. Caffeine added to energy drinks, sports drinks, sodas, and more comes without the benefit of antioxidants found naturally in cocoa, tea, and coffee.

Focusing on fiber

One thing you can almost never get too much of in your diet is fiber — and I'm not talking about the type that comes out of a drugstore container. Fiber that you find *naturally* in foods benefits your health in so many ways, and adding in more is easy when you know where to look for it.

TECHNICAL STUFF

Having enough fiber in your diet is important for good health. First, fiber can bind cholesterol and pull it out of the body through the small intestines (hence the claim on oatmeal products that it helps lower cholesterol). Second, it increases the bulk of fecal matter (your bowel movement) moving through your intestines, leading to greater regularity. Adults commonly get more constipated as they age or if they don't drink enough fluids. Eating adequate amounts of fiber daily along with taking in adequate water and other fluids helps combat constipation. Third, all types of fiber are important weapons in the fight against modern-day health problems that can keep you from living as well, including diabetes, heart disease, colon cancer, obesity, and high blood pressure.

Where to find fiber (hint: look for plants)

Most dietary fiber is found in plants — the closer eaten to nature the better. Many manufacturers now also add fiber to products like pasta, cereals, and breads. Be cautious about taking in too much of these "fake fiber" foods (some with more than 14 grams per item) as they can cause gas, bloating, constipation, and even diarrhea. On food labels, the "total fiber" listed on the label is the sum of the natural dietary fiber in foods plus any added fiber put into products during manufacturing.

TIP

Eat more of these foods to boost your fiber intake naturally:

>> All dry peas and beans (legumes), including navy, black, garbanzo, kidney, lima, and pinto beans, as well as lentils and soybeans

>> Vegetables, particularly green beans, snap beans, pole beans, beet greens, kale, collard greens, Swiss chard, turnip greens, spinach, peas, broccoli, Brussels sprouts, tomatoes, carrots, and corn

» Whole fruits (with skins, but not peels), including raspberries, blackberries, strawberries, blueberries, cherries, plums, pears, oranges, apples, bananas, kiwi fruit, and guava

» Dried fruits, such as apricots, figs, and dates (but watch your portions and how many carbohydrates you're eating because these can raise your blood glucose)

» Whole-grain foods, such as rye, oats, buckwheat, brown rice, whole-wheat breads and pasta, oat and wheat bran, milled flaxseed, high-bran-content cereals, soy flour, and popcorn

» Nuts and seeds, including cashews, peanuts, almonds, Brazil nuts, walnuts, pecans, pistachios, and sunflower seeds (but watch the calories in these foods because they add up fast)

Get enough fiber (hint: eat more plants)

Most people don't eat enough fiber for optimal health. At a minimum, you need at least 14 grams of fiber for every 1,000 calories you eat. Adult women need less than men because they eat fewer calories. After you reach age 50, recommended minimum fiber intake drops again for both men and women because you need fewer calories as you get older. Eating as much natural fiber as possible (even more than the minimum) should be your daily goal, no matter how young or old you are. Table 6-1 shows USDA's minimum recommendations for fiber intake.

TABLE 6-1

Recommended Minimum Daily Dietary Fiber Intake

Age	Men	Women
19 to 50 years	38 grams	25 grams
Over 50 years	30 grams	21 grams

WARNING

The only potential downside of eating up to 50 grams per day (besides going to the bathroom a lot), if you try to take in as much fiber as I challenge people to do, is that that much fiber may interfere with how easily your body absorbs some minerals like calcium and iron. For that reason, consider eating more foods with these minerals if you do consume large amounts of fiber, and drink plenty of water or other fluids to stay hydrated.

EMBRACING YOUR HEALTHY GUT BACTERIA

Current studies are focusing on the role of the *gut microbiome* — the bacteria that reside in your intestinal tract — on human health and disease. The human body hosts 100 trillion mostly benign bacteria, which help digest food, program the immune system, prevent infection, and even influence mood and behavior. The bacteria living on and in us make up an ecosystem that plays a role in many conditions that genes and environmental factors alone can't explain, including obesity, autism, depression, asthma, irritable bowel syndrome, and even cancer.

In fact, the type of bacteria you have can have a huge impact on whether you gain weight or stay slim, get diabetes or avoid it, and develop other chronic diseases or stay healthier. Although this research is ongoing, it's clear that fiber enhances the gut's abundance of the good bacteria that reduce inflammation. For no other reason, you should eat a diet naturally rich in fiber to keep your health-promoting gut bacteria happy and thriving.

Taking in carbohydrates

Having a healthful diet while eating carbohydrates is entirely possible if you keep a few concepts in mind. A balanced meal plan for the average person, according to the latest dietary recommendations from the Institute of Medicine of The National Academies, contains 45 to 65 percent of calories from carbohydrate, 20 to 35 percent of calories from fat, and 10 to 35 percent from protein. The American Diabetes Association does not recommend any particular intake of calories from each of these categories, and people with diabetes follow a variety of individualized meal plans.

A lower-carbohydrate intake, in addition to potentially lowering your blood lipids and your blood glucose, does help some people lose weight faster (at least initially) and keep it off, although how well this works varies by the person. Part of the confusion about how many carbohydrates you should eat when you have diabetes comes from the research itself. Many "low carbohydrate" meal plans studied are only as low as 40 percent of calories from carbohydrates, although some people follow extremely low-carbohydrate eating (less than 10 percent of calories). If you take insulin to manage diabetes, balancing calorie intake from all sources is likely as important or more important than just focusing on carbohydrate intake alone.

REMEMBER

Body weight is generally higher in people who consume carbohydrate-rich, highly processed foods that are rapidly absorbed and raise blood glucose. These are generally ones with a high glycemic index (the following sections delve farther into the glycemic index and glycemic load). Focus more on the types of carbohydrates you're eating than on the total amount.

Losing body fat is generally harder when your insulin levels are high, which they'll be after you release, inject, or pump enough insulin to cover your higher intake of carbohydrates, especially those that cause your blood glucose to rise rapidly. Because fat cells remain responsive to insulin, even when your blood glucose runs high, you'll gain fat weight when your liver converts some of that glucose into fat and stores it.

REMEMBER Take all carbohydrates you eat into account to manage your blood glucose.

WARNING Eating fewer carbohydrates doesn't necessarily lower the risk for type 2 diabetes if you replace the carbohydrates with a high intake of animal protein and fat. If you're following a low-carbohydrate diet, get your protein and fat in foods other than highly processed meats (lunchmeats, bacon, sausage, and the like).

Glycemic index (GI)

How rapidly a carbohydrate is digested, or its *glycemic index* (GI), affects your body's insulin responses and ability to manage your blood glucose. The more rapidly the body breaks down a food, the faster the carbohydrate is turned into glucose in your bloodstream. To manage the influx of glucose coming from carbohydrates, your body needs insulin. If you have diabetes or prediabetes, you may not be able to cover these glucose spikes with enough insulin.

GI values are usually scaled from 0 to 100, with glucose (the simple sugar, but also the same as what's in your bloodstream) having a GI of 100. The GI of a specific food can differ by person; other factors that can affect it include the following:

>> Type and amount of carbohydrate, fat, and protein a food contains

>> Amount of fiber and the nature of any starches in it

>> Preparation (raw or cooked)

>> Ripeness

>> Acidity

For example, thick linguine has a lower GI value than thin spaghetti. Overcooking in general raises the GI value of foods, so *al dente* pasta is always better. Highly acidic foods like vinegar can lower the GI value of another food when eaten in combination. Cold storage increases the *resistant starch* content (carbohydrates that are hard to digest) by more than a third, and the acid in lemon juice, lime juice, or vinegar will slow stomach emptying.

TIP

To lower your blood glucose spikes related to eating carbohydrates, consider eating pasta that is not overcooked, using vinaigrette as dressing on your salads (or oil and vinegar), and eating foods with more resistant starch (like cooled, cooked oatmeal).

TECHNICAL STUFF

The latest GI database is accessible through www.glycemicindex.com (search each food separately). High-GI foods have a GI value of 70 or higher, including almost everything with highly refined flour or added sugars like most breakfast cereals, pretzels, sugary candy, crackers, and bread. White potatoes may be natural, but they have a high GI. Other carbohydrates cause less of a spike in blood glucose levels and are generally easier for your body to handle in moderate amounts. Sweet potatoes, rice (white or brown), oatmeal, and white sugar have GI values in the range of 56 to 69, which makes them medium-GI foods. Most whole fruits, fructose (fruit sugar), dairy products, legumes (beans), and pasta (white or whole-wheat) fall into the low-GI category (55 and lower).

An excessive intake of high-GI carbohydrate foods can increase insulin resistance even in people without diabetes. The GI values of foods have mainly been determined in nondiabetic individuals, so a given food's effect may be exaggerated if your body releases less insulin or your insulin action is impaired. If anything, GI values may underestimate rather than overestimate the glycemic spikes caused by most carbohydrate-rich foods if you have diabetes.

TIP

Lowering the glycemic effect of your meals is generally beneficial to managing blood glucose spikes. Check your own response to your food by monitoring your blood glucose prior to eating and two hours after you start your meal.

In a study done in overweight adults, insulin resistance decreases when they eat a low-GI, whole-grain diet compared to a refined, "white" diet. In some studies, people with type 2 diabetes who follow a diet with a GI of less than 40 tend to improve their overall blood glucose, enhance insulin action, lower bad blood fats, and lose weight. Such positive results support the GI as an appropriate guide to eating, whether you have diabetes, prediabetes, or insulin resistance, or if you just want to stay healthy.

Glycemic load (GL)

For carbohydrates, portion size does matter. Glycemic load (GL) is a measure of both GI value and total carbohydrate intake in a typical serving. Paying attention to your GL is even more important with diabetes. A high-GI/GL diet will most likely worsen insulin resistance and overtax your body's ability to supply insulin, so limit your intake of foods with both a medium or high GI value and a high GL.

A GL of 20 or more is high, 11 to 19 is medium, and 10 or less is low. For a single serving of a food, having a GL over 20 means it is carbohydrate dense, even if the spike in your blood glucose may be slower or smaller (like when you eat most pasta). Though GI is defined for each type of food, GL can also be calculated for any size serving of a food, an entire meal, or an entire day's meals if you want to get a feel for how many carbs you're taking in.

TECHNICAL STUFF

Foods that have a low GL almost always have a lower GI value, with some exceptions: Watermelon has a high GI value (72), but the carbohydrate content per serving of this fruit is minimal, making its glycemic load (4) low. However, a serving of watermelon is just over a cup. Popcorn also has a higher GI value (72), but it takes a lot to equal a 50-gram serving with a GL of just 8.

Any carbohydrate-heavy meal with a high GL requires more insulin, but if the GI value isn't also high — as is generally the case with high-fiber foods — your blood glucose will stay lower. Legumes, which are rich in protein and fiber, contain carbohydrates with a lower GI.

A low-GL, high-fiber diet also raises circulating levels of *adiponectin*, an anti-inflammatory hormone released by fat cells that can increase your insulin action and improve your blood glucose. A low-GI/GL diet plan results in weight loss as well.

TIP

Use GI and GL together to lower your blood glucose:

>> Choose slowly absorbed carbohydrates, not necessarily just a smaller amount of total carbohydrates.

>> Use GI to identify your best carbohydrate choices, choosing lower-GI ones.

>> Limit your portion size when eating carbohydrate-rich foods like rice, pasta, beans, or noodles to limit the overall GL.

Cutting back on sugar

Foods that are higher in fiber are usually lower in added sugars, along with having less fat and fewer calories. White (table) sugar boosts your blood glucose less quickly than white potatoes do, but the negative effects of eating a lot of sugar and other refined carbohydrates can be significant, particularly given their lack of essential nutrients (besides calories). What's more, there is nothing inherently evil about fructose (fruit sugar), despite research suggesting that high-fructose corn syrup in beverages leads to a fatty liver. Taking in excess calories more likely leads to such health issues, not fructose by itself. That said, sugars (and carbohydrates) may be somewhat addictive as they cause the release of brain hormones like dopamine (in the pleasure center) in response to their intake.

TIP

You don't have to give up white and other refined sugars completely, but limiting your intake of them is a great idea. One of the easiest ways to start lowering the sugar content of your diet is to reduce or eliminate your intake of all regular soft drinks, juice, fruit juice drinks, and sugar-sweetened iced tea or lemonade. In place of sugary drinks and fruit juices, substitute water, diet soft drinks, or other beverages containing noncaloric sugar substitutes. Despite all the recent media hysteria over non-nutritive sweeteners potentially causing people to gain weight or end up with cancer, no scientific evidence backs up these claims if you're avoiding sugar to manage your blood glucose. Just practice moderation in your use of sweeteners of all types (natural or artificial).

TECHNICAL
STUFF

You can learn a lot by reading food labels and checking the ingredients. Food and drink manufacturers must list ingredients in order of descending weight. In many products, refined sugar would come first if companies didn't have creative ways to disguise it by adding four or five different sweeteners that then appear lower on the list of ingredients. "Added sugar" is a listing being included on food labels, but look for sugar equivalents, such as sucrose, dextrose, high-fructose corn syrup, corn syrup, glucose, fructose, maltose, levulose, honey, brown sugar, and molasses.

Boosting your health with protein

The latest nutritional fad is the high-protein diet, including protein shakes, supplements, and more. This approach isn't necessarily a bad thing. The major building blocks of protein are amino acids. About half of these 20 amino acids are essential, meaning you must eat those, but your body can form the rest. Protein doesn't cause rapid spikes in blood glucose levels. Eating protein also makes you feel full longer, whereas low-protein diets are associated with increased hunger. Consuming more lean protein together with more healthful fats may reduce your appetite and help you eat fewer calories and even lose weight if that is your goal. (The following section covers healthy fats.)

Your body metabolizes foods with lots of protein more slowly than it does carbohydrates, usually within three to four hours. Eating as much as 30 to 40 percent of your daily calories as protein, with a lower intake of carbohydrates and fats, may help with managing your blood glucose, losing weight, and keeping the weight off.

TIP

Because a high intake of protein from processed meats increases diabetes risk and can compromise your long-term health, pick high-quality sources of protein such as lean meats, soy products, legumes, fish, eggs, and nuts and seeds.

Some studies have shown that a diet rich in soy protein may be beneficial for people with type 2 diabetes. Soy protein consumption has a significant positive impact on heart disease risk and kidney problems in adults with type 2 diabetes with existing kidney disease. Eating soy protein lowered levels of blood glucose, blood fats, and C-reactive protein (an indicator of inflammation) and markers of kidney disease. Too much of anything — including soy — is not recommended, though.

Fitting healthy fats into your diet

Having diabetes — particularly when your blood glucose isn't well managed — can contribute to unhealthy changes in your blood fats. High triglycerides (mainly from dietary fat, but also formed in your body when you eat highly refined carbohydrates) and bad types of cholesterol play a major role in stimulating inflammation that can cause plaque to form in your arteries (a common occurrence in people with diabetes).

Not every type of fat is bad for you — although the nutrition world is still hotly debating the healthfulness of various fats — but a high intake of certain types of fat definitely can contribute to the development of insulin resistance and bad changes in blood fats as much as an excess intake of refined carbohydrates can.

Add omegas and other healthy plant fats

Two dietary polyunsaturated fats are essential: omega-3 and omega-6 fatty acids. Both are important to include in a healthy diet, particularly when you have diabetes and your nutrition is even more important in preserving your long-term health.

Omega-3 fats are abundant in dark green, leafy vegetables (for example, dark-colored lettuce, spinach, kale, turnip greens, and so on), canola oil, flaxseed oil, soy, some nuts (such as walnuts), fish, and fish oils. Only fish and fish oils contain larger amounts of two omega-3 fats called DHA (docosahexaenoic acid) and EPA (ecosapentanoic acid), which are critical for brain and nerve function, cardiovascular health, and more. Plant foods like walnuts contain mainly a third essential omega-3 fat called ALA (alpha-linolenic acid), which your body can convert into the other two if your intake of them is low. Omega-6 fats are abundant in the corn, sunflower, peanut, and soy oils that are used in making margarine, salad dressing, and cooking oils, and these oils may help lower inflammation. Because some studies have suggested that taking in too many omega-6 fats can lead to inflammation, just try to balance out your intake of the two types to optimize your health.

Diets high in certain types of fats — like the plant-based ones found naturally in avocados — may improve your body's insulin action. Even tropical oils like coconut that are minimally processed are now considered healthier options even though most of their fats are saturated.

TIP

The best advice is to simply cut down on the intake of unhealthier fats by eating more foods in their natural state, such as high-fiber vegetables, legumes, nuts and seeds, and fish.

It also now appears that unhealthful carbohydrates may impact your blood cholesterol and fats more than the fat that you eat. If you choose to eat a diet that falls within the general guidelines for all adults (20 to 35 percent of your total daily calories) and avoid lower-fat versions of snack foods that have added sugar and more refined carbohydrates in them, your blood cholesterol levels are more likely to go down.

Avoid trans and highly processed fats

Trans fats are mostly created by manufacturers when they hydrogenate or partially hydrogenate liquid oils to alter their texture. Consuming trans fats found in hydrogenated oils contributes to insulin resistance and makes keeping blood glucose and cholesterol levels under control more difficult. Their inclusion on food labels has led to fewer of them being added to foods by manufacturers, thankfully.

Found most abundantly in processed foods such as crackers, cookies, baked goods, and more, trans fats may be disguised as mono- and diglycerides, stearate, palmitate, lard, vegetable shortening, and hydrogenated or partially hydrogenated oils. Trans fats from natural sources, however, aren't unhealthy like the manufactured ones (you'll find a small amount in dairy products that is natural), and most foods contain very little of these anyway.

Eating even one meal high in manufactured trans or some saturated fats can interrupt the normal flow of blood through your arteries and veins for hours afterward and make your body's response to insulin sluggish as well. On the other hand, when you eat a high-fat breakfast that contains mostly a good fat like olive oil (rather than, say, sausage), your blood glucose and insulin levels stay lower. Your blood cholesterol should decrease as you reduce trans, saturated, and highly processed fats in your diet.

A WORD ABOUT CHOLESTEROL

Your body needs a certain amount of cholesterol, which is a waxy, fatlike substance important in cell and hormone composition, and your liver will simply make it if you don't eat enough. Cholesterol is found in all animal products, including meat, poultry, shellfish, fish, eggs, and dairy, but not at all in plants. The cholesterol found in eggs is no longer as maligned as it once was, and it's unlikely that the cholesterol in egg yolks is going to raise your blood levels of cholesterol.

Another fat to start watching out for is *interesterified* fat, which is also manufactured and now added to some processed foods in place of trans fats. This new type of altered fat is also heart-unhealthy, probably as much as trans fats, but it's hard to know how much is in foods because manufacturers don't have to report or list it on food labels yet.

What about fat in red meat, dairy, eggs, and nuts and seeds?

Although current research is unclear as to whether unprocessed red meats directly cause heart disease, more healthful choices are available, including fish, nuts and seeds, legumes, fruits, and vegetables. If you consume cheese and milk, pick lower-fat varieties — not because dairy fat is bad for your health but rather to take in fewer calories.

COUNTING ALL CALORIES, NOT JUST CARBOHYDRATES

For insulin users, estimating how much insulin is necessary to cover meals and snacks is frequently difficult but essential if they want to manage blood glucose well. Many individuals with type 1 diabetes have been taught to count carbohydrates, or try to estimate the amount of carbohydrates in grams that they're eating, and give themselves specific doses of mealtime insulin to cover that amount based on an individualized carbohydrate-to-insulin ratio. An example may be a 15:1 ratio, meaning that eating 15 grams of carbohydrate at a specific time of day takes one unit of rapid-acting insulin to cover it.

Though carbohydrate counting has been around a long time, more recent studies have recognized that estimating protein intake is also important in controlling spikes in blood glucose after meals because some of the protein is converted into glucose (although much more slowly than carbohydrates are). Protein takes three to four hours to break down and can raise your blood glucose a noticeable amount after it's fully digested, if you take insulin.

To complicate matters, eating a meal with more fat in it has also been shown to increase insulin needs in people with type 1 diabetes, even when carbohydrates are held constant, suggesting that more insulin is needed for higher-fat meals. Fat may slightly slow down the absorption of carbohydrate in your meal, but it doesn't change the overall blood glucose peak. However, eating a meal with either high protein or high fat increases your overall insulin needs, even when the carbohydrate content remains the same. In other words, all calories can raise blood glucose, not just those from carbohydrates, especially if you don't make enough of your own insulin or use what you make effectively.

Also, diets rich in the monounsaturated fats in nuts and seeds (as well as olive and canola oil) are heart-healthy and don't necessarily promote weight gain if eaten in moderation. Just don't eat the whole jar in one sitting!

Eating more healthful meals and snacks

Here are some easy tips for preparing and choosing more healthful meals:

>> Cook with olive or canola oil. Go easy on the oil (or use a cooking spray) and avoid frying foods.

>> Use lean cuts of meat, including beef with all visible fat removed; skinless chicken and turkey breast; and lean ground beef, ground chicken, or ground turkey, as well as fish, tofu, and soy protein.

>> Bake, broil, poach, or grill meat, fish, and chicken instead of frying them.

>> Limit or avoid highly processed meats (like bacon, sausage, and lunch meats) because the sodium and preservatives added to them are likely bad for your health. A high intake of highly processed meats also increases your risk for type 2 diabetes.

>> Lower-fat (and sugar-free, whenever possible) varieties of dairy products, including milk, cheese, sour cream, yogurt, and ice cream, may be good options simply to lower calorie intake.

>> Eat veggies raw, steamed, microwaved, or grilled, using only light seasonings or spicy peppers rather than drenching them with creamy, cheesy, or buttery sauces.

>> Steam vegetables in a small amount of water or grill them to prevent the loss of key vitamins and minerals.

>> Use mainly fresh or frozen vegetables and fruits; canned ones often contain added salt and/or sugar. If you must use canned fruit, purchase fruit packed in its juice. Choose canned vegetables with limited added salt or rinse well.

>> Keep fresh vegetables like baby carrots, broccoli, peppers, or cauliflower handy for snacks, and eat them with a healthful dip like hummus (chickpeas and sesame tahini) and fat-free or olive oil-based dressings.

>> Snack on whole fruits rather than manufactured products containing fruit, and keep a variety of fruits, such as grapes, apples, oranges, bananas, and seasonal fruit, on hand for healthful snacks (but watch how many carbohydrates you're eating).

>> Choose whole fruit over juice. If you drink juice, aim for 100 percent juice (not juice drinks) and limit your intake to one serving.

>> On salads, use balsamic vinegar or a limited amount of other dressings if you're concerned about your weight. Dressings containing oils of any type are still high in calories, while fat-free or reduced-calorie varieties often have added sugar, which can raise your blood glucose.

>> Add cut-up vegetables to stews, soups, or omelets to increase their nutrient value, water content, and fiber.

>> Buy only bread products that list whole grain as the first ingredient on the food label, and use other whole-grain products whenever possible.

>> Add extra fiber into recipes for baked goods, casseroles, and soups by spooning in a few tablespoons of oat bran, wheat bran, or milled flaxseed when you prepare them.

>> For baked goods, try using only one-half to two-thirds of the sugar called for by the recipe and use healthier margarines (also reducing the amount by a third if possible or using the "light" varieties). Eat baked goods and sweets in smaller portions or just have a bite.

Getting Your Vitamins and Minerals from Foods or Supplements

Obtaining nutrients naturally through your foods if you can is always best because they contain many important phytonutrients (such as flavonols, polyphenols, catechins, and lycopenes) that aren't available in an optimal form through dietary supplements. Taking large supplemental doses of any vitamins, minerals, or other nutrients can be counterproductive, though. For example, almost all anti-oxidant vitamins and minerals can actually cause damage when you take too much. Head to the later section "Antioxidants" for more on supplementing with these substances.

You can't overdose on antioxidants if you obtain them naturally through food, though, so get them that way whenever possible. The following sections discuss some of the most important vitamins and minerals for people with diabetes.

B vitamins

The vitamins in the B family include thiamin (B1), riboflavin (B2), B6, niacin, B12, folate, biotin, and pantothenic acid. These vitamins are involved in the digestion and metabolism of food, so it's not surprising that a deficiency in any of them can adversely affect your body's handling of carbohydrate, protein, fat, and more.

People with diabetes are more likely to be deficient in thiamin, and supplementing with this vitamin has been shown to prevent some diabetic complications and improve insulin action in adults with type 2 diabetes. Vitamin B6 and others in the B family may be effective in preventing the formation of harmful substances in blood (*advanced glycation end products*) associated with diabetes complications. Vitamin B12 deficiency is also quite common in people with type 2 diabetes or prediabetes, particularly if they take metformin, which can cause depletion of this vitamin over time (as well as symptoms of nerve damage). Low blood levels of vitamin B12 are associated with neuropathy-like symptoms that may be reversible with supplements.

REMEMBER

The American Diabetes Association recommends using supplements only if you're deficient in any vitamins or minerals. Getting adequate amounts of these through your diet is recommended.

TECHNICAL STUFF

Vitamin B12 deficiency, verified with a blood test, has been associated with a lower bone density in the spines of women and the hips of men. If you use metformin, you have a higher chance of developing this deficiency over time; you may want to ask your doctor to check your blood levels. Low intake of folate has been associated with an increased risk of fetal defects (related to neural tube development) in pregnant women, as well as a higher risk for thinning bones and heart disease in older adults.

Make sure that your daily diet contains at least 100 percent of all the B vitamins (their content should be listed on the label), and consider taking at least a general B vitamin supplement of 100 percent of the RDA if you have any deficiencies that can't be corrected naturally through your diet. Supplemental doses of B vitamins are generally harmless because you lose any excess through your urine, but taking megadoses of these vitamins isn't necessary or advisable. For example, taking large doses of supplemental folate can mask a deficiency of vitamin B12 and cause other symptoms like nausea, and too much B6 can cause permanent nerve damage.

If you have diabetes, you may want to talk to your doctor about supplementing with thiamin or benfotiamine, a derivative of vitamin B1 (thiamin) with additional antioxidant properties, because both have been used to treat neuropathic pain. They may also prevent other complications, improve insulin action, and lower your blood cholesterol levels.

Vitamin D

Vitamin D is unique in that it functions as a hormone. All the cells in your body have a receptor for it. Long associated with bone health, its effects are far-reaching: It can lower the risk of developing some autoimmune diseases, certain types of cancer, diabetes, infectious diseases, heart disease, asthma, and neuropathy. Having enough vitamin D in your body also lowers your risk of dying from any cause.

The body derives most active vitamin D (about 90 percent) from limited exposure to sunlight, which is why this vitamin is often called the "sunshine vitamin." Apparently, you need to get sunshine on your face and hands for a only few minutes a couple of times a week to create what you need in your body (depending on the time of year, of course, and where you live).

Still, many people with diabetes have low blood levels of this vitamin. Older adults also don't create as much vitamin D in their skin with sunlight exposure, and taking in enough through your diet alone is hard.

TIP

Some foods naturally high in vitamin D include fish oils, fatty fish (like salmon), mushrooms, beef liver, cheese, and egg yolks, but spending time outdoors likely works better to increase levels than eating more of these foods does (unless you're wearing excessive amounts of heavy-duty sunscreen). Because dietary supplements can raise blood levels of vitamin D, dietary experts recommend taking 600 international units (IU) of vitamin D if you're under 50 years old or 800 IU if you're older than 50.

Magnesium

Magnesium, an abundant mineral in the body, is involved in over 300 of the body's metabolic reactions. It improves your insulin action, so not having enough magnesium isn't good for your diabetes management. A magnesium deficiency can contribute to insulin resistance and raises your risk for developing type 2 diabetes (if you don't have it already). Low magnesium levels in adults with diabetes are also associated with eye disease, nerve damage, and depression. If you're getting muscle cramps frequently, you may be deficient in magnesium.

TECHNICAL STUFF

Magnesium greatly impacts your body's energy production, synthesis of genetic materials (DNA and RNA), protein formation, and bone health because it facilitates the enzymes and pathways that make these processes work. As a result, magnesium largely controls your blood pressure, regulates the rhythm of your heart, and prevents muscle cramps. In fact, magnesium deficiency has been linked to high blood pressure, stroke, plaque formation and heart disease, cardiac arrhythmias, alterations in blood fats, platelet stickiness, inflammation, oxidative stress, asthma, chronic fatigue, depression, and more.

This mineral is widely distributed in foods like unprocessed (whole) grains, nuts, legumes, and even dark chocolate (thank goodness for that!). You can lose some magnesium through urinating more when hyperglycemic or sweating excessively (such as during exercise).

Particularly if your blood glucose management could be better, you may want to consider taking a daily magnesium supplement, along with eating a more healthful diet. Taking too much magnesium can cause temporary diarrhea, but it's otherwise safe. But don't take more than 350 milligrams daily.

WARNING

If you have kidney failure, restrict your magnesium intake.

Deciding Whether You Need Other Supplements

Although diabetes can create a special metabolic situation that depletes certain vitamins and minerals from your body, you may be able to compensate with more healthful food choices, certain nutritional supplements, and improved blood glucose management. If you're getting the recommended daily amounts of vitamins and minerals in your diet, then you may not need any supplements — which are only beneficial if you're truly deficient. Insulin resistance and hyperglycemia can potentially cause certain deficiencies, but if you manage these conditions effectively, supplements are not universally recommended and could potentially be harmful.

Being cautious about supplements

If you decide to use home remedies or supplements, keep in mind that the term *herbal* or *natural* on a label doesn't mean that a product is harmless. In fact, many common poisons found in plants like hemlock and deadly nightshade are "natural." Some dietary supplements may have undesirable side effects; for example, certain forms of ginseng can raise blood pressure, and mugwort can cause dermatitis (skin inflammation).

Other "natural" supplements can interact with your prescribed medications to produce side effects or possibly negate the usual effects of the medication. For instance, people have been poisoned, in some cases fatally, by taking herbal preparations containing heliotropium while also taking a prescribed barbiturate. Also, there is no evidence showing how those supplements or herbs can interact with your current diabetes medications, so be extra careful with taking them.

To be on the safe side, tell your doctor about any herbal or "natural" supplements you use, especially if you take any prescribed medications.

Err on the side of caution when self-prescribing a supplement that can potentially improve your blood glucose, for a couple of reasons:

>> Most of the "natural" cures currently available online have no valid studies proving that they work, and many can be harmful.

>> Just because a supplement is supposedly helpful (like cinnamon to lower blood glucose), you should never assume that taking more of it is going to be more effective. You can take in toxic amounts of substances — even vitamins — if you self-prescribe large doses.

What's more, the supplements you buy may vary widely in their actual content. Some studies have shown no ginseng in products that are sold as ginseng supplements, and the packaging for many herbal preparations doesn't list the ingredients. Even when products do disclose the ingredients, the lists may not be accurate or complete. Up to 26 percent of all dietary supplements tested in one study contained contaminants sufficient to elicit a positive drug test in competitive athletes. Others may contain harmful and even potentially fatal contaminants.

Creatine

Creatine is a natural compound, normally found in muscle, that is involved in short-term energy production. It's well established as an effective supplement in weight lifters and other power athletes who are gaining muscle mass, but only when they're training. Taking creatine supplements in combination with doing resistance training may increase your strength gains from training and lower your insulin resistance, but doing so certainly isn't a requirement if you want to get stronger by doing such training. Talk to your doctor first about whether you should use creatine if you have any issues with the health of your kidneys.

Whey protein (essential amino acids)

Leucine, an essential amino acid found mainly in whey protein derived from cow's milk, is an important building block for muscles, and consuming adequate amounts of it is essential. Eating quality protein and getting enough calories are the preferred (and less expensive) method, but you can also find L-leucine (as well as creatine, which I discuss in the preceding section) as a dietary supplement in stores. You also get it as part of whey protein supplements or blends.

TIP

Take in adequate amounts of amino acids naturally through your diet by eating quality proteins (found in milk, egg whites, and more), but don't waste your money on expensive supplements. As you age, the most important thing to do for your muscles is to stay active and recruit all your muscle fibers (by doing heavier resistance work), not focus on taking amino acid supplements.

Carnitine

Many people with diabetes or undergoing renal dialysis are deficient in carnitine, which your body produces from amino acids. If your body makes enough, you don't need to supplement or to worry about consuming any carnitine in food. Having enough is important, though, because carnitine increases your insulin action and is essential for metabolizing fats and carbohydrates.

TECHNICAL STUFF

Carnitine is an important compound in your body because it transports fats into mitochondria of cells (the powerhouses) to produce energy. *Carnitine* is a generic term to describe L-carnitine, acetyl-L-carnitine, and propionyl-L-carnitine, but only the L-carnitine form, the one active in your body, is in food.

If you're deficient in carnitine, you can obtain it by eating meat, fish, poultry, and milk. It's most concentrated in whey protein (dairy products), but it's also safe to take as a supplement of L-carnitine or acetyl-L-carnitine, usually in 500- or 1,000-milligram doses.

Carnitine supplementation can improve insulin sensitivity by decreasing fat levels and glucose in blood. It may also help lessen some diabetes complications. In a study of 1,200 diabetic patients, researchers found that treatment of type 1 or type 2 diabetes with acetyl-L-carnitine (500-milligram or 1,000-milligram doses daily) for a year relieved diabetes-related nerve pain in feet and improved sensation of vibration. Thus, it may help delay progression of neuropathic pain or reduce its severity.

Antioxidants

One of the latest crazes is everyone taking antioxidants to stay young. Supplements containing antioxidants are supposed to be able to slow aging by preventing cumulative oxidative damage in the body. However, consistent research is lacking. Elevated blood glucose is one of the conditions that can trigger such damage caused by excess *free radicals* (compounds that cause oxidative damage and inflammation).

REMEMBER

Damage caused by free radicals in the body may contribute to the complications associated with long-term diabetes, including heart disease and eye, kidney, and nerve damage.

FINDING ANTIOXIDANTS IN FOODS

Some surprising foods and drinks contain large amounts of antioxidants. A typical cup of hot cocoa (containing 2 tablespoons of pure cocoa powder) has twice as many of these health-promoting compounds (like flavonoids) as red wine, two to three times more than green tea, and almost five times more than black tea. Drinking cocoa hot apparently releases more antioxidant power and may increase blood flow to the brain and improve memory (but use the sugar-free variety for better blood glucose management).

Normally, your body has enough antioxidant enzymes naturally to fight most or all the free radicals that are created. These radical compounds, if left unchecked, promote further insulin resistance and lower insulin secretion. Diabetes not only increases free radical generation when your blood glucose is elevated but can also depress your body's natural antioxidant defenses. (Exercise stimulates the production of these radicals, but it also enhances your body's natural antioxidant enzymes systems that get rid of them.) If your blood glucose levels aren't well managed, you're more likely to benefit from supplemental antioxidant therapies.

The antioxidants with the most potential benefit for anyone with diabetes are glutathione, alpha-lipoic acid, vitamin C, vitamin E, beta-carotene, selenium, copper, and zinc.

Glutathione is the main antioxidant enzyme found in all your cells, and, along with alpha-lipoic acid, is the most important antioxidant in your body. It protects the DNA in your cell nuclei from being oxidized. Having diabetes likely increases your need for glutathione and alpha-lipoic acid by depleting glutathione levels when your blood glucose is elevated, potentially leading to diabetes-related cataracts and other complications. Although your body can synthesize both from amino acids found abundantly in foods like asparagus, avocados, spinach, strawberries, peaches, melons, and citrus fruits, it may not always make enough to meet your body's needs.

Alpha-lipoic acid increases glutathione levels by helping cells absorb a critical amino acid needed for its synthesis, and it works to prevent stroke, heart attacks, peripheral nerve damage, and cataracts, as well as memory loss, cancer, and aging effects. Spinach (raw or cooked) is the best source of this nutrient, also found naturally in small amounts in broccoli, tomatoes, potatoes, peas, and Brussels sprouts. Spinach is especially touted for its ability to fight diabetic cataracts and macular degeneration (the leading cause of blindness in adults).

TECHNICAL STUFF

Diabetic complications like cataracts involve deficient glutathione levels within the lens of your eye, and nutrients like alpha-lipoic acid, vitamins E and C, and selenium can increase your levels of glutathione and its activity, allowing for better protection of your eyes and other tissues. A combination of vitamins C and E and the minerals magnesium and zinc may improve the good cholesterol in adults with diabetes.

Alpha-lipoic acid supplements may normalize diabetes-induced kidney dysfunction and damage to nerve cells, where they additionally promote nerve fiber regeneration and stimulate a substance known as nerve growth factor. In Germany, alpha-lipoic acid has been used for years to treat painful diabetic neuropathy in the feet and hands, and it can also improve *autonomic* (central nervous system) neuropathy. Most people can safely take 600 milligrams once or twice daily for relief of symptoms.

Chapter 7

Eating Right for Exercise

How well you fuel your body with food is a big deal when you're physically active. So are staying hydrated when you're exercising and refueling effectively after exercise. Doing all these things with diabetes as an added variable can be complicated, so the foods you eat can impact your body's response to physical activity. Knowing when and how to adjust your food intake before, during, and after exercise is important for keeping your blood glucose levels as close to your target range as possible. This is not always an easy feat to accomplish, but it does help if you understand more about how the macronutrients (that is, carbohydrates, protein, and fat) are metabolized and how quickly they are available for your body to use.

In this chapter, you discover how carbohydrates, protein, and fat play different roles in helping you achieve your exercise (and blood glucose) goals. Protein is critical for rebuilding muscles and maintaining strength as you age, and you find out how much you really need on a daily basis. On the other hand, fat isn't as important during all activities as you may think, so this chapter helps you focus on taking in adequate carbohydrates and making sure your fluid intake will keep you going. If you're a coffee lover, I also have some good news for you related to coffee and exercise.

Fueling Your Body with Carbohydrates

The most important energy source for all types of exercise is carbohydrate. At rest, your body typically uses about 60 percent fat and 40 percent carbohydrate. When you reach an exercise intensity harder than an easy walk, your body switches to higher carbohydrate use (even if your cardio machine says you're in a "fat-burning range").

REMEMBER

Carbohydrates are your body's fuel of choice for moderate or harder exercise. You must have them to fuel your muscles during most exercise sessions.

During exercise, your body uses a combination of carbohydrates available in your blood (glucose), muscles (muscle glycogen), and liver (hepatic glycogen). Any carbohydrates you eat are converted to blood glucose within five minutes to two hours. If you run low on carbohydrates during an activity, you'll have to slow down, you may "hit the wall" (and have to stop), or you may get low blood glucose. Eating a chronically low-carbohydrate diet can make it difficult for you to participate in an exercise that is hard or long at your highest potential level, but supplementing with carbohydrates during any activity helps you maintain your blood glucose.

REMEMBER

Always take in enough carbohydrate before, during, and after prolonged moderate- or high-intensity workouts to maintain and restore your muscle and liver glycogen (storage form of glucose in those tissues) and blood glucose, especially during that window of opportunity for glycogen repletion (30 minutes to 2 hours) right after you finish exercising. People doing longer duration exercise (more than an hour at a moderate or higher intensity) usually perform better when they eat carbohydrates during the activity, even if they don't have diabetes.

Carbohydrate intake during exercise

During longer athletic events in particular (like marathons or triathlons), taking in extra carbohydrates during exercise helps maintain your blood glucose levels, enabling you to keep going at a faster pace for longer without getting too tired. But supplementing with carbohydrates even helps you perform better during intermittent, prolonged, high-intensity sports like soccer, field hockey, and tennis.

There is a limit to how many carbohydrates you should take in during exercise, however. Studies have shown that trained cyclists without diabetes can only digest and use about 80 grams of carbohydrate per hour while doing fairly hard cycling. Having higher levels of insulin in your body may increase your supplemental carbohydrate use a bit compared to someone without diabetes, but it's unlikely to be by much when you consume carbohydrate during exercise because digestion is slower then due to greater blood flow to the muscles.

What types of carbohydrates should you consume during exercise? That depends on things like how long you'll be exercising, the intensity of your workout, and what your blood glucose and insulin levels are before and during the activity. If you have to supplement to prevent hypoglycemia (mostly insulin users), aim to take in carbohydrates with a higher glycemic index (GI), like glucose gels, because they're absorbed more rapidly and raise blood glucose levels more quickly. They're also easier to digest during exercise than most with a lower GI, such as beans. (The *glycemic index* is a scale for measuring how fast the body digests carbohydrates; flip to Chapter 6 for more information.)

TIP

Even if you don't routinely eat many high-GI carbohydrates, supplementing with them during activities is okay if you need them to prevent hypoglycemia or take some in during longer workouts or events.

High-GI carbohydrates you can use during exercise include sports drinks, sports bars, glucose tablets or gels, Gu, bagels, saltine or graham crackers, pretzels, hard candy, Smarties, and anything made with glucose or dextrose (another name for glucose). Any carbohydrates that are part of foods with a high fat content (such as potato chips or doughnuts) have a lower GI, will be absorbed much more slowly, and may not help you much during exercise.

REMEMBER

People with type 2 diabetes who don't take insulin or oral medications that cause insulin release are unlikely to need to supplement with any carbohydrates to prevent low blood glucose during most activities lasting less than an hour.

Normal daily carbohydrate needs

How many carbohydrates you should normally eat daily is hotly debated in the diabetes world. Your brain and nerves use about 130 grams of glucose daily as their primary fuel, so if you eat fewer carbohydrates than that every day, your body needs to convert some protein (or possibly fat) into glucose.

It's also much harder to restore your muscle glycogen levels between workouts on subsequent days if you don't eat at least 40 percent of your calories as carbohydrate (and eat enough calories in general). If you take in less than that, you'll be more likely to develop hypoglycemia overnight and during subsequent workouts.

TIP

Your typical daily carbohydrates should likely be lower on the GI scale than your exercise ones to make managing your blood glucose levels at rest easier.

Exercise carbohydrates for insulin users only

The general recommendations for grams of carbohydrate intake in Table 7-1 are just a starting place and apply solely during activity (based on duration and intensity), not before or afterward. They assume that you haven't taken any rapid-acting insulin recently for meals, snacks, or correction and take your starting blood glucose into account. People who don't use insulin don't need to take in exercise carbohydrates unless they do a really long event during which anyone — with or without diabetes — would eat or drink carbohydrates to supply extra fuels.

TABLE 7-1   **Recommended Carbohydrate Intake for Exercise (Grams) Based on Duration, Intensity, and Starting Blood Glucose**

Duration	Intensity	Starting Blood Glucose under 100 mg/dL	Starting Blood Glucose 100 to 149 mg/dL	Starting Blood Glucose 150 to 200 mg/dL	Starting Blood Glucose over 200 mg/dL
30 minutes	Low	5–10	0–10	None	None
	Moderate	10–25	10–20	5–15	0–10
	High	15–35	15–30	10–25	5–20
60 minutes	Low	10–15	10–15	5–10	0–5
	Moderate	20–50	15–40	10–30	5–15
	High	30–45	25–40	20–35	15–30

Adapted from Colberg, S. Diabetic Athlete's Handbook, Human Kinetics, 2009.

These carbohydrate intake recommendations also assume you're not lowering your basal insulin doses before or during the activity, but you may need to do both (that is, eat more and lower basal and/or bolus insulin) for longer duration activities. Determining what works best for you in every situation takes some trial-and-error.

Recommendations from the American Diabetes Association used to, but no longer, tell people how many carbohydrate grams to consume. This change is a good thing because the amount varies on a case-by-case basis and depends on several different factors. For example, your blood glucose can be affected by how long you plan to exercise, what type of exercise you do, its intensity, and even how hot or cold it is. You should rely on testing your blood glucose and trying various amounts of carbohydrate to figure out what works for you with exercise as an added variable.

TECHNICAL STUFF

You have a lot to juggle when you take insulin and want to be physically active. Most exercisers who take insulin also eat something before prolonged, less intense activities, but not necessarily before weight training, sprinting, or other hard, shorter workouts. The time of day also makes a difference because doing early morning exercise may not drop your glucose like doing the same activity later in the day does. Depending on all these factors, your personal cutoff level to eat carbohydrate before exercise should be whatever you find works best for you. If your blood glucose is normal or slightly low before exercise, you may also want to take in 10 to 15 grams of moderate- or high-GI carbohydrate without any insulin coverage right when you start, especially if your blood glucose levels typically start to drop during the first 30 minutes of activity. If you're wearing a pump, you may choose to use a temporary basal setting that lowers insulin delivery during exercise or even starting an hour or two before exercise, or possibly suspend your pump during exercise lasting an hour or less instead of eating. Or you may have to combine these strategies to prevent hypoglycemia.

TIP

If you're able to set a lower temporary basal rate on your pump or have low levels of circulating insulin due to the time of day, you may not need to eat anything. If your insulin levels are high in your bloodstream during exercise (usually at a time within two to three hours after you took your last insulin bolus for meals, snacks, or hyperglycemia corrections), you'll likely need to eat more to combat insulin's glucose-lowering effects.

WARNING

Some websites have recently attempted to create exercise "calculators" to estimate how many carbohydrates you need or how you need to adjust your insulin, but they generally can't give accurate recommendations, given all the factors that can impact your blood glucose when you're active. Getting a bad recommendation can often be worse than having no guidance at all, so do some trial and error on your own to figure out which adjustments you need to make. If you're unsure how to make your own adjustments, check with your diabetes care team about which changes may work best for you, including possibly increasing your carbohydrate intake and reducing your insulin doses to prevent exercise-related hypoglycemia.

TIP

Keep these points in mind when it comes to changing your carbohydrate intake for exercise, if you use insulin or take pills that cause your pancreas to release insulin (sulfonylureas or meglitinides; jump to Chapter 3 for more information on these):

>> When doing intense exercise (that makes it hard for you to talk during it), you may not need any carbohydrates during the activity, but watch out for hypoglycemia later.

>> Competitions have more of a glucose-raising effect (especially when you're nervous) than practices do, so check your blood glucose to see if you may need less carbohydrate.

» If you use a pump and reduce your basal rate prior to and during exercise, your carbohydrate needs may be significantly less.

» You may need extra carbohydrates before, during, and after activity (depending on intensity, duration, starting blood glucose levels, and so on).

» Consider whether you may need to consume some protein and fat after exercise and at bedtime to prevent lows later and overnight.

» Check your blood glucose more often after you experience a bad low or do hard exercise in the 24 hours prior to doing your latest workout.

» Doing new or unaccustomed exercise can cause hypoglycemia, both during and afterward, and you may need to take in more carbohydrates for that activity.

» If you take any insulin to cover what you eat within two hours after exercise, you'll likely need less insulin than normal.

» Prevent the lows that can occur 6 to 12 (and up to 48) hours following exercise with a balanced intake of carbohydrates, protein, and fat.

Glycogen repletion and carbohydrates

Muscle carbohydrate stores of glucose (glycogen) are replaced at a rate of only 5 to 7 percent per hour after a workout. The rate is slightly faster when stores are low, but it slows down as they start to fill up. Insulin action starts to wane, too, as your muscles restore their glycogen stores. On a positive note, the sooner your glycogen is replaced, the less likely you are to develop late-onset hypoglycemia, which can occur up to a day or two later.

WARNING

Not eating enough carbohydrate after exercise, or carbohydrate eaten without adequate insulin, may extend how long it takes your body to restore glycogen and result in late-onset hypoglycemia in insulin users.

After exercise, your muscles are using glucose to replenish themselves and continuing to burn calories, which can increase your risk of low blood glucose. Your risk for having a low afterward depends on what you did and which medications you're taking, but you won't know your risks unless you check your blood glucose levels to find out.

TIP

Especially if you use insulin, check your blood glucose within an hour of when you finish your workout and continue monitoring your levels at one-hour intervals for several hours to prevent lows or highs after exercise.

Take in adequate carbohydrate, along with sufficient (albeit likely reduced) insulin before, during, and after prolonged moderate- or high-intensity workouts to maintain and restore your muscle and liver glycogen and blood glucose. Doing so is especially important right after you finish exercising (within 30 minutes to 2 hours after).

Pumping Up with Protein

Protein is never a key exercise fuel, but it's critical for other reasons. During most exercise, protein contributes less than 5 percent of the total energy, although it may rise to 10 to 15 percent during a prolonged event like a marathon or Ironman triathlon. Taking in enough dietary protein is important because dietary protein allows your muscles to be repaired after exercise and promotes the synthesis of hormones, enzymes, and other body tissues formed from amino acids, the building blocks of protein. You should consume at least 12 to 35 percent of your daily calories as protein. For most people this means taking in at least 60 grams of protein daily.

TECHNICAL STUFF

About half of the 20 amino acids are considered essential in your diet, meaning that you must consume them or your body will suffer from protein malnutrition, which causes the breakdown of muscles and organs. Essential amino acids are found in meats, poultry, fish, dairy, eggs, and soy products; all plant-based foods besides soy are lacking one or more essential ones, but taking in combinations of plant sources (like rice and beans) can supply what you need. Your body can make the rest of the amino acids itself (they are the nonessential ones). But you need to have enough protein in your diet overall to synthesize body proteins after workouts, which is a critical time for increases in strength, aerobic capacity, or muscle size.

Protein intake for everyone

Because protein is important to overall health but isn't a major exercise fuel, you do need to worry about consuming enough, although it doesn't have to happen right before or during an activity. You'll get most effective restoration of liver glycogen if you keep your blood glucose levels in tight control after exercise. Consuming a small amount of protein along with carbohydrate (in a ratio of 1:4, or 1 gram of protein to every 4 grams of carbohydrate) after an activity may help you repair your muscles and get stronger more quickly.

REMEMBER

Typically, an ounce of chicken, cheese, or meat has about 7 grams of protein.

Protein intake for insulin users

Taking in more protein and slightly less carbohydrate after exercise can help keep your blood glucose more stable over time because protein takes three to four hours to be fully digested, and some protein is converted into blood glucose. You can eat protein strategically to prevent later-onset hypoglycemia, which insulin users are more likely to get. Have some in your bedtime snack (along with fat and carbohydrate) to prevent nighttime lows after a day of strenuous or prolonged activity, if you use insulin.

TIP

Taking in some protein along with carbohydrate right after hard or long workouts may help your body replenish its glycogen stores more effectively.

Maximizing protein for training and aging

Though anyone who is getting older — and that includes all of us — can benefit from taking in enough protein, supplements are usually not the optimal way to get enough. Let me explain why.

As you get older, your body may need more protein compared to when you were younger to form, maintain, and repair muscles and other body structures. Anyone who is doing regular exercise training also needs more protein to repair and build muscle, but you can usually get this amount (and more) when you're eating a balanced meal plan with adequate calories. To figure out how much you need, find the category that fits your age and training, and multiply your body weight (in pounds or kilograms) by the grams found in the corresponding Table 7-2 column.

TABLE 7-2	Recommended Protein Intake by Training Status and Age	
	Per Pound Body Weight	Per Kilogram Body Weight
Adults 19 to 50 years (inactive)	0.36 grams	0.8 grams
Adults over 50 years (inactive)	0.5 grams	1.1 grams
Endurance training	0.55–0.64 grams	1.2–1.4 grams
Strength training	0.68–0.77 grams	1.5–1.7 grams
Calorie deprived (diets)	0.73–0.82 grams	1.6–1.8 grams

The biggest myth about amino acid supplements, and protein in general, is that you must load up on them to gain muscle. That's just not true. The protein requirement for strength-training athletes may be about twice as high as normal, but most people in the United States already consume more than these higher amounts of protein in their daily diets.

To put it in perspective, to gain one pound of muscle mass a week (a realistic maximum), a strength-training athlete needs no more than 14 extra grams of quality protein per day. You can easily get this amount from these sources:

>> About two 8-ounce glasses of milk

>> 2 ounces of lean meat, chicken, fish, or cheese (which isn't much)

>> Slightly more than two eggs (only the whites contain protein)

Adequate intake of protein also helps to maintain lean body mass when you lose weight on a diet and can help you gain more muscle mass from exercise training.

Using Fat during Exercise

Although carbohydrate is the main energy source during exercise, fat is an important contributor, particularly during low-intensity or slower, prolonged activities like walking the dog or taking an all-day hike. It's also the main fuel that your body uses to keep your metabolism humming along during recovery from your latest workout. However, the body hardly uses fat at all during high-intensity aerobic and anaerobic exercise, both of which rely on carbohydrates for energy.

Your body has almost unlimited stores of fat, even if you're lean. However, consuming fat before or during exercise doesn't alter your body's use of stored carbohydrates. Taking in fat after exercise can help keep glucose higher later on because fat takes up to five to six hours to fully digest. When the digested fat that you ate earlier hits your bloodstream, you'll be more insulin resistant, which helps keep your blood glucose from dropping.

"Fat burns in a carbohydrate flame," meaning that your body can't use fat effectively during exercise after you've depleted your carbohydrate stores. You simply won't be able to continue exercising at the same intensity, or at all, if your blood glucose gets low or your glycogen is used up.

Both the fat stored in your muscles (triglycerides) and in your blood (free fatty acids) can provide some energy for muscle contractions. Fatty acids are stored in your adipose (fat) tissue as triglycerides and released by hormones (mainly adrenaline) to be circulated to active muscles. Not much of the fat stored in muscles is used during activities — unless they're extremely prolonged, lasting many hours — but later, when you're resting, those fats kick in some of the energy for recovery.

Fat use and intake for everyone

What effect does exercise training have on your body's use of fat as a fuel? Though you potentially have become better at using fat during exercise with training, fat use depends on how hard you're working out. If you work out at the same relative intensity before and after training (meaning that you pick up your pace as you get fitter and more trained), your fat use remains constant. Your body's use of fat as a fuel during exercise only increases after training if you're now working out at a relatively lower percentage of your maximal capacity (that is, the same pace as before training, even though you could now pick up the pace). Some evidence suggests that training while eating a lower carbohydrate diet with a higher fat content may increase your ability to use fat during the activity; however, relying on fat for fuel for the more serious athlete compromises speed.

REMEMBER

Being physically trained does lower any fat-induced insulin resistance, which makes it easier for you to restore muscle glycogen after workouts.

Eating high-fat foods for exercise (that is, fat loading) may be detrimental to your performance and isn't recommended. Also, any fat that you eat before and during exercise isn't digested and ready for use for many hours and may slow the digestion of any carbohydrate that you eat.

How much or how little fat your body uses as a fuel during exercise doesn't determine how much fat weight you lose from being active. Instead, it's entirely dependent on how many calories you expend, not which fuel your body burns. Fueling activity with more fat overall makes you use less blood glucose, which is why training reduces the carbohydrates you need to keep your blood glucose stable while doing the same activity at the same intensity (pace) after training. Limit your intake of trans fats and highly processed fats for better health, though.

Strategic fat intake for insulin users

Your blood glucose may stay more stable overnight if you eat a bedtime snack with a higher fat or protein content, such as ice cream, yogurt, or soymilk, on days when you've been particularly active. Fat provides an alternative energy source for your muscles for many hours after you eat it and some protein is converted into glucose before that, but even having a high-fat meal with the carbohydrates held constant increases insulin needs. Taking in more protein generally includes insulin needs as well.

Taking Caffeine or Drinking Coffee to Power Workouts

Do you need that cup of steaming java in the morning to start your day off right (or just to feel awake)? If so, you're not alone, and you're probably drinking it more for the effects of the caffeine than any other reason. *Caffeine* is a stimulant found naturally in coffee, tea, cocoa, and darker chocolates that stimulates the central nervous system and increases wakefulness. It also increases your body's release of adrenaline, which can mobilize stored fat and provide an alternate fuel to your exercising muscles.

Some people find that exercising feels easier with caffeine use. It's great for directly stimulating the release of calcium in muscles to increase the strength of your contractions. Feeling stronger or less fatigued is likely the most important effect as far as exercisers are concerned. It potentially increases performance in almost any event or physical activity that you choose to do, be it long or short, intense or easy.

A major concern of using caffeine is that taking in too much of it may increase your insulin resistance, but it's also likely that any such effect will be minimized during your actual workouts. When you get caffeine naturally through coffee, it may have less of an impact on insulin action than straight caffeine does (likely due to other compounds found in coffee). But the latest research shows that coffee may still raise your blood glucose (if you're not exercising), so watch how much you drink when you're just sitting around and not being active.

Another potential downside of caffeine is that it can exert a diuretic effect, meaning that when you consume caffeinated beverages while at rest, you may lose more water by urinating more than when drinking noncaffeinated drinks. Any caffeine you consume right before or during exercise has a minimal diuretic effect, however, so you don't have to worry about becoming dehydrated from using it then because it won't make you lose extra water during activities. The idea that caffeinated drinks will hydrate you less well than caffeine-free ones is only a myth, but this only applies to any drinks you take in during the activity. But too much caffeine can cause your bones to thin and decrease how well your insulin works, along with increasing your anxiety levels, heart rate, and risk for abnormal heart rhythms, so choose decaf options at least some of the time. You may also want to limit your intake to one large cup of coffee (containing about 150 milligrams of caffeine) before events to be on the safe side.

WARNING

Be cautious about maintaining proper hydration with water when ingesting caffeine before you work out, especially if you plan to exercise in a hot environment where you sweat more. The following section gives you more information on hydration.

Staying Hydrated with Fluids

Adequate fluid intake is essential to living well and feeling your best at any age. As you grow older, you may lose some of your normal thirst sensations, putting you at risk for dehydration unless you make a conscious effort to drink more. Adequate fluid intake is also by far the best constipation cure out there.

As a person with diabetes, you may have special concerns related to hydration. Many recommendations over the years have suggested people should drink at least eight 8-ounce glasses of fluid daily; however, this recommended amount hasn't been scientifically tested and you may need less if you're getting other fluids from the foods that you eat. If you simply drink when you're thirsty during the day, most of the time you'll stay hydrated. This works well until you're older and potentially lose your early thirst sensation with advancing age.

Fluids during exercise

Preventing dehydration without overloading on fluids is an individual balancing act. You shouldn't be gaining weight during a physical activity. You'll sweat and lose water in other ways, so your weight should go down (until you rehydrate). Replace only the weight that you've lost. After exercise, continue to use thirst as your guide, rehydrating after the fact with water or other fluids with no calories. If you must drink a lot of fluid during an activity, wait until you start to urinate before drinking any more.

For shorter physical activities (lasting an hour or less), plain water is fine unless you need some extra carbs to prevent hypoglycemia; then you can drink a sports drink like Gatorade or Powerade that contains some rapidly absorbed carbs. I discuss some of these other options in the later section "Using sports drinks, juice, and more."

REMEMBER

When you're active, consuming excessive fluid can also be harmful. If you drink too much water and other fluids during exercise, you increase your risk of diluting the sodium content of your blood, potentially causing a medical condition known as *hyponatremia,* or *water intoxication.* This condition puts you at risk for seizures, coma, and even death. This condition is more common in distance events such as marathons, and more common in persons who are running slowly (in the back of the pack).

To avoid overhydrating, swig a mouthful (about 1 ounce, or 30 milliliters), and drink that amount every 10 to 15 minutes or so. If you don't sense when you're getting thirsty, just start drinking about 15 minutes into your exercise session. This strategy may vary somewhat if your blood glucose has been running high; I discuss that scenario in the following section.

You don't need to worry about replacing electrolytes, like sodium, potassium, and chloride, unless you're exercising outdoors in hot weather for more than two hours at a time; even then, you can usually wait to replace electrolytes naturally with your food the next time you eat. The exception to this is people who sweat a lot and lose sweat with a high salt content. If you can lick your lips and taste lots of salt, or have salt on your jersey when you finish your activity, you should consult with a sports dietitian to discuss your hydration and electrolyte strategy.

TECHNICAL STUFF

In general, the fluids you drink should contain less than 10 percent carbohydrates (that is, 10 grams of carbs per 100 milliliters of fluid) to promote faster emptying from your stomach. Cold fluids are absorbed more rapidly than lukewarm ones. Keep the total volume below 500 milliliters at a time, or it will slow the rate of emptying and increase your risk for water intoxication. During exercise, start drinking at least a small amount of fluids before you feel thirsty because thirst isn't triggered until you've already lost 1 to 2 percent of your fluid body weight. Taking in a large mouthful (1 to 2 ounces) at a time usually suffices. The best way to stay hydrated during exercise with diabetes is to follow these guidelines:

>> Drink cool, plain water during and following exercise, especially during warmer conditions.

>> Take frequent breaks to have a chance to cool down, preferably out of the heat and direct sunlight.

>> To know how much fluid to replace, weigh yourself before and after a prolonged activity and only replace the weight you've lost (1 liter of water equals 1 kilogram, or 2.2 pounds) and no more.

>> If you prefer fluids with some flavor, try flavored waters or sports drinks that have no added carbohydrates or calories (with a pinch of salt to taste more like a sports drink).

What to do if your blood glucose is high

If you're exercising with any elevation in your blood glucose, drink slightly more fluids than you normally would because you can more easily become dehydrated. Elevated blood glucose can cause you to pee out more water, so your risk of losing extra fluids is greater when your glucose has been running higher.

Exercising itself compounds the risk by increasing sweating (thus loss of water), which can rapidly compound a dehydrated state. Because exercising during hot weather can be especially dangerous for older individuals — who may not release heat as effectively as younger adults — adequate fluid replacement and frequent rest breaks need to be high priorities.

Having *autonomic neuropathy* (central nerve damage related to diabetes) can also compromise your ability to release heat and stay hydrated, so be more cautious and drink more fluids during exercise if you have this complication.

Using sports drinks, juice, and more

During longer workouts or a long sports event, supplementing with carbohydrates is key. During marathons or triathlons — and even intermittent, prolonged, high-intensity sports like soccer, field hockey, and tennis — taking in extra carbohydrate helps maintain your blood glucose levels, enabling you to keep going at a faster pace for longer without fatiguing. It also provides your muscles with an alternative source of carbohydrate (besides muscle glycogen).

With so many sport drinks, gels, and other sport-related supplements to choose from, how do you know which is best, if any? Simply keep in mind that more concentrated ones will not empty from your stomach or raise your blood glucose as quickly during exercise.

As far as food supplements go, it's a personal choice. More people use ones with a balance of carbohydrate, protein, and fat during longer bouts of exercise, or they may just use glucose tablets or gels (even athletes without diabetes often do this). For workouts lasting less than an hour, you may not need any extra carbs in solid or liquid form.

Don't fill your stomach with too many solid foods when your exercise level is going to be hard, or you may feel queasy or get an upset stomach.

Fruit juices are usually more concentrated than 10 percent. They're not the best thing to take in during exercise, but if you do drink juice while exercising, add some water to it to dilute it so you can digest it faster. But remember that their glycemic effect is usually lower than many other choices. You may also want to avoid juice simply because drinks with high amounts of fructose (fruit sugar) may cause abdominal cramps or diarrhea. Fructose is absorbed more slowly than glucose and pulls water into your stomach when you consume it in high concentrations, especially during exercise.

3 Getting Up and Moving

IN THIS PART . . .

Choose which activities are best for you to do and get started doing them.

Find out more about cardio training and how to fit more of it into your day.

Become stronger (not just fitter) with some resistance training.

Focus on getting better balance to stay on your feet, stretch to become more flexible, and mix it all up for best results with cross-training.

Chapter 8

Setting the Stage for Getting Active

I f you haven't been physically active recently (or ever), this chapter is for you. To set up a lasting fitness routine, pick the activities that work well for you and choose the right gear to wear from the start. Establishing a fitness routine takes some prior planning and some commitment, but it's worth the effort.

In this chapter, you discover the tricks that help you set up a routine and stick with it for the long haul. That usually means scheduling activity into your day, keeping track of your efforts, and changing up your workouts from time to time. You also pick up strategies to keep yourself motivated to maintain your new exercise habit and get past the obstacles between you and being physically active. Finally, I bust some common exercise myths, some of which you may have heard before and some of which may be complete news to you.

Finding the Right Activities

What kind of activities should you pick? There are so many fitness fads out there to choose from, including CrossFit, HIIT (high-intensity interval training), yoga, functional fitness, kettlebell workouts, and group personal training. It's hard to figure out what's right for you, both in the short run and over the long haul (your real goal). This section is your guide to what's recommended for fitness and what you should consider when choosing how to be more physically active.

REMEMBER

The goal when setting up your fitness program is to design it around physical activities that you can adopt and enjoy for the rest of your life, not ones that you hate doing or that get you injured and make you stop being active.

Getting "fit" according to the latest guidelines

How much activity and what types of exercises do you need to reach an acceptable level of fitness? According to updated physical activity guidelines released by the U.S. government in 2008, all healthy adults ages 18 to 65 years need to do moderate-intensity aerobic physical activity (for example, brisk walking or bicycling on level terrain) for at least 150 minutes a week or vigorous-intensity aerobic activity (like running or uphill bicycling) for at least 75 minutes weekly. The American College of Sports Medicine (ACSM) has issued similar recommendations for adults of that age range.

In addition, the federal guidelines and ACSM strongly recommend that all adults do some type of resistance or weight training at least two days each week. You should do these planned physical activities in addition to your usual activities of daily living, such as basic self-care, casual walking, grocery shopping, gardening, housework, and taking out the trash.

Goals are the same for all individuals with the exception of modified guidelines for those 65 years and older or people between 50 and 64 years of age who have chronic conditions or physical functional limitations that affect their ability to move or their physical fitness. If you have a physical impairment, such as arthritic joints, that makes it harder for you to be active, you may need to modify your goals a bit to be as active as you can be under the circumstances.

REMEMBER

Maintaining your physical functionality is an important benefit of exercise and even more important as you age. Keeping some level of fitness makes it easier for you to keep doing your everyday activities, such as carrying groceries, cleaning the house, taking out the trash, or just taking care of yourself. Keeping fit to live long, well, and independently should be your goal, not just staying alive a long time without good health and the ability to do (most of) what you want to do.

TIP

For older people or those with limitations, engaging in resistance training is especially important to prevent loss of muscle and bone mass. Working on flexibility and doing exercises can improve balance and lower the risk of falling.

Standing up more

Most people's calorie use during the day comes more from daily movement than from a formal exercise plan. Just standing up for two hours a day rather than sitting can expend upward of 350 calories daily and may be the difference between remaining lean and gaining excess body weight.

Homing in on your favorite workouts

One thing people forget to consider when designing a fitness program is enjoyment. Do you think the people you see grunting and groaning during agonizing workouts are truly enjoying themselves? Due to human nature, if the activities you pick are simply not fun for you, you're likely to stop doing them at some point.

Choosing an activity that's a workout

Another thing to keep in mind is that you have to work out at a certain intensity to gain fitness. That means your activity usually has to be moderate or vigorous to really boost your fit factor.

However, what you need to pick to boost your fitness depends largely on your starting fitness level. A brisk walk may be moderate or easy for someone who is adapted to doing harder workouts, while people who are sedentary and just starting out may not need an activity any harder than walking to gain greater fitness and endurance.

Tricking yourself into finishing

Even when you start on a new exercise program with the best intentions, slipping up on doing it becomes easy as time goes on. On those days when you simply lack the motivation to exercise, make a deal with yourself: You'll start your workout with the goal of doing at least half of it, and when you get to the halfway point, you can choose to stop or continue. Amazingly, you may find that most of the time when you reach that first goal, you're feeling more physically energized and mentally ready to complete the whole workout.

TIP

If you just can't finish your workout on any given day, see if you can do five more minutes before calling it a day.

GETTING EMOTIONALLY FIT THROUGH ACTIVITY

Another reason to be physically active involves your mental health, not just your physical well-being. Exercise is vitally important in alleviating feelings of stress, anxiety, and depression. Everyone — people with and without chronic health conditions — can use regular exercise to relieve mild to moderate symptoms of depression and anxiety, as well as to improve mood and self-perceptions.

If you're physically active, particularly if you're a woman (which already makes you more prone to depression), you'll experience better mental and physical health and less depression than someone who is physically inactive.

Becoming physically active can also positively affect your self-perception and benefit your self-confidence, self-concept, and self-esteem. Everyone is susceptible to bodily misperceptions because of television. Overweight teens who spend more time watching soap operas, movies, music videos, and sports reportedly have an even greater bodily dissatisfaction and drive for thinness than those who don't. Bodily dissatisfaction is associated with lower self-esteem, especially for women and girls. If you perceive yourself as fat and out of shape, you're particularly vulnerable to a negative self-image. Exercise can improve your body shape and size and, consequently, raise your self-esteem and improve your bodily satisfaction, regardless of how much you weigh.

Remember: Exercise can not only improve your short-term mental state and mood but also increase your overall sense of well-being long-term.

You can also set smaller goals at the beginning (for example, doing the first five to ten minutes of your workout at an easier pace than normal) and end up finishing more than you thought you could or would. Often, you can get rid of that sluggish, lethargic feeling that comes from being inactive and from having higher levels of insulin resistance. Just get moving on any given day and see how much better you'll feel.

Picking Workout Clothes and Equipment

Clothes, shoes, socks, and other exercise gear can make being physically active easier for you. Consider what activities you'll be doing when selecting what you need to wear or use to do them.

Dressing right

What you choose to wear when you're physically active is important, but it's not more important than getting moving itself. If you can buy clothes you feel good exercising in, then by all means do that. If not, just pick some loose-fitting clothes that allow for maximal movement of your joints in all directions and that let air movement help keep you cooler. (Leggings are comfortable, but they can make you feel hot because of their tight fit.)

TIP

Avoid wearing pure cotton socks because they tend to get wet and stay wet, which may promote damage to your feet. Wear polyester, cotton-polyester blends, or specialized athletic socks to prevent the formation of blisters and keep your feet dry during exercise.

Also keep in mind that darker clothes can absorb more heat from any direct sunlight while you're exercising outdoors. Dress in white or light-colored clothing, if possible, to keep from getting as hot from the sun.

Choosing the right footwear

Wearing appropriate shoes is critical to preventing problems with your feet and legs. The best choices vary with the activity; walkers and runners generally need some cushioning, while tennis players require footwear with greater stability for side-to-side movements. For most physical activities, you benefit by picking your shoes based on whether you rotate on your feet toward the arch of your foot or the outside edge.

TIP

To determine how you step, look at the wear pattern on the bottom of your shoes.

Exercisers who are *pronators* — that is, they *overpronate,* or rotate their feet too far to the inside — or have flat feet or are overweight wear out the insides of their soles first. If you have this problem, motion-control shoes may help. Overpronation can place extra stress on your knees, hips, and ankles and cause injuries if your shoes don't compensate for it. Conversely, *supinators* usually have high arches and more rigid feet and wear out the soles of their shoes on the outside edge. If you're a supinator, you'll generally do better in highly cushioned shoes with plenty of flexibility to encourage foot motion. If you have normal arches, aim for shoes with moderate control, such as a two-density midsole.

TIP

If you're unsure which type of arches you have, get your feet wet and make a footprint on the ground to see how much of the arch region of your foot shows. Based on that, any sporting goods or specialty running shop should be able to guide you in your selection of a particular brand or style of workout shoes that work best for your feet.

If you have any loss of sensation in your feet (from peripheral nerve damage due to diabetes), picking appropriate shoes for activities is even more critical. For this condition, athletic shoes with silica gel or air midsoles work better to cushion your feet. An ill-fitting shoe can rub your feet and contribute to irritation, calluses, and even ulcers, which you need to avoid and treat quickly to prevent the possibility of gangrene and amputation. Many athletic stores have employees trained to help you choose appropriate footwear. You can also talk with your podiatrist or diabetes healthcare team about the best shoes to wear on your unique feet for keeping fit.

WARNING

You (or someone else) must check your feet daily for signs of trauma (redness or irritation) and aggressively treat any irregularities you find to prevent worsening of the problem. Place a mirror on the floor and hold one foot over it at a time to see the bottom if you can't check your feet easily otherwise.

Getting the equipment you need

The equipment or gear you may need to work out varies by the activity. Specialists for every type of sport exist, so check with some of them if you need to buy special stuff to do your activity right. For example, getting a soft mat on which to do yoga, stretching, or floor exercises can help prevent irritation to your hips, back, and other joints. You can find out more about your equipment needs for specific activities in the discussions about those activities in the chapters to come.

Staying Motivated to Be Active

What is your biggest excuse for not being more physically active? If you answered "motivation," you're not alone.

A lot of tools exist to help you stick with being more active, including tracking your progress using the latest technology. You need to find the technique that works best for you.

Starting (or jump-starting) your motivational engine

Most people with diabetes aren't active at recommended levels, and many lack access to behavior change programs to help them get started. To motivate or remotivate yourself, try some of these suggestions:

>> Fit exercise in whenever you can, even if it's for ten minutes at a time.

>> Schedule exercise time into your daily life (and keep to your schedule).

>> Avoid getting injured by starting out at an appropriate exercise level (not too long or hard) and progressing slowly.

>> Include balance exercises to avoid falls and stretching to prevent injuries. (See Chapters 12 and 13, respectively, for more on these exercises.)

>> Pick activities you enjoy doing (like dancing) and do those to stay more engaged and motivated to be active.

>> With all the potential health benefits from being active with diabetes, use the promise of better health as part of your motivation.

>> Keep your body in motion all day long in any way possible.

Tracking your progress

Sometimes the biggest obstacle to staying motivated is the feeling that your exercising isn't getting you anywhere. That's where keeping track of stats like your daily step counts can be a valuable tool; the actual numbers may paint a much more positive picture than the one in your head. The following sections give you a few options for monitoring how many steps or step equivalents you take each day.

Using a pedometer

Wearing a *pedometer* (step counter) is a simple way to remind yourself to take more daily steps. If you don't have one, you can easily get an inexpensive device that gives you a better feel for your daily activity. Becoming more conscious of how active you are (or aren't) during the day may spur you to add in more steps whenever possible. Studies have shown that instructing sedentary, overweight women to walk 10,000 steps per day (monitored by a pedometer) is more effective for increasing their daily exercise than asking them to walk 30 minutes most days of the week.

Count how many steps you take and then set daily goals for yourself. Anyone will benefit immensely from taking at least 10,000 steps each day. But taking even 2,000 more steps every day than you are now can make the difference between gaining more weight and losing some. (For most adults, 2,000 steps equals about one mile of walking, but stride length, accuracy, and more factors can affect recorded step counts.) Taking more steps can also give you more energy to make it through each day.

TIP

To get the most out of your tracking device, keep the following in mind:

» Pedometers and most accelerometers (a similar device) can count your steps during walking, jogging, and running only; they don't account for your movement during cycling, rowing, upper body exercise, swimming, and other activities. Use online calculators to get step equivalents for any activity for which steps or motion can't be directly measured. (The later section "Using a step equivalency calculator" has more on this approach.)

» On average, 3,100 to 4,000 pedometer-counted steps are equivalent to 30 minutes of moderate-intensity walking for most people.

» Go for a simple but accurate tracking device and mostly ignore all the bells and whistles like functions that indicate calories burned; these values tend to be less accurate.

» Attach your device where it can correctly count steps (firm waistband in an upright position for pedometers). For a larger abdomen, place the device at the small of your back, or use one that works in a pocket, on your wrist, or another stable location.

» To test your device's accuracy, do the following:

   • Walk and count 20 steps at a typical walking pace; the device should record between 18 and 22 steps to be considered reasonably accurate.

   • If it repeatedly fails this test, consider getting another type.

Calculating and increasing your average daily steps

TIP

Just taking more daily steps can help improve your blood glucose; control your weight, cholesterol, and blood pressure; and make you feel less fatigued overall.

Follow these steps to calculate your average daily number as a baseline:

1. **For seven days, use a tracking device (such as a pedometer) to count the number of steps you take each day and record the number.**

   Remember to reset the device every morning.

2. **Add up all the steps you took in seven days and divide that number by seven to get the average number of steps you take daily.**

   Use this formula: Total number of steps in seven days ÷ 7 = average daily steps.

   So if your total weekly step count is 23,100, the math looks like this: 23,100 ÷ 7 = 3,300 average daily steps.

3. **Aim to add 500 steps to your daily average every two weeks.**

If your current daily average is 3,300, your goal should be to take 3,800 steps each day for the next two weeks. Then repeat the process with that period's results and set a new goal.

Using a step equivalency calculator

If you don't have access to a device that can count your steps or you're doing an activity for which counting them isn't possible, estimate the number of daily steps based on the activity. Many online tools help you do this, or you can use Table 8-1 to estimate the steps for your total minutes of each activity you do.

TABLE 8-1 **Estimate Your Activity Step Equivalents**

Activity	Steps per Minute	Activity	Steps per Minute
Aerobic dance, low to high intensity	115 to 190	Martial arts, judo	185
Ballroom dancing, slow to fast	55 to 100	Running, 5 to 10 miles per hour	185 to 350
Bowling	55	Shopping	70
Canoeing, leisurely	70	Stair climbing	160
Climbing, rock or mountain	273	Stationary cycling, moderate to vigorous	212 to 318
Cycling, 5 to 20 miles per hour	55 to 200	Step aerobics	145
Fitness club exercise, general, slow to fast	90 to 270	Swimming laps, moderate to vigorous	120 to 290
Gardening, weeding	73	Swimming leisurely	90
Golf, with and without a cart	70 to 100	Tennis, singles or doubles	160 or 110
Housework, general	90	Water aerobics	100
Jogging	185	Weight lifting, moderate to vigorous	121 to 182
Jogging, on mini-trampoline	136	Yoga and stretching	100

TIP

Search online for "step conversion calculator." Multiply the one-minute step equivalent by the number of minutes you do an activity to get your step count.

Using mobile technology to get fit

In today's mobile technology world, you have a lot of choices for tracking your daily activity and monitoring it online and on the go. It may motivate you to stay on top of your diabetes management as well.

In one study, using a diabetes-related smartphone application (Glucose Buddy) combined with weekly text-message support from a provider vastly improved blood glucose management in some adults with type 1 diabetes. Many people with type 2 diabetes don't have access to programs to help them make lifestyle changes, but using technology tools, mobile applications, social media (like Facebook), and video games (Wii Fit) are proven tools for behavior change that work.

Often taking advantage of built-in accelerometers and GPS data, many exercise and fitness apps can monitor and measure factors like calories expended, miles covered, heart rate, and more. Others are simply programs that help guide you doing exercise programs (for example, resistance training or CrossFit workouts). Others are focused more on diet and weight loss.

Hundreds of mobile apps for smartphones and other devices, as well as online websites, can work for you. Here are just a few of the more popular ones:

>> **MyFitnessPal:** Very popular free calorie counter that allows you to track your diet as well as your daily exercise.

>> **Endomondo Sports Tracker:** Traditionally used by runners, it has been acquired by Under Armour, which also picked up MyFitnessPal under its umbrella to go with this tracker.

>> **DigiFit iCardio:** Works with a heart rate monitor purchased separately.

>> **Fitbit:** Tracker that works with Fitbit devices and many smartphones.

>> **Polar Beat:** Polar makes heart rate monitors (watches and sensors)

This list of apps is by no means all inclusive. For example, the "Zombies, Run!" app is an audio adventure and game rolled into a running workout. You listen to a story about zombies and keep running to complete missions as they come up in the story — silly, yes, but engaging, especially if you aren't motivated by seeing all the data from your activities. An alternate is "The Walk," which also uses audio storytelling to add some adventure to your walking workouts. As you walk, you hear a story and are tasked with completing different missions, which may be all the motivation you need to stay active.

TIP

Quite a few apps exist that focus on ways to monitor blood glucose and diabetes management as well as fitness and diet, such as One Drop. Look for them online.

Assessing and Overcoming Barriers

What keeps you from being active, even if you know it's good for your health and your diabetes management? Why can't you get yourself up off the couch and out the door? It sounds like you need to assess the barriers standing in your way and devise some strategies to triumph in your quest to get and stay fit.

What keeps you from being more active? Your barriers likely fall into one or more of seven distinct categories:

>> Lack of time

>> Social influence

>> Lack of energy

>> Lack of motivation

>> Fear of injury

>> Lack of skill

>> Lack of resources

A good first step in staying on track is to pinpoint what's getting in the way of your being more physically active to boost your health. The following sections help you figure out which group(s) your personal obstacles fall in and give you some suggestions for getting past common issues.

Finding out what your barriers are

Take this CDC quiz to see which areas you need to focus on to get yourself moving in the right direction. You can also access the quiz online at www.cdc.gov/diabetes/ndep/pdfs/8-road-to-health-barriers-quiz-508.pdf.

The quiz lists common reasons people give to describe why they don't get as much physical activity as they think they should. Read each statement and indicate how likely you are to say each of them (very likely = completely agree; very unlikely = completely disagree).

Using the following scale, give yourself the score that corresponds with your answer for each statement. Write your number down next to each question to use for final scoring at the end.

Very likely: 3   Somewhat likely: 2   Somewhat unlikely: 1   Very unlikely: 0

1. My day is so busy now; I just don't think I can make the time to include physical activity in my regular schedule.

2. None of my family members or friends likes to do anything active, so I don't have a chance to exercise.

3. I'm just too tired after work to get any exercise.

4. I've been thinking about getting more exercise, but I just can't seem to get started.

5. I'm getting older, so exercise can be risky.

6. I don't get enough exercise because I've never learned the skills for any sport.

7. I don't have access to jogging trails, swimming pools, bike paths, and so on.

8. Physical activity takes too much time away from other commitments, such as work, family, and so on.

9. I'm embarrassed about how I will look when I exercise with others.

10. I don't get enough sleep as it is. I just couldn't get up early or stay up late to get some exercise.

11. It's easier for me to find excuses not to exercise than to go out to do something.

12. I know of too many people who have hurt themselves by overdoing it with exercise.

13. I really can't see learning a new sport at my age.

14. It's just too expensive. You have to take a class, join a club, or buy the right equipment.

15. My free times during the day are too short to include exercise.

16. My usual social activities with family or friends don't include physical activity.

17. I'm too tired during the week, and I need the weekend to catch up on my rest.

18. I want to get more exercise, but I just can't seem to make myself stick to anything.

19. I'm afraid I may injure myself or have a heart attack.

20. I'm not good enough at any physical activity to make it fun.

21. If we had exercise facilities and showers at work, then I would be more likely to exercise.

To score your quiz,

>> Enter the number you rated for each question in the corresponding blank (so the number for statement 1 goes on the line marked 1, statement 2 on line 2, and so on).

>> Add the three scores on each line. A score of 5 or above in any category shows it's an important barrier for you.

___ + ___ + ___ = _____
1   8   15   Lack of time

___ + ___ + ___ = _____
2   9   16   Social influence

___ + ___ + ___ = _____
3   10   17   Lack of energy

___ + ___ + ___ = _____
4   11   18   Lack of motivation

___ + ___ + ___ = _____
5   12   19   Fear of injury

___ + ___ + ___ = _____
6   13   20   Lack of skill

___ + ___ + ___ = _____
7   14   21   Lack of resources

Getting past your unique barriers

Barriers — perceived or real — greatly reduce the chances that you'll participate in regular exercise. A great number of potential hurdles exist, but they largely come in three main flavors: physical, environmental, and emotional. In the following sections, I explain how these groupings relate to the categories in the preceding section and give you some tips for working around them.

REMEMBER

Most American adults with type 2 diabetes or prediabetes don't exercise regularly, even less so than the rest of the adult population. People with type 1 diabetes also exercise less often than others, likely because managing their blood glucose can be a daunting task with activity. You may need additional strategies, such as the ones I discuss in Part 2, to get fit with diabetes.

Physical health barriers

These include things like lack of energy and fear of injury. Making improvements in your lifestyle can lead you to be more active and have better blood glucose management. Overcoming barriers that interfere with having a more physically active lifestyle is especially critical when you have health issues like nerve, kidney, or eye damage from diabetes.

REMEMBER

If you have physical impediments to exercising, joining a supervised exercise program to get started may help. The individuals running the program can encourage you to participate and aid you in monitoring your signs and symptoms, exercise responses, and blood glucose.

If you've been mostly on the couch because of physical issues, start out with easy or moderate activities rather than hard ones. Doing so helps you overcome two of the main reasons why people drop out of exercise programs by preventing injuries and potentially making exercise more enjoyable when it's easier at the start. Starting out at an exercise intensity that is too hard for your fitness level is usually not something that feels good or is enjoyable, and it can also get you injured.

TIP

Start out at a lower intensity and work up slowly to harder exercise over time — but only if you really want to.

Environmental barriers

Environmental barriers include many things, such as bad weather that keeps you from walking outdoors. Not everyone has access to the same exercise opportunities or facilities or resources, and your barriers may include limited or no access to exercise facilities in your budget (or any facilities at all).

High crime rates in your neighborhood, lack of access to child care, and fear for your personal safety during outdoor walking or other activities can make you less likely to get moving. You may not have any parks, walking trails, fitness centers, or community recreational centers located nearby.

TIP

Always have a backup plan, such as walking in the mall or doing an alternate activity like an exercise video at home that day. Home-based programs are another great option. If you have a seldom used piece of exercise equipment in your house (or can borrow one from someone), start using it regularly. You can do so much while working out at home, like talking to someone else (in person or on the phone), catching up on your reading, listening to music, or watching your favorite show. Having a distraction makes the time pass quickly. You owe it to yourself and your health to take this time for yourself.

Emotional barriers

Barriers in this category can be along the lines of lack of motivation, lack of skill, and social influences. Developing confidence in your ability to exercise safely is important, along with gaining support for your new exercise habit from family, friends, and health care and fitness professionals. Even being told to do culturally inappropriate activities is a barrier — like if someone wants you to exercise in public wearing exercise pants, but your religion requires you to always wear dresses or skirts. If you lack confidence in your ability to be physically active (especially if you're overweight) or lack the support and encouragement you need from your immediate family or close friends, find people who will support you. For example, include others in neighborhood walks.

REMEMBER

The most common reason adults give for not exercising on a regular basis is a perceived lack of time, meaning that they don't think they have time to fit it in. The first thing you need to do is to stop thinking of exercise as only planned activities and instead try to move more throughout the day. You'll be amazed at how much more active you become and how little time you sacrifice to do it. Any movement you do adds to how many calories you use daily.

If your self-motivation is lacking, seek out support from more-motivated people. Making your activities more social, such as exercising at a gym, in groups, or with friends and family, can help you stick with them. Try scheduling your physical activity in your calendar (like appointments) to make it more likely that you'll follow through.

TIP

Insulin users may be afraid of getting low blood glucose during exercise. The chapters in Part 2 have more information about how to prevent and treat hypoglycemia caused by exercise, a key consideration for participating in that case.

Setting some SMART goals

You need to build confidence in your ability to exercise with diabetes and set exercise goals that won't sabotage you from the start. Particularly when you have diabetes, specifically planning your exercise and tracking goals to see your progress is helpful.

TIP

Set some appropriate physical activity goals that are SMART, meaning that they're specific, measurable, attainable, realistic, and time-frame specific:

>> **Specific:** Set goals that are as precise as possible related to exercise frequency, duration, intensity, and type of activity.

>> **Measurable:** Choose goals you can quantify so you can accurately track, measure, and identify progress.

>> **Attainable:** Set goals that are challenging, but reachable, to increase your confidence and your likelihood of setting even more challenging future goals.

>> **Realistic:** Even goals that are attainable may not be helpful if they're for something you aren't likely to complete, so develop goals that are relevant to your current situation and that you can realistically accomplish in the time frame you choose as a goal.

>> **Time-frame specific:** Putting a deadline on your goal helps keep you working toward it. Set short-term goals that provide more immediate feedback on your progress, such as one week.

You benefit most from setting realistic and practical goals for getting and staying fit. Goals that are too vague, too ambitious, or too distant don't give you enough self-motivation to maintain your interest over the long haul.

Table 8-2 illustrates some less effective goals with SMART versions of those goals.

TABLE 8-2   **Less Effective versus SMART Goals**

Goal type	Less Effective Goal	SMART Goal
Specific	I will eat more healthfully.	I will eat two servings of non-starchy vegetables at every meal.
Measurable	I will be more active.	I will exercise for 30 minutes a day 5 days a week.
Attainable	I will know whether my blood glucose is low after I exercise if I start feeling symptoms, and then I'll drink some regular soda.	I will check my blood glucose before and after exercise and treat any lows by taking the glucose tablets I'll have on hand.
Realistic	I will lose 30 pounds in a month.	I will lose one to two pounds a week.
Time-frame specific	I will increase how long I exercise when I get more fit.	I will add five minutes to each walk this week, check my progress at the end of the week, and possibly set a new goal.

TIP

Create a plan for yourself for this week that includes what you plan to do (using SMART goal statements), potential barriers, an action plan for overcoming your unique barriers, and a later evaluation of what worked and what didn't work. When you get the hang of setting and using SMART goals, you'll never go back to using vague ones.

Debunking Common Exercise Myths

Separating myth from fact will help you down the road to getting fit faster and staying that way. The following sections set some of these misconceptions straight.

No pain, no gain

The pain part of exercise results from the build-up of acids in active muscles (like lactic acid), and acids drop the pH of your muscles and sensitize pain receptors. Usually, it's just a sign that you're working hard or that your muscle is fatiguing.

However, you can certainly have gains in your strength and endurance without pushing yourself to the point of having a lot of pain in the process. The more fit you become, the more easily your body can clear out those excess acids produced by physical activity.

TIP

Feeling too much pain during an activity may be a signal that you're likely to get injured. Back off to keep yourself injury free.

Exercise makes you tired

Although you may feel somewhat tired during a workout, when you're done you usually feel more invigorated for a while afterward. Doing regular physical activity is guaranteed to raise your overall energy levels. If you're having trouble concentrating at work or the stress of your day is getting you down, the best remedy is a short walk or other physical activity to raise your energy levels, clear your mind, and decrease your stress.

REMEMBER

Doing regular physical activity also helps you sleep better at night, leaving you more refreshed and energetic during the day.

To lose fat, you have to be in a fat-burning range

Exactly what is "fat-burning" range? First, you must understand what fuels your body uses during rest and exercise. Typically, 60 percent of your energy needs are supplied by fat (stored or eaten) during rest, with the other 40 percent coming from carbohydrates.

As soon as you start to do any type of physical activity, though, carbohydrates go up to a much higher percentage of your total energy supply. Even during brisk walking, you use very little fat and mostly carbohydrates. During more vigorous exercise, your body gets almost all energy from carbohydrates. You use plenty of fat during recovery from exercise, though.

TIP

Try to expend as many calories during exercise as possible without worrying about being in a fat-burning range. This range really isn't relevant.

If you don't use your muscles, they turn into fat

It's physically impossible for inactive muscles to turn into fat. When you work your muscles out regularly, they can increase in size or simply look more toned; if you stop using them, the muscle fibers will atrophy and disappear — like what happens with aging if you don't fight against it. Then if you don't start eating less, you'll gain weight as fat that then can be stored under your skin.

Lose weight first, because weight training will bulk you up

Women are often especially worried about bulking up and getting bigger arms or legs. However, if you're losing fat all over (including from under your skin) while you're gaining muscle mass, you'll stay about the same size. If you gain muscle without losing fat, you may look slightly bigger, or simply more toned. Either way, it's not a big deal because most people don't gain enough muscle from weight training to ever look bulked up.

Lifting weights more slowly builds larger muscles

If you try lifting weights more slowly, you'll certainly feel the pain, but it absolutely doesn't mean that your muscle size gains will be more. On the contrary, lifting weights slowly when you can lift them more quickly will build more muscular endurance, while lifting the heaviest weight as quickly as possible will recruit extra muscle fibers and cause you to build bigger muscles.

TIP

If you're lifting a weight slowly but could lift it more quickly, you either need to pick up the pace or try a heavier weight.

Working on your abs will make your belly flat

As much as you want to pick and choose where you lose your fat, spot reducing just isn't possible. Doing hundreds of crunches won't make you lose stomach fat any faster than you lose it from anywhere else.

If you want a flat belly, you can work on toning up your abdominal region, but focus more on simply burning off excess calories. Doing harder workouts also builds more muscle, and having more muscle increases your daily caloric needs. One side benefit of including abdominal exercises is that having toned abs makes pulling in your stomach easier, so your belly can look flatter even if you can't spot reduce.

You can't exercise too much

As with anything, excessive exercise has a limited benefit. When you do more than 60 to 90 minutes of aerobic exercise daily, you're much more likely to develop overuse injuries such as stress fractures, tendinitis, bursitis, and other joint issues. You don't want to get injured, because then you'll have trouble working out. You're better off doing slightly more intense exercise for less time, which you can do with any type of interval training to gain the same benefits (or even more) from your workout.

To gain muscle, eat more protein

It's true that you have to eat some protein to gain protein in your body. (Muscles are made of amino acids, the building blocks of protein.) And, yes, physically active people do need more protein than sedentary ones, but not that much more. No athlete needs more than 1.6 to 1.7 grams of protein per kilogram of body weight (about 0.75 grams per pound), or just twice that of a sedentary person.

Does that mean you need to take protein supplements or up the protein in your diet? Probably not. Most Americans already eat well over their recommended amount of protein per day just by eating normally, mostly from meat, poultry, fish, and other animal sources like dairy and eggs. Having a glass of milk or some yogurt after a workout may be an easy way to take in a good combination of carbohydrate and protein to help your muscles rebuild. Some athletes have actually touted chocolate milk as the ultimate recovery drink following workouts.

TIP

If you want to take in extra protein naturally, try eating more egg whites or drinking milk of some type post-exercise.

If you're not sweating, you're not working out hard enough

Everyone equates sweating with working hard, but that simply isn't always the case. People's sweating rates vary. Being physically trained improves your ability to sweat more and to start sweating sooner, but men always tend to sweat more than women.

Sweating is related to not only exercise intensity but also the environment you're in. If it's hot and humid, you're going to sweat more, even if you're not working out that hard. You also sweat less if you start out dehydrated or lose too much fluid while you're working out.

IN THIS CHAPTER

» Finding ways to be more active all day long

» Getting an overview of various kinds of exercise

» Understanding the importance of warming up and cooling down

» Establishing a routine

» Being aware of activities that may not work for you and treating injuries that do occur

Chapter **9**

Setting Your Workout Up for Success

This chapter is all about getting moving in ways that are appropriate for you. You may love jogging but hate aquatic activities, while someone else may feel most at home in the pool. I explain which activities are recommended for people with diabetes or prediabetes (and why) and give you advice on easing into your workout and avoiding injuries. Keeping yourself from getting sidelined by overuse or acute injuries related to exercise is critical for staying active.

Adding in Spontaneous Physical Activity

Any daily activities you choose to do benefit your health no matter what they are. The best advice is to pick ones you enjoy that you're more likely to do regularly. Simply sitting too long at one time is now a recognized health hazard, so getting up regularly from a seated position is important, too.

Unfortunately, most people naturally try to do as little activity as possible. How many times have you driven to a store and then circled around the parking lot or waited a long time to find a spot close to the door rather than just parking farther away and walking? When you do that, you're missing out on an opportunity for *spontaneous physical activity,* or SPA.

Besides the fact that calling it "SPA time" makes is sound more appealing and fun, adding in more daily movement in any way possible is likely to benefit your health in countless ways. SPA can happen when you get a few more steps by parking farther away or when you stand up or walk around while talking on the phone instead of sitting down.

Identifying the benefits of SPA time

If you get and stay more active every day by doing more SPA, you undoubtedly enhance and maintain your overall health, vitality, and youthful vigor more effectively. Doing easier activities like standing or walking around, even if they don't make you break a sweat, uses up calories and helps you keep your weight stable. You won't get as fit from doing most SPA activities like these. But when matched for number of calories burned, doing easy or moderate spontaneous activities for more total time during the day works as well for improving your blood glucose and your aerobic capacity as doing harder, planned exercise for less time does.

REMEMBER

Doing activities of any intensity benefits your diabetes management. If it's an easier activity like SPA, you just have to do it for longer (or more total time during the time) to get the same glucose benefit.

Adding a dozen extra steps here and there can add up to a lot of calories burned over the course of the day, week, and year and prevent weight gain. But doing anything — even fidgeting — makes your metabolism work better compared to sitting continuously for long periods of time, so remember to keep your SPA time going strong. (The following section has more on using SPA to break up sedentary time.) The more, the better, so think of creative ways to add more movement into each and every day.

TIP

Easy activities like cleaning, washing dishes, grocery shopping, gardening, playing with your kids or grandkids, walking the dog, standing, or any other activity can help lower your blood glucose and keep you more fit and active. Here are a few more options:

>> Pace or stand while talking on the phone instead of sitting.

>> Always take the stairs instead of the elevator or escalator.

>> Window shop at the nearest mall.

- » Wash your car by hand (and wax it, too).

- » Put on some music and dance.

- » Set up a basketball net in your driveway and shoot some hoops.

- » Walk to a nearby school when school is out of session and use its playground equipment.

- » Hide the remotes for the TV, stereo, and other devices so you have to get up to adjust the settings.

- » Walk in place, dance, move around, or even just stand up while watching TV — at least during the commercials.

- » Limit your TV and home computer use to no more than two hours per day. If you can't get down to that little, try lowering your current at-home screen time by 30 minutes to start.

Taking a stand against being sedentary

Simply standing up more expends a lot more calories on a daily basis than you can imagine. In one study that compared lean and overweight adults, the main difference in their lifestyles was that the lean ones stood up for two hours a day longer than the ones who were carrying too much body fat.

If nothing else, just keep yourself from sitting for long periods of time. Break up those times with frequent periods of standing or walking around for a few minutes. Doing so can lower your blood glucose.

REMEMBER

Try to remember to get up and stand or walk around for 3 to 5 minutes after every 30 or more minutes you've been sedentary. Longer standing time is associated with a lower risk of dying for any reason.

Getting thinner by doing spontaneous activities

Even though you consume hundreds of thousands of calories a year, your body can maintain your body weight within a pound or two — a truly amazing feat. So what's making people gain so much weight these days despite this inborn ability to autoregulate body weight? They're likely using up too few calories through physical movement.

You don't gain all your excess body fat overnight. You may gain a few extra pounds during the holiday season and never lose them. Or you may be gaining weight slowly over a few months or several years.

Either way, small lifestyle changes have a big impact on your body weight over time. For instance, if you eat just 50 fewer calories a day than you need (equal to only a small apple, a small piece of chocolate candy, or a few bites of most meals), your total weight loss from skipping those calories alone will be 5 pounds of body fat a year. And you'll lose those 5 pounds easily without giving it much thought and with minimal effort.

But wait! You can double your weight loss with added SPA time: Combine taking in 50 fewer calories a day with using up an extra 50 calories by adding in bits of activity throughout the day. You can do so with a little extra walking, stretching, or other easy activity, even just standing longer. Then you'll lose 10 pounds in a year without dieting or trying that hard.

Choosing the Best Training for Diabetes

For fitness gains and blood glucose management, daily spontaneous physical activity helps, but it may not be enough. You likely need to do both more daily SPA and some cardio, resistance, or other exercise training to keep fit with any type of diabetes or prediabetes. (Check out the earlier section "Adding in Spontaneous Physical Activity" for more on SPA.)

TIP

If your workouts are short, work harder to gain more fitness. Do at least one longer workout each week to build greater endurance.

Table 9-1 lists the four categories of exercise recommended for people with diabetes, along with some basic guidance on intensity, duration, and so on. When it comes to resistance training, in case you're not current on the lingo, *repetitions* are the number of times you do the move (like a push-up) and *sets* are how many times you repeat those repetitions (such as three sets of doing 12 repetitions of push-ups). The following sections discuss each of these categories in more detail.

REMEMBER

Any exercise you do during the day counts, not just your planned workouts.

TABLE 9-1

Recommended Planned Activities for Diabetes

	Aerobic	Resistance	Balance	Flexibility
Examples (what to do)	Walk, run/jog, cycle, row, swim, or use cardio machines Continuous or interval training	Free weights, bands, machines, and/or body weight as resistance	Stand on one leg, balance equipment, tai chi, or lower-body and core resistance exercise	Static or dynamic stretching, other stretches, or yoga
Intensity (how hard)	Moderate to vigorous (somewhat hard to very hard)	Moderate to vigorous (somewhat hard to very hard)	Light to moderate	Stretch to point of tightness or minor discomfort (but not pain)
Duration (how long)	At least 150 minutes per week (30 minutes at a time is ideal, but it can be shorter or longer) for most; if you're more fit, 75 minutes weekly (ideally doing at least 15 to 20 minutes at a time) of harder exercise okay	At least 8 to 10 exercises, 1 to 3 sets, and 10 to 15 repetitions to near fatigue per set on every exercise	Any duration	Hold static or do dynamic stretch for 10 to 30 seconds; repeat 2 to 4 times per stretch
Frequency (how often)	3 to 7 days a week; don't go more than 2 days in a row without cardio exercise	At least 2 days weekly, but 3 days is better; take at least 1 day off in between	2 to 3 days weekly; daily is okay	2 to 3 days weekly; daily is okay
Progression (how to keep getting fitter)	If you want to get more fit, focus more on doing harder exercise and/or intervals	Increase work, lower repetitions to 8 to 10; add more sets next, another day per week last	If you're over the age of 40, do balance training for longer and/or more often	Stretch for longer and/or more often over time

Cardio (aerobic) and interval workouts

Cardio training is what most people think of when they decide to start an exercise program. It certainly can include walking, but also a lot of other activities like swimming, cycling, and others. Adding in or doing faster intervals is a newer fad, but one that can increase fitness more quickly than doing most cardio training at a slower, continuous pace.

TIP

For more on how to choose your cardio activities, refer to Chapter 10.

Walking through some aerobic exercise options

Most adults with type 2 diabetes who exercise simply get active by walking regularly. Studies have shown that increasing aerobic activity by 38 minutes per day — walking just an extra 4,400 steps, or about 2.2 miles — lowers your blood glucose, blood fats, and blood pressure, even if you don't lose any weight. Adding in even more physical activity during your leisure time also lowers your chances of having a stroke by at least 25 percent if you have diabetes. You gain the same benefits if you have type 1 diabetes.

If you consistently take at least 10,000 steps daily (about 5 miles of walking) or do the equivalent, you'll likely be able to take lower doses of your prescribed medications, even without changing your diet. (Chapter 8 has more information on the step equivalents of many activities.) Maybe walking isn't your cup of tea, and you'd rather take a bike ride around the nearest park. That's fine (though keep in mind that cycling expends only about a third of the energy you use walking the same distance). What matters most for your health is burning off those extra calories in any way because that helps you manage your blood glucose as well as your weight. Simply pick the activities you like best and are most likely to stick with doing.

Getting fit faster with interval training

REMEMBER

You can also get more fit in less time by adding some harder *intervals,* where you increase the intensity of your exercise for short periods of time, into any aerobic activity. The options for adding interval training into your workouts are endless and the benefits to your fitness and overall health almost limitless.

In addition to getting you fit faster, doing intervals of any type uses more calories, makes you feel more tired when you finish (in a good way), and likely allows you to increase your general walking speed due to the extra conditioning. Many people experience major gains in their endurance after doing only six to eight minutes of harder exercise a week.

To do intervals when you're walking, speed up slightly for a short distance (such as between two mailboxes) before slowing back down to your original pace. During your walk, continue to include these short, faster intervals occasionally and, as you're able, lengthen them so that they last two to five minutes at a time (although you may want to start out doing only 15 to 30 seconds of faster walking at a time). If you're on a cardio training machine, choose to do one of the interval profiles that make your workout harder from time to time.

Resistance (strength) and core training

If you only have time to add in one planned activity to your life, make it some type of resistance training. Why, you ask? The following sections explain.

TIP

See Chapter 11 for more on what exercises to do and how to resistance train effectively.

Revving up your insulin, muscle, and strength

As far as insulin action goes, nothing is more important than how much room you have in the muscle gas tank you use to store dietary carbohydrates. Doing some resistance work is critical if you want to keep the muscle you have now and possibly gain more.

REMEMBER

It's also the only way to prevent losses of muscle and strength as you age. Even though everyone loses some muscle mass over time — even active individuals — being sedentary accelerates your losses of this insulin-sensitive tissue, and diabetes appears to speed up how fast and how much you can lose. It truly is a case of "use it or lose it."

Although aerobic training can help you keep your muscle mass, only the muscle fibers that you actively recruit and use regularly remain over time. Moderate activities like walking don't bring all your muscle fibers into play, just the slower and intermediate speed ones in most cases. Only more intense workouts or very hard interval training can engage the rest, so you must include some resistance and/or sprint training in your exercise plan to preserve your faster, more powerful muscle fibers.

Having more muscle not only enhances how well your insulin works but also revs up your metabolism, helps control your body weight, makes you stronger, and improves your self-esteem and satisfaction with your body. Who doesn't want to look more toned and fit?

After you start doing resistance training, your strength can increase a lot in just the first couple of weeks from neural changes, which occur before your muscles appear to have expanded. Most strength gains that happen after the first few months come from building bigger muscles, though. If you have physical barriers to weight training, get an appointment with a physical therapist or fitness professional to help design a program for you. If you do not know how to get started, enlist the help of a personal trainer available at most fitness facilities.

TIP

Major strength gains and muscle fiber retention can occur even if you just train one day a week, but two to three days are recommended for optimal results.

Focusing on getting a fit core

Core training is just specialized resistance training that focuses specifically on increasing the strength of your core muscles — primarily your abdominal and back muscles but also your butt and upper leg muscles. Having a strong core makes doing a variety of daily activities and preventing falls easier.

TIP

Chapter 21 features ten easy resistance exercises you can do anywhere that build a strong core.

Balance exercises

You may think your balance is fine. More than likely, though, you may start feeling less steady on your feet as time passes. Try tying your shoelace by lifting that foot while standing solely on the other one to find out how good your balance really is.

REMEMBER

If you're over 40, your balance is already on the decline. It's not your fault; it's just a natural result of getting older.

You can fight back and get better balance. Studies have shown that doing balance training can reduce your risk of falling, even if you've more unstable on your feet due to losing some of the feeling in your feet from neuropathy. Group exercise classes, including resistance and balance training and tai chi, reduce falls by almost 30 percent in older adults with diabetes.

You can also try to boost your balance with alternative training like yoga and tai chi, both of which can also improve blood glucose, cholesterol, and body fat, at least in adults with type 2 diabetes. Tai chi — which is the foundation for all martial arts forms — may even help with your symptoms of neuropathy and improve your quality of life.

Lower-body resistance training also doubles as a type of balance exercise, so include exercises that target your legs and body core.

TIP

Chapter 12 has many more easy balance exercises, but you can start doing this very simple balance exercise anytime:

>> Hold onto a table or stationary chair with both hands while standing on one leg. When you feel stable in this position, slowly release one of your hands. Stand there until your leg muscles feel tired. Do this exercise two to three times a day on alternating feet, and within a couple of weeks or months, your balance will rapidly improve.

> » If this exercise is too easy for you, try holding on with just one fingertip or not at all. If you're still not challenged enough, try doing it with your eyes closed (with or without hands).

Flexibility training

Losing some of the flexibility in your joints is expected as you age. Using your muscles regularly can cause them to get stiff and sore afterward. It helps to do either static or dynamic stretching exercises to loosen your muscles and improve your joint flexibility. Having a greater range of motion around your joints can help avert injury and keep you on your feet by preventing falls. Use a full range of motion around your joints during all activities, if possible.

REMEMBER

The best time to stretch is when your muscles are warm. Stretching is separate from warming up and cooling down for your aerobic exercise.

Older adults with diabetes often suffer from limited joint mobility. If your blood glucose goes higher than normal, it can cause you to lose flexibility faster than normal aging alone does, which is all the more reason to not only stretch frequently but also manage diabetes as best you can.

Though stretching exercises improve your flexibility, in most cases doing them regularly isn't enough to make your blood glucose better. But doing yoga or tai chi as a stretching activity may help manage your diabetes.

TIP

You can get started with doing more stretching by following the stretches in Chapter 13.

Cross-training for optimal fitness

Cross-training is basically just mixing up your exercise routine during the week by including alternate activities on different days. By the time you add in all four types of recommended activities during the week, you're essentially already doing cross-training. It helps keep you from getting injured and makes your activities more enjoyable overall because they're varied.

TIP

Chapter 14 covers a lot more about doing cross-training.

KEGEL EXERCISES FOR WOMEN (AND MEN, TOO)

Stress incontinence (that is, when a small amount of urine is forced out of your bladder when you're active) occurs more often in women whose bladder neck has *prolapsed* (slipped from its usual position) outside the abdominal cavity. It's particularly common in women who have gone through childbearing, even when they're still in their 20s and 30s.

When they cough, sneeze, bounce, or jog with this condition (all of which are potential stressors), they often experience increased pressure on their bladder, but not on their internal sphincter, resulting in urine leakage even if they've just peed. Men can also experience some of the same problems, and weak pelvic floor muscles can also lead to a less strong erection and premature ejaculation.

A simple treatment for both women and men consists of pelvic muscle training called *Kegel exercises*. A side benefit of these exercises is that your increased muscle strength is likely to enhance your sexual pleasure, which largely depends on the training of these muscles because they're the ones that contract during orgasms.

These exercises may feel hard to do at first, but the more often you practice them, the easier they get. Seeing big improvements may take up to eight weeks. For best results, contract these muscles 50 to 100 times daily by doing as many repetitions as you can several times a day. To minimize stress incontinence, also contract these muscles before coughing or sneezing.

Easy Kegel exercises include the following:

- During urination, try to stop and start your urine flow; at the end of the exercises, make sure you empty your bladder totally (men and women).

- Tighten your anal muscles as if stopping gas from coming out. Then shift muscular tightness from your rear to your front area (men and women).

- Variations include contracting and holding these muscles for about ten seconds at a time (instead of rapidly contracting and relaxing them), with five-second rests between extended contractions (women and men).

- Tighten your vaginal muscles around two fingers inserted into your vagina or around a tampon inserted halfway (women only).

- Get an erection and hang a washcloth or small towel on your penis. Then try to contract your pelvic muscle to lift the towel several times (men only).

Warming Up and Cooling Down

Most workouts consist of ramping up to doing the activity, completing it, and cooling down before you stop exercising. The recommended exercise times included in Table 9-1 earlier in this chapter refer to the part of your workout that is sandwiched in the middle of a warm-up and a cool-down, or the *conditioning phase*, such as walking at moderate intensity for 30 minutes.

The *warm-up* consists of doing an easier exercise before your cardio or resistance workout to increase blood flow and get oxygen to your muscles. It lasts four to five minutes. If walking is your exercise for the day, to warm up you can walk at a slower speed first. If you're doing resistance training, start out doing movements with little or no resistance added, or you can do a cardio warm up to get your heart pumping faster and your blood flowing.

The *cool-down* is the last phase of your activity, during which you slowly reduce your heart rate; in the walking example, you'd cool down by walking at a slower pace for another three to five minutes before ending. Neither the warm-up nor the cool-down technically counts as part of your target workout time because you do them at a much lower intensity than your conditioning phase.

REMEMBER

Some stretching usually follows the cool-down, but you can also do it after your warm-up. Or you can stretch any time your muscles or joints start to feel tight during an activity or later in the day.

Carving Out a Fitness Routine

I don't know who originally said that half the battle is just showing up, but this line certainly applies to finding time to be regularly active. The tips that follow not only help you find that time but also get the most out of any training you do.

Finding time every day to be active

A good practice is to aim to do both SPA and planned exercise every day, although it can vary with the day and your schedule. If you run into a barrier that keeps you from doing a planned workout, simply shift your focus to doing more unplanned activities like standing up, taking more steps, and moving all day long.

TIP

If you're stuck waiting in an airport, walk around and stand up while waiting. If you're bogged down with meetings at work, try to schedule some walking ones (if you can), or find a way to stand up frequently during them. Take the stairs to your next meeting instead of the elevator. Get others around you to join in with SPA time.

Creating a personalized workout plan to keep you accountable

Just like when you schedule an appointment and put it in your calendar, you're a lot more likely to follow through on anything that is penciled in. Do the same with your physical activities. If you've set SMART goals (see Chapter 8), convert them into a weekly plan for this coming week, and then keep doing so week after week. You'll be more successful in being active if you plan it out in advance and stick with the plan to the extent that you can. (That said, don't beat yourself up when life happens and gets in the way sometimes.)

You can use Table 9-2 as a template for making your own weekly workout plan.

TABLE 9-2 **Your Weekly Workout Plan**

	Aerobic (3 to 7 days a week; no more than 2 days in a row without any)	Resistance (2 or 3 days not in a row)	Balance (2 to 7 days a week)	Flexibility (at least 2 to 3 days)	SPA (every day)
Monday					
Tuesday					
Wednesday					
Thursday					
Friday					
Saturday					
Sunday					

Changing up your routine with hard and easy days

You benefit from purposefully varying your exercise intensity from day to day by doing hard and easy days of training. By alternating workout intensities (easy, moderate, or hard), you get both the enhanced fitness and strength benefits of harder workouts and the healing effects of greater recuperative time between them.

Staying active on alternate days doing more laid-back activities makes managing your blood glucose easier for you. For many people with diabetes or prediabetes, just doing easy or moderate activities is enough for them to keep fit, especially if they're way out of shape to start.

TIP

Try to never let more than two days pass between workouts if you want to keep your insulin action revved up.

Varying how hard you work out also helps prevent *overuse syndrome,* which is caused by overstressing your body with repeated heavy workouts and may cause more frequent colds, chronic tiredness, and joint and muscle injuries.

REMEMBER

Aim to get one day of rest a week, even if on that day you simply do a different activity, have an easy workout day, or stay active with SPA.

Getting enough beauty sleep

Getting enough sleep — seven to eight hours a night for most adults — gives your body time to rebuild and recuperate. If you don't sleep enough, you'll be physically stressed and release stress hormones like cortisol that trigger your liver to produce more glucose and increase insulin resistance. That's bad news for your blood glucose and a pretty compelling reason to try to get enough quality sleep every night.

Progressing (slowly) over time

Your fitness routine isn't a race to the finish. Remember that many people drop out of exercise programs because they're too hard. To stay active for a lifetime, start out slowly and progress slowly over time. Don't overdo it early on if you want to stay active for years to come. For example, unfit adults who want to start running should begin with walking until they raise their fitness enough that jogging or slower running is doable.

REMEMBER

The best exercise program for you personally is the one that you're able to keep doing for the rest of your life.

Steering Clear of Certain Activities

Not all activities are equally good for everyone. If you have a major joint or foot problem that limits walking, don't feel obligated to start walking. That could make your problem worse and keep you from being active doing anything. Stationary cycling or another seated activity may be a better cardio option for you.

Keep these other pointers in mind when evaluating potential activities:

>> **Running isn't for everyone.** You may not want to hear this if you're an avid runner, but running isn't a lifetime activity for most people. Doing this activity causes a lot of wear and tear on your joints over time, especially if you have to run on less-than-optimal surfaces or with worn out shoes. Certainly, consider doing other activities — especially ones that get you off your feet like cycling — if you have a lot of issues with your knees or hips.

What can you do instead if you have to give up running or you just don't like doing it in the first place? For most overweight adults with diabetes, walking and adding in some faster pace intervals works fine to get them fit.

>> **Choose seated activities if you're unstable on your feet or are wheelchair bound.** This is also a good option if you have other issues impacting your feet or legs. You can do myriad activities seated if you have mobility issues, feel unstable on your feet, or are wheelchair bound. Chair dancing is an aerobic exercise option that is fun for many. You can find a way to do most resistance exercises sitting or lying down instead of standing, and stretching in a seated position is also possible. Some balance exercises involve standing but using something to stabilize yourself while you're on your feet. Chapters 10 through 13 list various other cardio, resistance, balance, and flexibility exercise options.

>> **Avoid overusing your joints.** Steering clear of repetitive activities — particularly if they aggravate your joints at all — is a good practice for cross-training. (Head to Chapter 14 and the earlier section "Cross-training for optimal fitness.") If you stick with doing different activities on varying days of the week, you're a lot less likely to develop any injuries from overusing your joints. You want to use your joints, just not abuse them. The later section "Preventing and treating overuse injuries" has more on these types of ailments.

>> **Remember that diabetes can make you more prone to exercise injury.** Although everyone gets stiffer with age, diabetes accelerates how quickly you lose flexibility when your blood glucose runs high. (See the later section "Recognizing what causes overuse injuries" for details on how diabetes affects joints.) The best prevention of all these issues is optimal blood glucose management and regular stretching to maintain a greater range of motion around your joints.

Preventing and Managing Injuries

Getting injured when being active happens often enough that you need to know how to prevent and treat injuries when they occur. When you start doing regular training, you increase your risk of injuring yourself or developing an overuse injury over time.

The best medicine is prevention. The more you know about how to handle and prevent injuries before they develop, the better off you'll be because you won't have to worry as much about having to take time off from exercising and side-tracking your fitness program.

Identifying common injuries

Having intense or lasting pain during or after exercise isn't normal. Acute injuries can happen when you use improper exercise techniques or experience an accident, such as dropping a dumbbell on your foot. Overuse injuries result from repeated physical movements that lead to irritation and pain.

Here's a quick look at some of the most common injuries that can occur during activities or because of overuse:

>> **Ankle sprain:** If you've ever "turned" your ankle when walking or running, you may have experienced an *ankle sprain.* This injury is a painful stretching or tearing of a ligament. *Inversion ankle sprains* are the most common and occur when your foot twists inward. The outside ligaments are then stretched or torn.

>> **Plantar fasciitis:** If you have pain in your heel when standing or walking, you may have *plantar fasciitis.* This condition is due to inflammation in the *plantar fascia* (found along the arch on the bottom of your foot). It can be caused or aggravated by wearing shoes with poor arch support or very stiff soles and not stretching your calves and back of your legs after exercise.

>> **Heel spur:** A *heel spur* is an abnormal bone growth on the heel that results from untreated or prolonged plantar fasciitis — that is, chronic inflammation at the point where the ligaments or fascia attach to your heel bone. Spurs protrude out from the back of the heel or right under the heel, beneath the sole of the foot, and they can cause pain.

>> **Shin splints:** Though they aren't an easily defined injury, *shin splints* occur when you put too much force on your shinbone and the connective tissues that attach your muscles to the bone. Their symptoms are indistinct but include sharp pain along the lower leg (shinbone) while exercising. They're believed to be caused by inflammation of the shin bone and possible stress fractures of the tibia or fibula (lower leg bones).

>> **Achilles tendinitis:** Caused by inflammation and swelling of a heel tendon, *Achilles tendinitis* can cause swelling, redness, pain, aching, and stiffness before, during, and after exercise. The pain gets worse when you walk uphill or climb stairs. You may get this condition from tight calf muscles, poor stretching habits, running on hard surfaces and hills, overuse, or wearing worn-out shoes.

Avoiding other acute injuries

Taking a few important precautions can help you avoid the following acute injuries when you're active:

>> **Knee injuries:** Avoid rapid changes in direction or be careful to keep your knees steady when landing from a jump, progress exercise slowly, choose safe activities, always warm up and cool down, and stretch your leg muscles on both sides of the joint. In addition, choose exercises that help strengthen the knee muscles, such as cycling, leg press, and chair squats.

>> **Lower back injuries:** Avoid heavy weight lifting, minimize making rapid changes in direction, choose activities that don't stress your low back, progress exercise slowly, always warm up and cool down, and stretch your lower back and thigh muscles.

>> **Intense pain:** If you ever have joint, muscle, or chest pain, stop and possibly check with your health care provider if the pain doesn't subside immediately or recurs when you exercise. Explore other, less painful options for your exercise.

Treating acute injuries properly

Treat your acute injuries properly with R.I.C.E.:

>> **Rest:** Stay off your feet as much as possible and use crutches if necessary.

>> **Ice:** Cover the area with a towel and place a bag full of ice on it for 10 to 20 minutes several times a day for two to three days to reduce swelling.

>> **Compression:** Use a pressure bandage (like an Ace bandage that you can wrap around the affected area) to help reduce swelling.

>> **Elevation:** Elevate your foot slightly higher than your heart to help reduce throbbing pain and reduce swelling.

If you properly care for your injuries, they should get better within a week. If they're not improving, or if you have a single point of intense pain, you should probably see a physician. (For leg injuries in particular, look for a podiatrist who has expertise in foot, ankle, and lower leg problems as well as diabetes.) He or she should be able to pinpoint the cause of your discomfort with an X-ray, bone scan, or MRI. You may need physical therapy or rehabilitation for persistent problems.

REMEMBER

Judicious use of ibuprofen (Advil or Nuprin) or naproxen sodium (Aleve) can help control pain and inflammation associated with acute or chronic injuries. These medications are not recommended if you're having health problems with your kidneys, though.

TIP

As soon as the injury improves, ease slowly back into your exercise routine. Don't rush it, though, or you may suffer a relapse.

Common causes of all injuries

When it comes to exercise-related injuries, the following are common culprits:

» **Footwear:** No arch support, shoes too tight or too big

» **Exercise errors:** Excessive exercise, progressing too quickly to higher exercise intensities, no stretching, no warm-up/cool-down

» **Faulty biomechanics:** High/flat arches, muscle tightness

» **Environment:** Exercising on slick, muddy, wet, icy, or uneven surfaces

Preventing and treating overuse injuries

Ever had an injury that ended in "–itis"? You likely had an overuse one.

Overuse injuries are characterized by inflammation of an area, soreness, and swelling, and they're nagging and persistently uncomfortable. Using the same joints and muscles in a similar way over weeks or months doing excessive training, or doing too much too soon, can cause them.

REMEMBER

Doing more exercise is good — but only up to a point. You're more likely to get exercise-related overuse injuries like inflamed tendons or stress fractures by doing more than 60 to 90 minutes of moderate or hard exercise daily, particularly if you're doing the same activity day after day.

Recognizing what causes overuse injuries

The onset of overuse injuries can often be linked to changes in athletic endeavors or techniques. For example, if you've been running 3 miles (5 kilometers) several days a week at a moderate pace and you start running 5 miles (8 kilometers) six days a week at a faster pace than before, you're setting yourself up for an overuse injury. Exercise causes damage to your muscles and joints that ultimately strengthens them, but only if you give them time to rest and recuperate.

TIP

Don't increase your amount of training by more than about 10 to 20 percent per week after you start, or you may open yourself up to an overuse injury.

Joint damage is another cause of overuse injuries. Aging alone can cause you to lose cartilage in knees, hips, and other joints — leading to osteoarthritis and joint pain — but having diabetes also potentially speeds up damage to joints. Reduced flexibility limits movement, increases your chance of injuries, and can cause many joint-related problems associated with diabetes. Although everyone gets stiffer with aging, diabetes accelerates it by changing the structure of collagen in the joints, tendons, and ligaments. In short, glucose sticking to joint surfaces and collagen makes people with diabetes more prone to overuse injuries like tendinitis and frozen shoulder, and their joint injuries may also take longer to heal properly, especially if blood glucose is high.

REMEMBER

Tendinitis is specifically inflammation of tendons that attach muscles to bones. You get it when a tendon rubs repeatedly against a bony structure, ligament, or another tendon or when it's being impinged. For instance, tennis elbow is a type of tendinitis on the outside of the elbow common in tennis players but also in rowers, carpenters, gardeners, golfers, and other exercisers that repeatedly bend their arms forcefully.

Uneven body alignment, such as knock-knees, bowed legs, unequal leg lengths, and flat or high-arched feet, can also cause injuries. Even prior such issues lead to a greater likelihood of overuse injuries, along with factors like the type of athletic shoes you use, the terrain (hilly, flat, or uneven), and whether you work out on hard surfaces like concrete roads or floors or softer ones like grass, dirt or gravel trails, asphalt, and cushioned floors.

Preventing overuse injuries

Try these tips to prevent overuse injuries:

>> Always warm up and cool down, and stretch regularly to stay limber.

>> Make gradual increases in training intensity, duration, and frequency.

>> Give your joints a rest if you have nagging aches and pains.

>> Adopt a hard/easy workout schedule and vary your workouts by the day.

>> If your problems are anatomical, fix what you can (such as getting orthotics to correct differences in your leg lengths).

>> Wear proper shoes to prevent most lower-extremity and foot problems.

>> Do activities that lower injury risk, such as working out on an elliptical trainer a few days a week instead of doing outdoor running on asphalt.

>> Keep your blood glucose levels as close to normal as possible.

TIP

To prevent the recurrence of an injury after you can resume your normal activities, work on strengthening the muscles around the affected area. To keep from getting the same shoulder injury again, for example, do resistance exercises using all sections of the shoulder, upper arm, upper back, and neck muscles.

Also train doing other activities to maintain your overall fitness while your injury recovers. If you have leg issues, you can still work out your upper body with activities that allow your legs to rest and recuperate. Try alternating weight-bearing activities like walking or running with non-weight-bearing ones, such as swimming, upper-body work, and cycling, to avoid injuring something else. You may also want to seek out the assistance of a physical therapist in choosing the best activities to get on top of your enduring injuries.

Expecting some muscle soreness from exercise

Whenever you start a new exercise, expect mild soreness or stiffness in the next day or two. Stretch out tight muscles and joints after workouts. If you feel sore the day after, try some gentle warm-up and cool-down exercises.

If you're so sore you can barely move a day or two later, you likely have *delayed-onset muscle soreness* (DOMS). Although DOMS is unpleasant, only time can treat it. You'll often feel better if you do light exercise, stretch, gently massage the affected muscles, and take a hot bath or get in a hot tub or sauna. Luckily your body responds by building stress proteins into the repaired muscles, making reaching that same level of soreness in the same muscles very difficult for six to eight weeks afterward, even if you overdo it again.

Dealing with muscle cramps

Painful, involuntary contractions of your muscles are called *muscle cramps.* They're most common in muscles that cross two joints, such as your calf muscle (*gastrocnemius*), quadriceps and hamstrings (the front and back of your thighs), and feet.

They can feel like a slight twitch to severe cramping that makes the muscle feel rock hard, lasting from a few seconds to several minutes. They can also ease up and then cramp again before disappearing.

They're likely related to poor flexibility, muscle fatigue, or new activities. Athletes get more cramps in the preseason when less conditioned and more fatigued. Cramps often come on near the end of intense or prolonged exercise or the night after. Exercising in the heat can cause cramps from dehydration and depletion of electrolytes lost in sweat.

To deal with them, stop your activity. Gently massage the cramp and stretch it out until it stops. To prevent cramps, increase your fitness level, avoid excessive fatigue, warm up before intense workouts, stretch regularly, and stay hydrated.

Chapter **10**

Including Cardio Training

N ot all types of cardio, or *aerobic*, training are equal, and most can be done at varying intensities. Some people like to walk or jog, while others can benefit from working out on indoor cardio training machines, such as elliptical striders, rowers, cross-trainers, and more. You may not have access to all these machines, and some you may like to do more than others.

If you have some training machines in your house already that are dusty and holding up your clothes, it's time to dust them off and put them back into service to boost your health and fitness. If you have access to a pool and want to swim or participate in other aquatic activities, now is the time to get started on those. For some, cycling outdoors is the way to go — fresh air, sunshine, and exercise to boot. There's usually no wrong way to increase your endurance and overall fitness with regular cardio training.

TIP

The bottom line is that you need to include some type of cardio training to stay fit, even if it just consists of walking daily or taking more steps.

Getting Started with Cardio Training

Though any activity that uses your large muscle groups in a rhythmic way over a period of two minutes or more is considered aerobic, feel free to pick the activities that best suit you. What works for you now may need to be shifted to another activity or a variety of training as time passes.

Considering which activities you should do

Any activity that you do continuously for two minutes or more is primarily cardio training, although some are a mixture of aerobic and more intense anaerobic activities when they involve a lot of stop-and-start movements (like tennis and basketball). Some examples of mostly aerobic activities include walking, jogging or running, cycling, rowing, swimming, arm biking, aerobic exercise classes, aerobic machines such as the elliptical trainer, recumbent or cross-trainer bike, conditioning machines, circuit training, and dancing.

REMEMBER

Doing any type of aerobic activity has the potential to get you more fit. The key is to pick activities that you can do safely to improve your endurance. Try to include a wide range of activities to increase your overall fitness. As you become more successful and confident at being active, you can add in or substitute other types of activities to expand your exercise options.

Looking at amount, intensity, and duration

To follow the latest guidelines (including those in Chapter 9), all healthy adults who are 18 to 65 years old should do at least 150 minutes of moderate cardio training or 75 minutes of vigorous exercise per week (or a combination of both). This recommendation also applies to all adults with type 1 or type 2 diabetes.

Because most people with type 2 diabetes have a low aerobic capacity, doing 150 minutes of moderate (or harder) cardio training each week is particularly beneficial. If this scenario describes you, focus on getting in enough exercise to get fit, with the added benefit of possibly burning some extra calories to help you lose weight or keep your weight down.

TIP

If you've been mostly sedentary, start with mild or moderate exercise. Then progress slowly to higher intensities or longer durations to avoid getting injured, losing your motivation to exercise, or having any possible problems with your heart or blood vessels.

Decoding the difference between moderate and vigorous

Moderate-intensity activities make you feel like you're working "somewhat hard," but you should be able to talk while exercising (but not sing). Examples of moderate exercises include brisk walking, swimming laps at a steady pace (but not pushing too hard or sprinting), and cycling on level terrain. Take advantage of any strong physical attributes you have when you pick your activities. Low-impact or non-weight-bearing types of activity, such as cycling, swimming, and aquatic or chair exercises, may be more appropriate for those with complications or coexisting conditions like peripheral or autonomic neuropathy. (Head to Chapter 16 for more on exercising with diabetes and other health conditions.)

Vigorous- or *high-intensity* activities challenge you physically and feel "hard" due to your more rapid breathing and greatly elevated heart rate. During them you may have trouble talking due to heavy breathing. Some examples are race walking, jogging or running, water jogging, bicycling uphill, gardening with a shovel, and playing competitive sports like soccer or lacrosse. For individuals without lower-body joint limitations or other limiting health conditions, jogging and running are acceptable high-intensity activities. (Flip to the later section "Jogging or Running Indoors or Outdoors" for more on these options.) In general, two minutes of moderate-intensity activity is the equivalent of one minute of vigorous-intensity activity in terms of calories burned and fitness gained.

REMEMBER

As a rule of thumb, if you're doing moderate-intensity aerobic activity, you can talk but not sing during it. If it's vigorous, you may not be able to say more than a few words without pausing for a breath.

Breaking up exercise into shorter periods

You can break up your planned aerobic activity into smaller bouts during the day — as long as it's a minimum of 10 minutes at a time — and achieve almost the same fitness gains as doing a longer workout. (However, even doing 5 minutes at a time to start is likely beneficial if that's all you can do. Doing enough 15-second walks during the day to reach your aerobic exercise goal, though, would be ludicrous.) Sometimes having the option to do 10 minutes here and another 10 minutes there and having it accumulate to meet your goal for the day keeps you from skipping your planned exercise entirely when life gets in the way of your doing a longer workout.

TIP

If it's hard for you to do a full workout at one time when you start out, you can split your sessions into two or more shorter bouts of 10 minutes (or less) each and work up to longer sessions.

Remembering to warm up and cool down

Easing your way into and out of the more demanding part of your workout is important. The best way to do that is to spend at least three to five minutes doing an activity at a lower intensity before ramping it up to your desired one. Do an easier activity for another three to five minutes when you're getting ready to stop to cool down. Remember that your body clears out any lactic acid that has built up more effectively during an active cool-down compared to just resting. After cooling down can also be a good time to do some stretching since all your joints are more nimble then and it's easier to flex your joints through their full range of motion.

Determining whether to see a doctor first

Brisk walking and other mild and moderate activities are generally safe to start on your own. But if you want to do vigorous activities and you have been sedentary, it's recommended that you see your health care provider first just to be on the safe side.

WARNING

If you haven't had your annual checkup this year, getting one prior to starting harder exercise than you're currently doing may be a good idea. At the same time, your doctor can check for any possible health issues that make being active less safe or less effective and help you manage those. The goal is to be as active as you can possibly be without getting injured or demotivated.

Walking Your Way to Better Health

Brisk walking is likely the best medicine for both the prevention and treatment of type 2 diabetes and for your overall health, and it's more sustainable as a lifelong activity than many others. Walking is a great exercise for people with type 1 diabetes as well.

Walking is the most common type of physical activity done by adults with diabetes and often the most convenient. Your self-confidence may improve after you start a walking program because you'll likely find you are better at being active than you thought, which may lead you to additional physical activities.

TIP

Trick yourself into walking more by incorporating it into other activities, such as walking farther than you need to when you shop. Walking can be the gateway to more vigorous exercise, which can further increase your overall health benefits. Getting in some additional aerobic work, especially to avoid spikes in your blood glucose after meals, never hurts.

Walking correctly to avoid injury

To lower your chances of developing an overuse injury from regular fitness walking, you need to adopt the proper form. Really, it's all about lining up your body parts, standing tall, and not taking strides that are too long.

Here are some tips to walk correctly for fitness:

>> **Try to stand up straight, keeping your shoulders pulled back.** Align your head and your neck with your spine, and tighten your abdominal muscles (or at least keep them pulled in).

>> **Walk heel-to-toe.** Use your behind foot to push off your toes, and land on the heel of your forward foot, rolling onto your toes last.

>> **To use your whole foot, try to let your ankle flex and move freely from back to front during each stride.**

>> **Don't over-stride.** If you want to walk faster, simply take more steps per minute rather than longer strides.

>> **To get the most help from your arms, bend both your elbows at about a right angle and use them to propel you forward by swinging them next to your sides.** Swing them from your shoulders, but don't overswing them.

>> **Keep your hands somewhat loose at the ends of your arms.** Clenching them feels like more work and doesn't help you walk faster.

>> **Don't lean forward or backward on hills.** People tend to lean forward going uphill and back going downhill, which can strain the back. Keep your posture erect and use your toes (push off them more going uphill) and knees (relax them more on the downhill portions) on hills.

>> **Stretch regularly, particularly your lower legs.** Also do some strength training with your legs to get them stronger.

Planning out your walking routine

Walking indoors on a treadmill is fine, but studies have shown that exercising outdoors has additional emotional benefits for everyone. So if you can walk outside, try to do it at least sometimes. (Always have an indoor backup plan for when the weather isn't conducive, though.)

Choose to do your outdoor walking either for a certain amount of time or a given distance. Having a planned route helps you mentally deal with how far you've gone and how far you have left to go to finish.

TIP

When walking outdoors, always carry a mobile phone with you in case of emergency, along with supplies to treat a blood glucose low just in case.

For your planned walks, also make sure you're wearing proper shoes and socks if you're going to walk more than ten minutes. Athletic shoes are best because they're made to help cushion your lower leg joints and your feet and make you more stable on your feet. Having the right shoes also helps prevent overuse injuries. Make sure to change to a new pair before the old ones completely wear out and lose their cushioning ability. Chapter 8 has more info on choosing your footwear and other exercise garb.

You don't have to necessarily plan for unstructured walking, especially if you take steps all day to reach your target. Just keep in mind various ways to add in extra spontaneous physical activity (which I discuss in Chapter 9), and you'll end up taking more daily steps.

Jogging or Running Indoors or Outdoors

Running isn't for everyone. If you have any lower leg issues that get aggravated by jogging or running, simply pick other activities that don't bother your joints or muscles in that way.

Jogging (which is running at a slower pace) is also not the best exercise to start with if you've been sedentary. Start with walking first and then progress to slow jogging for short periods until you can run continuously without walking or stopping. You may not be ready to progress further for weeks or months.

If you want to start jogging or already do it regularly, make sure you progress realistically with your training and don't overdo it. Nothing is worse than starting a running program and then getting sidelined by a nagging injury or blister.

Examining outdoor jogging versus indoor treadmills

Running on hard surfaces like concrete and asphalt can take a toll on your joints. Those surfaces aren't designed to absorb the impact of your stride, and the force each step causes is a little different from the last due to unlevel surfaces and other changes in the terrain. Outdoor running can also come with wind resistance that makes you work harder when running into it and less hard when it's pushing you from behind.

On the other hand, most treadmills are built with padding beneath the moving belt that softens your landing, reducing the stress on your leg joints and feet. This feature is especially good if you have knee, leg, or foot pain or are recovering from an injury.

Treadmills tend to give you a less challenging workout if you don't vary the settings — which you can do whether you choose to jog, run, or just walk. Use incline settings to simulate going up hills. Doing so helps you use up more calories and get fit faster. You can still get overuse injuries from running on the smooth surface of a treadmill belt, though.

TIP

Alternating between indoor and outdoor running gives you the potential benefits of both types of workouts.

Perfecting your technique

Perfect running form apparently varies from person to person, but everyone should avoid certain form errors. One is hitting the ground with the back of your heel first. Some experts suggest that you should learn to run in shoes like you'd run barefoot, meaning that you land more on the front part of your heel or mid-foot before rolling forward to your toes. Just thinking about how you're landing on your feet with each stride can help you develop better form.

TIP

Running barefoot isn't advised for most people with diabetes. For better form, simply try to run in athletic shoes like you'd do if you were running barefoot.

Every runner can improve his or her running or jogging technique. Try these additional suggestions to improve your stride and avoid injuries:

>> Train by varying workouts on different days: shorter distances, interval runs, tempo (near-race pace) runs, and longer-distance training runs.

>> Correct common muscle imbalances like tight hip flexors (muscles that lift the thigh up) caused by too much sitting.

>> Use flexibility and muscle-strengthening exercises to improve hip joint mobility, and stretch out your calves to limber up your ankles. (Chapters 11 and 13 offer some suggestions for resistance and flexibility activities, respectively.)

Keeping your joints and feet healthy with footwear

Regardless of which types of surfaces you're running on, you should buy running shoes that provide the right kind of cushioning and stability for your foot type at a specialty store to keep this activity from ravaging your joints. Replace your shoes every 400 to 600 miles — or sooner if they've worn down a lot in fewer miles than that. Having uneven bottoms and less cushioning in your shoes sets your joints up for more wear and tear. Once again, get some help with selecting the right shoe for your feet.

WARNING

If you have some loss of sensation in your feet due to nerve damage and still want to jog or run, wearing the right shoes and socks is critical to preventing injuries to your feet that can progress into something even more serious. (Flip to Chapter 8 for more on sock choices.) Also, check your feet daily for redness, blisters, calluses, and other signs of irritation and treat them sooner rather than later. It may be better to pick a less impactful exercise, though, for the long-term health of your feet.

Speeding through a workout plan

You can benefit from alternating easier and harder days and varying the type of training you're doing. Back in the early days, long, slow distance was all the rage, but now the running experts recommend doing faster intervals or even sprint training some days, which helps increase fitness more. (For details on working with intervals, check out the later section "Including Some Interval Training.")

TIP

To boost your running fitness or safely train for specific events, follow these training tips:

>> Before you start your workouts, always warm up with a slow jog or brisk walk to get the blood flowing in your muscles and your joints more limber.

>> For most people, training 8 to 30 miles is a good range; more than 30 miles may raise your chances for getting overuse injuries.

>> To keep from getting injured or sick from overtraining, never increase your mileage by more than 10 to 20 percent in a single week.

>> If anything hurts in your feet, shins, knees, hips, or back, take some time off from running and substitute another activity (like aquatic activities).

>> Train harder or do faster intervals one day a week to boost your fitness level or prepare for a running event.

>> Add in another day where you train slower but longer.

>> Include at least one day a week of rest — or, barring that, one day when you substitute other physical activities in place of your usual ones.

If running or jogging are activities you enjoy and you're motivated to do a 5-kilometer (5K), 10-kilometer (10K), or longer running race, make sure you train appropriately to avoid injuries. You can search online for many recommended workouts — such as the Couch to 5K ones — and follow their training suggestions. You should take at least two months of consistent training to be ready for even a 5K event. Plan ahead and leave plenty of time to train right for your event. For additional considerations for longer events, race to the next section.

Gearing up for a longer event

If you're training for a prolonged event like a half or full marathon, include some longer workouts to enhance your endurance capacity. They don't all have to be long, though. In fact, most people only do one long training run a week that's not even the full length of their upcoming event. Increasing your exercise beyond 60 minutes doesn't increase your endurance gains enough in most cases to justify risking an overuse or other joint injury from training longer most days of the week.

TIP

If you don't have time to fit in longer training, you can benefit by pushing yourself a little bit harder for less time, such as adding in some faster intervals.

Including Some Interval Training

Interval training — or doing more intense activities even occasionally or intermittently — benefits diabetes management by giving you the greatest blood glucose and weight loss benefits from your activities. Some of the potential benefits you can gain from doing interval training include the following:

>> Burns more total fat and glucose than steady-pace aerobic training

>> Improves your blood glucose management

>> Builds endurance and speed

>> Strengthens your heart muscle

>> Gets the workout over with more quickly if you're working to a preset distance or route, which may make exercise less boring and fit into your schedule better

>> Extends the calorie-burning power of muscles after workouts

To get started with any type of interval training, simply increase the intensity of your exercise for short periods of time. That may just mean picking one of the interval profiles on fitness training machines or walking faster between two mailboxes from time to time when you're out for your daily walk.

Continue to include these short, faster intervals during your walks or other activities, and lengthen them to last 2 to 5 minutes each (or even up to 30 minutes, as done in the PUP study described in the following section). You end up more fit, feel more tired when you finish (in a good way), and likely discover that your walking speed has increased due to the extra conditioning. The same intensity principle applies to almost every kind of exercise you do, from walking to cycling to gardening.

REMEMBER

Even competitive athletes generally plateau at a certain level unless they do some version of interval training from time to time.

Investigating more ways to do interval training

The options for integrating interval training into your workouts are endless, and the benefits to your health are almost limitless, assuming you respect your health limitations and don't start on this type of training before you're physically (and mentally) ready to take it on.

WARNING

You can add moderate intervals into easier activities, but high-intensity intervals aren't an appropriate starting point if you're unfit, sedentary, or obese.

The effects of interval training have been studied in some people with type 2 diabetes. In one study, active adults with type 2 diabetes who were already walking over 10,000 steps a day began *pick up the pace* (PUP) training, which involved some faster-paced walking during a normal workout. They measured their usual walking speed (in steps taken per minute using a pedometer) and then began walking for 30 minutes, three times a week, at a pace that was only 10 percent higher than normal. That means if their usual pace was 90 steps per minute, they upped it to about 100. Twelve weeks of PUP training for 90 minutes a week improved how well their insulin worked and increased their fitness level without requiring them to take any extra steps.

Another way to do intervals is just to vary the way you're doing an activity. With walking, you may alternately take longer and then shorter strides for short periods of time. This method may not be as effective in terms of aerobic fitness as doing harder training, but it may encourage you to use a wider range of motion, which can help enhance the flexibility of your joints. Adding in arm movement, such as pumping your arms in an exaggerated manner while walking, can also benefit both fitness and your upper-body flexibility.

Hitting on whether high-intensity intervals are for you

Another training fad is doing *high-intensity interval training* (HIIT) or the related form *sprint interval training* (SIT). Though popular, high-intensity interval training is an inappropriate and potentially dangerous activity to start with if you're sedentary, especially if you're overweight or obese. After you've been doing other training for a reasonable amount of time (at least three to four months), or if you're a younger, more fit person, such training may be an appropriate choice, however.

REMEMBER

Recent research has shown that HIIT can improve blood glucose control and cardiovascular health in individuals with type 2 diabetes, assuming they safely implement it and use it as an adjunct to more traditional exercise approaches. Although some researchers have shown this type of training to be safe for the exact people studied, more research is needed to determine its safety in all individuals with diabetes, particularly anyone who has more health complications. For example, although some individuals with type 2 diabetes and nerve damage have safely undertaken HIIT, these results can't be generalized to everyone with diabetes.

Note, too, that HIIT isn't necessarily as efficient as it may sound. Some studies have had people do ten 60-second intervals as near maximal as possible, with one-minute active rest periods in between. That only adds up to 10 minutes of near-maximal exercise, but it takes nearly 25 minutes to complete when you add in a warm-up, cool-down, and rest periods, so it's not much of a time-saver. Plus, people report that intense intervals lasting 60 seconds or less are more enjoyable than ones lasting longer.

REMEMBER

HIIT also has the potential to aggravate joints and result in overuse injuries, particularly if you're not used to being active.

Putting Indoor Cardio Machines to Use

At first, all you could use indoors to exercise was a treadmill or a stationary cycle. Over the years, the fitness industry has come up with many different exercise training machines to keep everyone interested and engaged in working out (not to mention all the various workouts themselves, such as Pilates and kettlebell training). Try them out if you haven't already.

You can buy machines to use at home (see the nearby sidebar "Getting a deal on home training machines"). However, if you can join a health or fitness center that has club-grade machines or use some at your neighborhood community center, those options are likely higher quality to work out on than the ones you can afford to put in your home.

Exploring elliptical machines

Elliptical trainers have some advantages over treadmills. Because your feet are in constant contact with the foot pedal of an elliptical machine, using one is less stressful on your knees, hips, and back than walking or running on a treadmill. This benefit is particularly advantageous if you've had to stop running due to joint issues; many people who can't run anymore have no problem "running" on elliptical machines. It's also a full body exercise like walking or jogging on a treadmill if you use an elliptical that has arm levers while doing your leg movements.

Even though elliptical training is kinder and gentler to your leg joints, it still allows you to do a weight-bearing exercise that promotes bone health.

Another benefit of elliptical striders is that you can easily choose an interval profile to follow for your workout, which can automatically take you through short periods of higher work, followed by easier segments. Most treadmills simply allow you to change your speed and the incline on them manually. Ellipticals also let you choose which parts of your lower body to focus on working harder by changing the incline of the foot pedals to get a workout for your calves all the way up to your glutes (butt muscles).

Surveying stair-steppers and other cross-trainers

Stair-stepping machines came on the scene before most elliptical ones (see the preceding section). Their workouts can be intense for many people, though, and aren't the best place to start out if you're sedentary. They also can irritate your knee and hip joints if walking up stairs usually bothers you.

In recent years, some hybrid cross-trainers have combined the forward movement of ellipticals with a stair-stepping motion. You can now find cross-training machines that allow you to mimic jogging, walking, running, and climbing a staircase at multiple levels of resistance and intensity. Most also have arm levers that let you get an upper and lower body workout at the same time. Many also have various profiles you can choose to add in harder intervals of some sort. All have the same benefits of reducing lower body joint stress, which is very helpful if you already have joint issues or are carrying a lot of extra body weight.

Cycling indoors as an alternative

If you have an underused stationary bike, it's time to clean it off and put it to good use. Otherwise, you may want to consider investing in a newer model or using one at a fitness facility. You can choose between traditional ones and others that have *recumbent* seats (that have a back and allow you to sit normally), which are more comfortable for many people with low-back pain or other issues. The newer stationary ones also have hill and interval profiles that you can choose to increase fitness faster.

Overall, if you're less stable biking outdoors than you used to be, using a stationary cycle can take away any concerns you may have related to falling over on your bike or crashing while riding. Indoor cycling is also recommended if you have impaired vision. It's an activity that doesn't make you bear your weight, which may work better if you have some mobility issues or have arthritis in some of your lower leg joints.

REMEMBER

You can always fit in an indoor cycling workout, regardless of the weather or time of day. Watching TV, talking with someone or on the phone, or reading while you're cycling also make the time pass quickly.

Rowing to get fitter

One of the best things about using a rowing machine is that you can do a full-body exercise that doesn't make you carry your own body weight (unlike treadmills, elliptical machines, and other cross-trainers). Cycling only works the lower body muscles. Rowing is low-impact (putting little pressure on joints) and works your legs, hips, and buttocks in the lower body and your back, shoulders, and arms in your upper body. You can adjust most rowing machines to create a harder resistance to pull against, and you can vary your workout by changing the rate at which you pull.

REMEMBER

Good form is important when you row. When you're rowing with good form, about 60 percent of your power comes from pushing back with your legs, 20 percent from keeping your abdominals tight, and 20 percent from pulling with your arms. Try to keep your back straight throughout the rowing movement. Push back with your legs first, and then pivot backward at your hips so your shoulders pass and are slightly behind your pelvis (a slight lay back). Finally, pull your arms into your chest with your hands returning about where you'd put them for a bench press or near the bottom of your rib cage. When your hands are pulled into your chest, reverse the order and repeat.

GETTING A DEAL ON HOME TRAINING MACHINES

Some of the machines sold for use at home may be inexpensive, but many are low quality as well. Is it any wonder that most of them end up shoved in the back of the garage?

Some gyms are willing to sell older club machines at a huge discount when they're getting ready to replace the ones they have with newer models. Many of these machines have a lot of wear and tear on them from being used by so many people, but most still hold up well and are worth looking at as a (reasonably) inexpensive purchase for your home use. Check the original prices on any you're considering buying used, and don't pay more than about 20 percent to 25 percent of the original price for an extensively used one.

Cross-country skiing indoors

Cross-country skiing is well-known as one of the best exercises for increasing your endurance and overall fitness. If you're looking for a full-body workout that is weight-bearing, then using a cross-country skiing machine may be for you. It fully engages both your legs and your arms during the skiing movement, and you don't have to worry about snow sticking to the bottom of your skis and slowing you down. The coordination you need between the movement of your arms and your legs can be tricky to work out at first, but soon you'll be skiing like a pro on one of these machines.

Other Activities to Get Aerobically Fit

Swimming and outdoor cycling are other popular activities and as good for getting fit as brisk walking, jogging or running, and using cardio training machines. Each activity has its own unique benefits and drawbacks, but they're worth considering as well.

Swimming your way to better health

Swimming is good for you for so many reasons, and it's a full-body exercise. If you're carrying a lot of extra weight, have mobility issues, or want to exercise off your feet for any reason, swimming or other aquatic exercise in a pool is a great choice. Most aquatic classes offer a blend of cardio, resistance, and flexibility training given how your body moves through water.

TIP

Water supports up to 90 percent of your weight, making it an appropriate activity during recovery from most injuries as well.

One of the biggest issues people have with working out in a pool is that they have to wear a bathing suit in public (unless they have their own in their backyard). The good news is that after you're in the water, most of your body is largely hidden by the water and not that visible to others either in the pool or out.

Another barrier to doing aquatic activities is finding a pool to use, especially year-round. Even if you have your own backyard pool, you may only have access to it during the warmer seasons. Look around your area to find out about pools in local fitness clubs, community centers, senior centers, nearby schools, or other recreation centers. Most such places with pools likely also offer classes if you prefer aquatic exercises to swimming on your own.

Biking outdoors

Cycling outdoors gives you most of the same benefits you can get from using a stationary cycle indoors (see the earlier section "Cycling indoors as an alternative"). If you love being outdoors and feel stable enough to stay upright when riding a bike, outdoor cycling may be an ideal activity for you to do. Prices and types of bicycles (road, mountain, and triathlon) vary widely so talk with a reputable bike dealer prior to purchasing a bike to make sure you get the right one for you.

Considering cycling clothing and gear

Do you need to wear skin-tight cycling shorts or buy special clothes to cycle outdoors? Honestly, you can ride a bike without any special clothing at all. Your regular clothes are fine when you're not going far or fast on your bike.

But if you're going to be taking longer rides or cycling outdoors during nastier weather, you'll be a lot more comfortable in cycling clothing. It's cut to fit better when you lean over your handlebars, allows for more natural movement overall, and wicks sweat away from your skin due to its synthetic materials. The padding in cycling shorts cushions you against the bike seat and lowers your risk of getting blisters or saddle sore during longer rides. Wearing cycling gloves also takes some stress off the palms of your hands.

Investing in cycling equipment

How much you want to invest in a road cycle is up to you; they come in all price ranges. For simple rides around the neighborhood for exercise, an inexpensive bike from the big-box store may work just fine. For more serious cycling or racing, you're talking about a lot bigger investment.

Cycle aside, make sure to invest in a helmet that fits your head well to protect against serious head injuries if you take a tumble on your bike at some point. Having an attachable water bottle or hydration pack is also recommended to make it easier for you to stay hydrated on longer rides (over an hour).

TIP

A big worry many cyclists have while cycling outdoors (other than avoiding getting hit by traffic or crashing your bike) is getting stuck on the road out in the middle of nowhere with your bike needing repairs. Luckily, you can make most bike repairs with a few easily portable tools. Always be prepared. The most likely repair is fixing a flat tire. For that, carry a spare inner tube or two with you, tire levers, and an air pump or CO_2 cartridge. You also want a small tool kit with a selection of Allen wrenches and other essentials that you can easily stow in a jersey pocket or saddle bag. Also carry a mobile phone with you for emergencies related to your bike or your diabetes.

Mapping out your cycling route

If you're into online programs and apps, an abundant number now exist that allow you to map out your routes (before or after you take them) to calculate your exact mileage and other features. Most smartphones are GPS-enabled, and apps are also available that use that feature to track not only your mileage but also your speed.

If you live in a bike-friendly area, you may be able to pick up some local print maps that highlight area trails, bike lanes, and roads with less traffic more conducive to cycling. You can also use Google maps and click on the cycle icon to get the best routes to take when cycling.

Trying Easy Aerobic Activities

You can do a number of easy cardio moves either seated or standing, as described in the sections that follow. For people with foot or balance issues — or for anyone who is wheelchair bound — many of these can provide safe alternatives to the cardio options already covered.

Seated march

If you like to march but without standing on your feet, this exercise is for you. Figure 10-1 shows you what to do.

1. Start by sitting upright and marching your feet in place, right foot and then left foot.

2. Swing your arms back and forth with your elbows bent while you march.

3. Continue marching for about one minute.

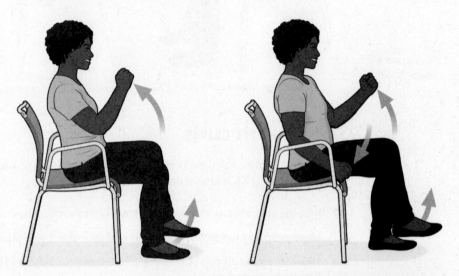

FIGURE 10-1: Seated march.

Illustration provided by the American Diabetes Association and David Priess.

Seated foot drill

This activity is marching to a faster beat, so to speak. Feel free to hold on to the sides of your chair with your hands (as shown in Figure 10-2) while you keep up this faster pace.

1. Do the seated march exercise from the preceding section, picking up the pace by tapping your feet faster.

2. Continue sitting upright.

3. Keep tapping for 45 seconds.

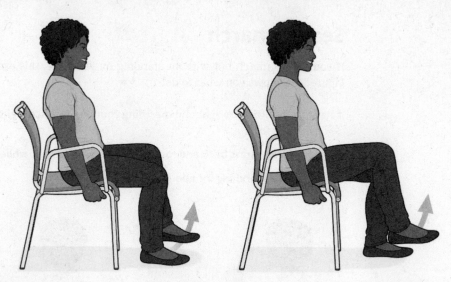

FIGURE 10-2:
Seated foot drill.

Illustration provided by the American Diabetes Association and David Priess.

Seated arm curls

This activity (Figure 10-3) rests your legs and gives your arms a workout. You'll find you can easily do this anytime and anywhere.

1. Keeping your elbows at your sides, start with your fists beside your legs.

2. Move your fists in front of your body and up toward your shoulders.

3. Make sure your elbows stay firmly planted at your sides and bring your fists back down to your legs.

4. Repeat the arm curls for 30 seconds (about 30 arm curls).

Seated overhead punches

These overhead punches will not only give your shoulders a workout, but they'll also let you vent your frustrations in a healthy way. Follow Figure 10-4 to get started.

1. Start with your fists in front of your shoulders.

2. Punch your right fist up overhead and bring it back down.

3. Punch your left fist up overhead and bring it down.

4. Alternate right-side and left-side punches for 45 seconds (about 20 times for each arm).

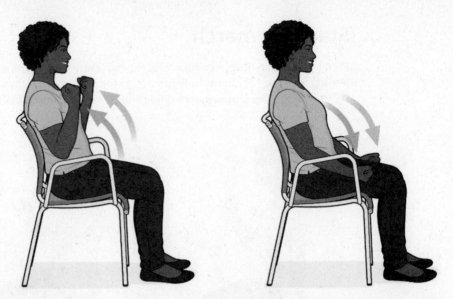

FIGURE 10-3:
Seated arm curls.

Illustration provided by the American Diabetes Association and David Priess.

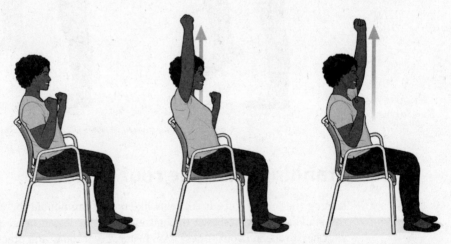

FIGURE 10-4:
Seated overhead punches.

Illustration provided by the American Diabetes Association and David Priess.

Standing march

Doing your marching standing will expend even more calories than doing it sitting. So try it (as shown in Figure 10-5) for 45 seconds either as the next step up from doing the seated march (Figure 10-1) or as an additional activity.

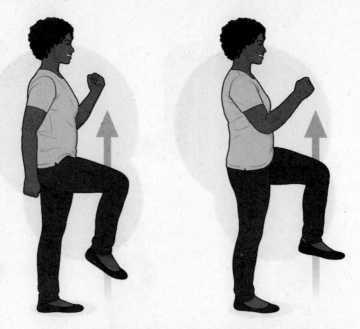

FIGURE 10-5:
Standing march.

Standing raise the roof

Raising the roof (Figure 10-6) feels like more than double the workout of doing the standing march (shown in Figure 10-5), but it can be so good for raising your heart rate and your fitness level faster. Try it today and practice it as often as you can.

1. **Marching in place, bend your elbows and push both your hands toward the ceiling.**

   Your palms should be up while you straighten your elbows.

2. **Bring your hands back to shoulder level and then push them back up toward the ceiling.**

3. **Repeat Steps 1 and 2 for about 45 seconds.**

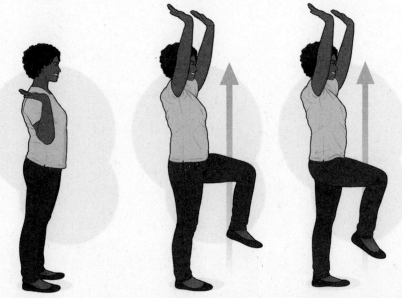

FIGURE 10-6: Standing raise the roof.

Illustration provided by the American Diabetes Association and David Priess.

IN THIS CHAPTER

» Seeing how resistance training affects your strength, insulin action, and so on

» Considering sets, reps, and equipment for your resistance training

» Approaching resistance training correctly and safely

» Building up your body core with training

» Trying some simple resistance exercises

Chapter **11**

Building Strength through Resistance

Nowadays when people say they're too busy to fit more than one type of exercise into their lives, the best advice is to go with some resistance training. The reasons are many, but most revolve around your muscle mass — keeping it and gaining more as you fight against the effects of the inevitable march of time. Having more muscle mass also allows your insulin to work better.

REMEMBER

Because women have less muscle mass and more body fat than men, resistance training is even more important for them to get more muscle and lose fat — which helps with blood glucose and burning more calories every day. Increasing your muscle mass also helps you burn more calories all day every day.

This chapter gives you multiple options on how to get started with or continue doing resistance training. You can even do it at home without any special equipment. You can do it standing, seated, or, in some cases, lying down. What more can you ask for? Use good training techniques and form, and make sure you get your core strong while you're at it for best results.

Maximizing Your Muscle Strength to Supercharge Your Health

The benefits of resistance training to your health — especially if you want to live a long, healthy, and independent life — are practically endless. Your health improves because resistance training

>> Increases your metabolism

>> Burns stored fat and glucose

>> Helps with weight loss

>> Lowers insulin resistance

>> Improves blood glucose and A1C

>> Builds muscle strength and mobility

>> Reduces the need for various medications

>> Tones your muscles (also making you look better)

>> Improves your posture

>> Raises your mood and state of mind

Due to the stress of the muscles pulling on the bone, resistance training has also been shown to build stronger bones; it's also beneficial in protecting your joints and preventing injuries by strengthening the muscles around them.

REMEMBER

If you have any physical limitations, working on your strength helps prevent loss of muscle mass and bone strength. Keeping your physical function is important as you age, and doing any type of resistance work makes doing everyday activities and practicing daily self-care easier.

Strength gains are also the key to preventing injuries, particularly from falling. You're more likely to fall the older you get, but as I explain later in the chapter, doing resistance training may be able to keep you on your feet.

Recruiting all your fibers to keep your muscle

Muscle fibers run the spectrum from being very aerobic (slow-twitch fibers) to being mainly recruited for heavy lifting or near-maximal exercise (fast-twitch fibers), and all types of fibers can exist within a single muscle. For easy work, you use only the very aerobic fibers in the muscles you're using. But if you increase your workload, you recruit not just the slow fibers but also some of the intermediate-speed ones.

REMEMBER

A maximal weight lift brings your slower muscle fibers into play, along with the very fastest ones that created the most power in the shortest time. Why is it so important to recruit all your muscle fibers? Like so many biological systems in your body, if you don't use these fibers, you lose them over time.

REMEMBER

Anyone past the age of 25 is slowly losing muscle mass, which in turn reduces glycogen storage capacity and lowers insulin action.

To keep your insulin working well and your diabetes better managed, you need to retain as much of your muscle mass as possible — and potentially gain more muscle. You can lose body fat at the same time even though you're eating more and improve how well your insulin works. You can have major gains in your strength even if you train just one day a week, although training two to three nonconsecutive days a week generally works better.

Note: Although training keeps you from losing muscle, expect any noticeable gains in the amount of muscle you have to take more than six weeks. You can tell when it happens — you get more definition in your muscles when you're working out regularly. It may take doing heavier lifting to get the full effects on muscle mass gains and insulin action (see the later section "Enhancing your insulin action and health").

Training when you're on a diet

If you're on a diet, you really, really need to resistance train. Going on a diet without exercising can cause you to lose muscle, not just fat weight. Being inactive makes the problem worse. Think of muscle atrophy as leading to a smaller gas tank to store carbohydrates that fuel active muscles; not only are you losing more muscle faster by not using it, but your smaller gas tank also remains full without doing training.

Having muscles that are packed full of glycogen makes you more resistant to insulin, whether it's naturally released, pumped, or injected. Carbohydrates that can't be stored in muscle or the liver raise your blood glucose and get stored as fat.

Normally when you exercise, your liver releases enough glucose to keep your blood levels optimal. The glucose travels through the bloodstream and enters the muscle cells without insulin. Having more muscle also means you burn more calories doing anything (which only adds to any calorie cutting that you may be doing with your diet).

Enhancing your insulin action and health

Keeping the muscles you have as you age or gaining more muscle can help you manage your blood glucose, as well as your overall health, more effectively. For example, among older Hispanic adults with diabetes, resistance exercise improved their muscle quality, whole-body insulin action, and blood glucose management while lowering the low-level inflammation around the body often associated with heart disease.

If you're a woman 65 years of age or older with type 2 diabetes, combining aerobic and resistance training may give you even greater improvements in your insulin action. Doing both types of training results in more gains in your muscle mass and bigger loss of abdominal fat than aerobic training alone.

TECHNICAL STUFF

In people with type 2 diabetes, four to six weeks of moderate intensity (40 to 50 percent of maximal) resistance training improved their insulin sensitivity by 48 percent without causing any significant changes in their body fat or muscle mass. Similarly, newly diagnosed type 2 diabetic men who did 16 weeks of progressive resistance training (the resistance lifted was increased over time) just twice a week gained muscle mass, lost body fat (particularly in the abdominal region), and greatly enhanced their insulin action — all despite a 15 percent increase in the number of calories they consumed.

Resistance training can bestow extra health benefits, such as a higher metabolism, greater self-esteem, feelings of accomplishment, and greater strength in as little as one to two weeks (from neural changes that occur before increases in muscle size). This type of training involves repetitive muscle contractions that increase the transport of glucose into your cells, leading to better sensitivity to insulin and blood glucose. These changes are good news because they have the potential to lower the total amount of medication you need.

WARNING

You may need to ask your health care provider about adjusting your medication doses as you begin your training. (Check out Chapter 3 for information on adapting medication usage for exercise.)

DOES RESISTANCE TRAINING BULK WOMEN UP?

Getting "bulked up" from resistance training is unlikely if you're female because women are lacking the high levels of testosterone men have that promote big gains in muscle. But doing resistance training can improve how your muscles look, making you appear more toned and fit rather than flabby and out of shape. As a woman, your muscles simply become toned, your waist and hips get slimmer, and you lose inches instead of turning into the Incredible Hulk.

Getting the Most Out of Your Resistance Training

The goal of resistance training is increased muscular fitness, both in terms of muscular strength and endurance. *Muscle strength* is the muscle's ability to exert force, while *muscle endurance* is the muscle's ability to continue to perform without fatigue.

Resistance training is recommended for diabetes, with age and experience as prime considerations in program development. Regardless of what you choose to do, remember that engaging in any type of resistance training is always better than doing none.

Warming up

You don't necessarily have to do resistance exercises with aerobic activity, but warming up your muscles before starting any resistance exercises is still important. The best way to warm up if you're not also doing an aerobic workout is to go through the same motions that you'll be using for your workout, but without any resistance. Stretching some after you warm up or after you finish working out also works as your muscles and joints are more pliable then.

TIP

Take the time to stretch any muscles that feel tight during workouts; that helps increase both your flexibility and your strength.

REMEMBER

If you have mobility issues, feel unstable on your feet, or have to stay in a wheelchair, you can still do resistance training. Usually, you can also do many of the exercises that are done standing while you're seated. Check out some of the seated activities in the later section "Working Out with Easy Resistance Exercises at Home or Work" to get started.

Mixing it up with resistance bands, hand weights, weight machines, and more

You have many different options for your type of resistance and exercises. Choose among using resistance bands, free weights (dumbbells, barbells, or household items), resistance machines, or your own body weight as resistance (for example, doing planks or lunges). The main difference among the options you choose is the intensity of your training. You don't even have to join a gym to make this type of training happen.

TIP

For each workout, try to do at least eight to ten different resistance exercises (at least six to start) that work your full body musculature (upper body, lower body, and core).

The following sections delve into the options you have to choose from when it comes to doing your training. You may choose one over another due to convenience, or you may simply pick one because you find it easier to start with. Whatever your reason, you can't go wrong with doing some type of resistance training.

Trying out resistance bands

The benefit of using resistance bands is that they're inexpensive, easy to use, and very easy to travel with. Some bands are like wide strips of a flexible, rubbery substance that you can grip with your hands or tie. Other bands look more like thin rubber tubing and may come with attached handles, and some are like big rubber bands or figure eights.

You can purchase resistance training bands, such as Dyna-Bands or other rubber tubing, from almost any sporting goods store, certain superstores, chain drugstores, and from multiple online sites. You can also use resistance bands sold for Pilates and other workouts to do your resistance exercises.

For many varieties of bands, you can progress your training by using ones of varying resistance (usually colored coded so that you can tell which ones offer easy, medium, or hard resistance). If you tie the band during certain exercises, use a simple bow or a square knot.

TIP

You can make any type of resistance bands work for you, so pick whichever ones you feel most comfortable with.

Getting a handle on hand weights

If you prefer to use more traditional dumbbells to hold in your hands during exercises, pick up an inexpensive set of small ones. If you're just starting out, get a set that ranges from 1 to 10 pounds, or possibly a smaller range, like 1-pound, 3-pound, and 5-pound weights.

If you're strong enough that small weights are extremely easy, you may want to either invest in a costlier set of heavier weights or consider joining the nearest gym or workout facility to have access to heavier loads and resistance machines (see the following section).

REMEMBER

If you'd rather not invest in any weights, you can get creative using household items of varying weights that you can easily grasp in your hands. See more ideas of items to use in the later section "Working out with household items."

Looking at resistance machines

The main difference between using free weights and machines is that machines isolate and target one main muscle or muscle group at a time, while free weights also make you use your core muscles (to stand or sit upright).

The choice of whether to use free weights or resistance machines to work the same muscle groups is a personal one, but using a combination of both is one way to add variety to your workouts. Whether you do a machine that isolates your biceps muscle, for example, or use dumbbells or bars to curl up instead, your biceps muscle itself gets a similar workout.

Some people find it easier to use one or the other. Most advanced resistance workouts end up having you use some type of free weight training and not just machine exercises.

TIP

By using both hand weights and machines, you can get even more strength gains or variety in your workouts. By working your biceps with free weights one workout and a machine the other, or doing one set with free weights and a second set with machines during the same workout, you can vary your use of your core muscles. Do multiple sets on a muscle by including different exercises that work the same one (such as doing your first set with a machine, your second set with dumbbells) if you find that more enjoyable.

Working out with household items

Try using full water bottles and soup cans held in your hands if you don't have hand weights. Lifting a 5- or 10-pound bag of flour can be added resistance. Look around your house for other potential items you can use while doing your resistance work. Just watch your back and lift correctly if you start lifting your kids or grandkids.

Using your own body weight as resistance

If nothing else, start doing strength training exercises using your own body weight as resistance. It's become a fad in recent years, so you want to consider joining in on exercises like planks, side planks, lunges, wall push-ups, chair push-ups, bridging, and many more.

TIP

If you find that your own weight is more than you can lift when you start doing some of these exercises, find ways to modify them to make your resistance less. You can do wall push-ups rather than regular ones, or do push-ups from your knees rather than from your toes.

Getting in plenty of reps and sets often enough

Adults should ideally do resistance exercises that maintain or increase muscular strength and endurance at least two (preferably three) nonconsecutive days each week. Working the same muscle groups on a daily basis doesn't allow adequate time for recovery and muscle repair between workouts, but if you want to resistance train more than three days per week, you can alternate muscle groups when you train on consecutive days.

REMEMBER

No specific amount of time is recommended for muscle strengthening, but you want to get in enough reps and sets to tax yourself. Strength comes from pushing your muscles to work hard.

You can gain or maintain strength by doing anywhere from 3 to 15 *repetitions (reps)* per set on each exercise. Also aim for one to three *sets*, with at least two minutes of rest between multiple sets.

Generally, doing 8 to 12 reps and two to three sets is recommended, although you can gain strength from just doing a single set particularly if the set is a challenge for you and difficult to finish. You should feel the specific muscle or muscles working hard during the last 3 to 4 reps in each set. Try to do each exercise to the point where you'd have trouble doing even one more rep without help, at least on the final set.

TIP

If you complete the set without feeling somewhat fatigued, choose a heavier resistance or weight. If you can't complete your goal number of repetitions, try using a lighter amount.

The actual resistance you should be using is usually determined by your *1-repetition maximum* (1-RM), or the most weight you can lift just one time. This number is particularly important to know if you're using free weights or resistance machines, but it's less critical if you're using various resistance bands or your own body weight as resistance.

To be truly effective, your training should be either moderate (50 percent 1-RM) or vigorous (75 to 80 percent 1-RM) for optimal gains in strength and insulin action. But doing lighter work still brings you some gains and may be the place to start if you're really out of shape or haven't resistance trained for a long time.

Knowing how much, how often, and how to do resistance training correctly

Here are a few tips as you start resistance training:

>> Do two to three sets of 10 to 15 reps per exercise.

>> Start with a goal of one to two workouts per week of six to eight exercises. Eventually work up slowly to three days per week and 10 to 12 exercises.

>> Don't resistance train the same muscle groups more often than every other day.

>> Gradually increase resistance or weight over time.

>> Do exercises with slow, controlled movements.

>> Extend and use the full range of motion around each joint you're working.

>> Breathe out throughout the exercise, preferably during exertion, and always avoid holding your breath.

>> Stop exercise if you experience dizziness, unusual shortness of breath, chest discomfort, palpitations, or joint pain.

Getting stronger and stronger over time

If you're just starting out or returning to resistance work after an extended period without doing any, start out on the lower end of the intensity scale to help prevent injuries as you begin to work out more regularly. Your frequency, number of exercises, and repetitions should slowly increase until you're up to doing 10 to 12 exercises on three nonconsecutive days per week.

REMEMBER

If you're already doing quite a bit of resistance work, using heavier weights or resistance machines helps take you to the next level of strength and muscle mass gains.

Varying your routine

If you vary your routine it will make your exercise more fun over time and work a variety of muscles, making it a better choice. Making progress in terms of your resistance, either by using heavier weights or by increasing the number of repetitions and sets, is also important.

Mix it up with some easy days, where you do more reps with lighter weights, and some hard days, when you lift heavier weights fewer times. When you do each depends on how motivated you feel on a given day and how much time you have to train.

Increasing reps and sets

If you stop overloading your muscles, your strength gains will plateau or start reversing. When you can do more than the number of reps you're aiming for (that is, if you can do 13 or more reps on your hardest set when your goal is 8 to 12), you're ready to increase the weight or resistance.

REMEMBER

If you do it correctly, resistance training never feels any easier, but you know you're getting stronger because you can lift more weight and do many things in your daily life more easily.

LIFTING AS MUCH AS YOU CAN HANDLE

If you want to get the best benefit for your diabetes management you can from resistance training, some studies suggest that you need to bring on the heavy weights. Lifting moderately to vigorously is critical if you want to bring all your muscles fibers into action.

The best way to keep the muscle you have and to gain more is to recruit not only your slower muscle fibers but also as many of the faster ones that you can as well. If you use up more glycogen when training, your insulin action stays enhanced for longer and is higher overall.

So bring on the heaviest weights (or resistance) that you can stand for the best results — both with your diabetes and your overall health. Enhancing the size of your muscle glucose tank benefits you in more ways than one.

Avoiding injuries

To avoid injury, progress slowly in intensity, frequency, and duration of training sessions. Most progressive resistance training has you increase weight or resistance first — and only after you can consistently exceed the target number of repetitions per set — followed by a greater number of sets and lastly by increased training frequency.

Eyeing where your training should be in six months

For most people, progressing over six months to training three times per week is appropriate. On those days, you do three sets of 8 to 10 repetitions at 75 to 80 percent of 1-RM on eight to ten exercises.

If you have joint limitations or other health complications, simply aim to complete one set of exercises for all your major muscle groups. Start with 10 to 15 reps and progress to 15 to 20 reps before adding extra sets.

Working Out the Right Way

Getting stronger and fitter with resistance training requires you to know what to do and how to do it. Using bad form or the wrong technique can get you injured. Picking the right plan to follow is also important.

Using the right technique

Perform each exercise using slow, controlled motions and a full range of motion. That means you should move your joints gently and slowly through the entire range of whatever motion you're doing, but don't push past the point of comfort. As you increase your flexibility, your range of motion increases.

WARNING

Jerky movements can put too much stress on the joint and cause injuries. You should be in control of your motion throughout every resistance exercise you do.

If you move too quickly, momentum takes over, and you lose some of the benefits of working against gravity. Good posture helps ensure that your joints and muscles are in correct alignment and that you're getting maximum benefit from the exercises.

When you're resistance training, be sure to breathe out during the exertion part of each exercise. If you can't perform the exercise without holding your breath, it's too hard, and you need to use less resistance. Holding your breath increases your blood pressure.

REMEMBER

If you experience pain in your joints, stop the exercise you're doing and try an alternate one. You can work each muscle multiple ways, so finding another exercise that doesn't cause discomfort, joint irritation, or injury is always possible.

Pulling your weight with the right plan

If you want to get the most out of your training, follow a plan like the one in Table 11-1. It needs to progress appropriately so you get as much benefit from it as you can.

TABLE 11-1

Progressive Resistance Training for Diabetes

Week	Training Day 1 (%1-RM)	Training Day 2 (%1-RM)
1	Baseline 1-RM testing	50%, 1 set, 10–15 reps
2	50%, 1–2 sets, 10–15 reps	50%, 1–2 sets, 10–15 reps
3	50%, 1–2 sets, 10–15 reps	50%, 1–2 sets, 10–15 reps
4	50%, 1–2 sets, 10–15 reps	50%, 1–2 sets, 10–15 reps
5	60%, 1–2 sets, 8–10 reps	60%, 1–2 sets, 8–10 reps
6	60%, 1–2 sets, 8–10 reps	60%, 1–2 sets, 8–10 reps
7	60%, 1–2 sets, 8–10 reps	60%, 1–2 sets, 8–10 reps
8	60%, 1–2 sets, 8–10 reps	60%, 1–2 sets, 8–10 reps
9	70%, 1–2 sets, 8–10 reps	70%, 1–2 sets, 8–10 reps
10	70%, 1–2 sets, 8–10 reps	70%, 1–2 sets, 8–10 reps
11	70%, 1–2 sets, 8–10 reps	70%, 1–2 sets, 8–10 reps
12	70–80%, 1–2 sets, 8–10 reps	70–80%, 1–2 sets, 8–10 reps
13	70–80%, 1–2 sets, 8–10 reps	70–80%, 1–2 sets, 8–10 reps
14	70–80%, 1–2 sets, 8–10 reps	70–80%, 1–2 sets, 8–10 reps
15	70–80%, 1–2 sets, 8–10 reps	70–80%, 1–2 sets, 8–10 reps
16	70–80%, 2–3 sets, 8–10 reps	70–80%, 2–3 sets, 8–10 reps

TIP

Going forward, you can progress your training by introducing different resistance exercises, doing additional sets per exercise, or adding in a third training day.

Choosing the right exercises

Select strengthening exercises that involve the major muscle groups in your upper body, lower body, and core. These groups include your back, legs, hips, chest, shoulders, arms, and abdomen. If you work the muscles on one side of a joint, make sure to work the ones on the other side as well (like biceps and triceps muscles in the upper arm or the quadriceps and hamstring muscles in your thighs).

Some sample resistance training exercises include

>> Seated row

>> Bench press

>> Leg press

>> Triceps extension

>> Seated biceps curl

>> Leg curls

>> Leg extension

>> Shoulder press

>> Abdominal crunches

For ideas on other exercises to include in your training regimen, see the following section and Chapter 21.

Incorporating More Core Training

Core stability training is a series of exercises aimed at developing strength in abdominal and low back areas, or the body *core*. Your core strength allows you to stabilize yourself during all types of movement and prevent falls and other injury during motion.

Knowing what core training can do for you

Core strength and stability training are components of physical health that often get overlooked with aging and weight gain. Having a strong body core is the key to being able to get around when you're older and take care of yourself. Maintaining a strong core also improves your ability to do walking and other everyday activities.

Core training can greatly benefit your health while making you more fit by

>> Strengthening and stabilizing your trunk

>> Supporting your spine and boosting your posture

>> Preventing or reducing low back pain

>> Giving you a strong base of support for all movements

>> Lowering your risk of getting injured during exercise and other activities

>> Helping you coordinate full body exercises and movements

>> Improving your balance and coordination

>> Tightening and shaping your core muscles around your waist and hips

Strengthening your core lowers your risk of falling, even if you have nerve damage in your feet that makes you less stable. When you've experienced even one fall that injures you, you may become less active to avoid falling again, even though being inactive increases your risk of falling. Start training now to stay active later.

TIP

Start working to preserve your core strength before you ever lose it so you can keep doing everything that you want to do in life.

Discovering which core exercises to do

Many core exercises use only your own body weight as resistance, with no special equipment needed. By figuring out which exercises you can easily do on your own, you equip yourself to stay strong and agile enough to live independently throughout your lifetime.

Although many core exercises are possible to do depending on how fit you are, some examples targeting the hips, lower back, and abdominal muscles are

>> Planks

>> Knee planks

>> Side planks

>> Knee side planks

>> Crunches/crunches with a twist

>> Twists with medicine ball

>> Bridging/bridging with a single leg raise

>> Leg lifts

>> Core ball transfers

>> Knee fold tucks

Staying Safe by Taking Precautions

You may need to follow some precautions when doing resistance training with diabetes or prediabetes. You want to gain benefits from being more active, not get injured or demotivated. You can stay safe, but you may need to be more careful than someone who doesn't have diabetes to contend with during training.

TIP

To keep yourself in good health when you do resistance exercises:

>> Consult with a physician prior to exercising if you have any of these conditions:

- Proliferative retinopathy or prior retinal hemorrhage that has not fully cleared out (see Chapter 16)

- Neuropathy (nerve damage), either peripheral or autonomic (central)

- Foot injuries (including ulcers)

- High blood pressure (especially if not well controlled)

- Serious illness or infection

>> Have a blood glucose meter handy to check your blood glucose before, during, and/or after exercise or anytime low symptoms occur.

>> Immediately treat hypoglycemia with glucose tablets, regular soft drinks, or other rapidly-absorbed carbohydrates.

>> Stay properly hydrated with frequent intake of small amounts of cool water during activities, especially during hotter conditions. Chapter 7 has more on hydration.

» If you have high blood pressure or unstable proliferative retinopathy, prevent excessive increases in blood pressure by avoiding heavy resistance, head-down, and jumping or jarring exercises.

» Never exercise with active retinal bleeds (visible bleeding that is ongoing into the middle of the eye), and stop exercise if visual changes occur.

» Wear proper footwear (to minimize trauma) and socks (preferably not pure cotton ones) that keep the feet dry.

» Check your feet daily for signs of trauma, such as blisters, redness, or signs of irritation, and get problem areas treated early on.

» Place a mirror on the floor and hold your foot over it if you can't see the bottom of your feet by yourself.

» Seek immediate medical attention for chest pain or any pain that radiates down the arm, jaw, or neck that may be a sign of a heart attack.

Working Out with Easy Resistance Exercises at Home or Work

You can do quite a few exercises using your own body weight as your resistance, which is the trendy way to train anyway. Try some or all of these exercises at home or at work to get stronger.

Sit-to-stand exercise

Do the exercise shown in Figure 11-1 to build strength in your legs and torso. (This is also great practice to ensure you can get off the toilet on your own as you age.)

1. Sit toward the front of a chair so your back is not touching anything.

2. Fold your arms across your chest, keeping your back and shoulders straight.

3. Lean forward slightly and use only your legs to stand up slowly.

4. Sit back down, finishing with your back straight again.

5. Repeat Steps 3 and 4 about 15 to 20 times at your own pace.

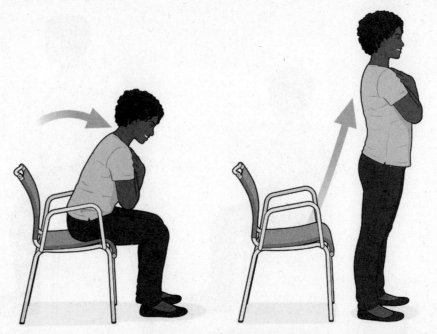

Chair push-ups

You can build more strength in your arms and upper body practicing the move shown in Figure 11-2. This is an easy move to do while you're at work without anyone noticing.

1. Sit in a chair and grasp the arms of the chair.

If you don't have a chair with arms, hold onto the sides of the chair.

2. Slowly push your body as far as you can up off the chair.

3. Hold your weight and then slowly lower yourself back down.

4. Repeat Steps 2 and 3 15 to 20 times.

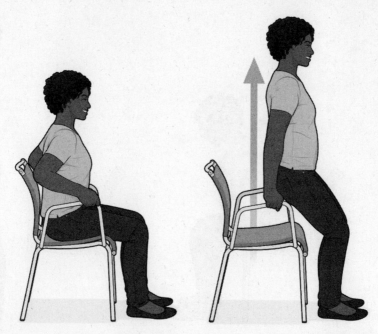

FIGURE 11-2:
Chair push-ups.

Illustration provided by the American Diabetes Association and David Priess.

Chair sit-ups

While easier to do than sit-ups while on your back, the chair version of sit-ups shown in Figure 11-3 can still increase the strength in your torso. Try this at work or at home.

1. Sit up straight in a chair with your feet on the floor and hands to sides for support.

2. Bend forward, keeping your lower back as straight as possible and moving your chest down toward your legs.

3. Slowly straighten up, using your lower back muscles to raise your torso.

4. Repeat Steps 2 and 3 20 times.

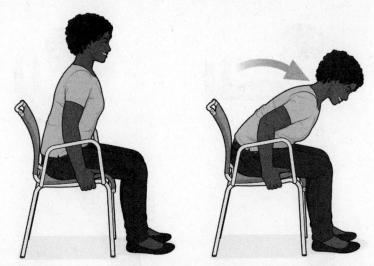

FIGURE 11-3:
Chair sit-ups.

Illustration provided by the American Diabetes Association and David Priess.

Wall push-ups

Push-ups against a wall (as shown in Figure 11-4) are easier to do than normal push-ups, but this is a great place to start if you haven't been doing any at all. If you are unable to stand, skip this exercise.

1. **Stand about 2 feet from the wall and place your hands on the wall about shoulder-width apart.**

2. **Keep your body in a straight line and start to bend your elbows, bringing your head toward the wall.**

3. **Straighten your arms and push your body back from the wall.**

4. **Repeat Steps 2 and 3 about 20 times.**

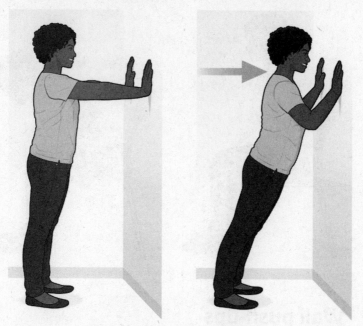

FIGURE 11-4:
Wall push-ups.

Illustration provided by the American Diabetes Association and David Priess.

Standing leg curls

This exercise (shown in Figure 11-5) helps build up strength in the back of your thighs. Stand up and do this at different times during the day to take an exercise break from sitting.

1. **Place your hands on the back of your chair or on the wall, more than shoulder-width apart, and then bend your right knee.**

2. **Keeping your knees close together, smoothly lift your right heel up toward your bottom.**

3. **Hold your heel as close to your bottom as you can lift it for a few seconds before returning your foot slowly to the floor.**

4. **Repeat Steps 2 and 3 15 times with your right leg, and then switch to the left and repeat from Step 1.**

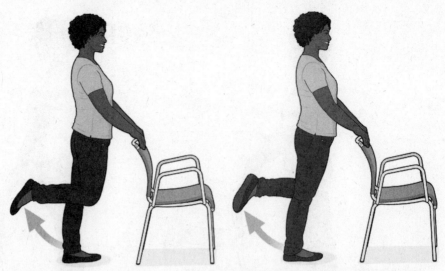

FIGURE 11-5:
Standing
leg curls.

Illustration provided by the American Diabetes Association and David Priess.

Standing calf raises

Increasing the strength in your calves doing the exercise shown in Figure 11-6 will help you walk up any stairs with more power. It also doubles as a way to improve your balance ability (see Chapter 12). For a more challenging exercise, stand with your toes on the edge of a step when you do these. Holding a weighted object, like a dumbbell or full water bottle, in one or both hands can also increase your workout.

1. Stand behind a chair with your feet about shoulder-width apart.

2. Keep your fingertips on the chair as you raise your heels off the ground.

3. Slowly lower your heels back to the ground.

4. Repeat Steps 2 and 3 20 times.

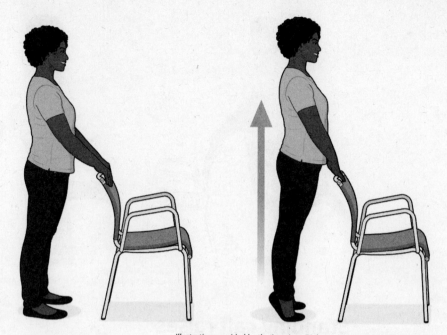

FIGURE 11-6: Standing calf raises.

Illustration provided by the American Diabetes Association and David Priess.

» Homing in on how to increase your balance

» Adding balance training into your daily life

» Practicing balance with some simple exercises

Chapter 12

Finding Your Balance

When you talk about balance in the diabetes world, it's usually related to your blood glucose. This chapter, however, is about physical balance — that is, how to stay on your feet and avoid falls.

People with diabetes have an elevated risk of falling, and falls can lead to injury or even death. Having some loss of sensation in your feet from long-term diabetes, aging, chemotherapy, or another cause increases those risks.

Staying flexible and doing exercises that improve your balance as you age is key. Even though having a strong core is important (see Chapter 11), the best way to prevent falling and its related injuries is to include balance training as part of your regular workouts. Thankfully, you can improve your balance with simple exercises, at least some of which you can fit into your busy schedule.

REMEMBER

When you have diabetes, your risk of falling is even greater, especially if you have some nerve damage to your feet. But doing strength and balance training lowers your risk and may keep you from falling.

WARNING

Make sure you always have something you can grab onto to keep from falling when doing any balance exercises. If you're very unstable, you may need to have someone stand close by in case you ever feel unsteady, especially with your eyes closed, when doing balance exercises.

Examining the Effects of Aging and Diabetes on Balance

Think your balance is terrific? If you've been working on it regularly, it may be. If not, you may have lost more of your balance than you know. Even if you started out as a gymnast or just someone steady on your feet, you may be surprised to find out how much time has taken its toll on your balance ability.

Understanding that your balance declines as you get older

Sadly, due to the normal effects of getting older, everyone's ability to balance begins to decline past the age of 40. Even as soon as you reach 30, your balance and posture start to become more important. Poor balance is associated with an increase in falls and injuries like wrist and hip fractures, even in people who are only at the midpoint of life (middle-aged).

REMEMBER

Even if you don't have balance issues yet, it's never too early to start working on your steadiness. Regardless of your age, you can regain much of your ability to balance with practice.

Recognizing that diabetes adds to loss of balance

Having diabetes increases your risk of losing your balance and falling for many reasons. Some people sustain damage to their central nervous system (brain and spinal nerves) that makes them unsteady on their feet. Even losing the feeling in your feet (through peripheral neuropathy) affects your ability to balance and walk correctly.

As I discuss in Chapter 9, having spikes in your blood glucose can change the structure of joint surfaces, making them more brittle and prone to injury and less flexible over time. Having diabetes speeds up the declining flexibility that comes with aging because no one's blood glucose is perfectly normal all the time. Being less limber makes you less able to recover your balance when you start to fall while walking or during another activity.

Checking your own balance

So how can you tell whether your balance has declined? To see where your balance currently stands, try this exercise:

1. **Stand on one leg.**
2. **Shut your eyes.**

Don't try this test without something nearby to grab onto if you need it.

If you can't stand steadily on one leg for at least 15 seconds — with or without your eyes closed — then you need to start practicing as soon as possible to improve your balance, regardless of how young you are.

To balance effectively, you need adequate strength in your ankle and hip muscles, good feedback from the nerves in your feet (to help your brain with its *kinesthetic*, or position, sense), and a functioning *cerebellum* (part of the brain that fine-tunes your movements). You rely more heavily on your eyes to compensate for negative changes in your ability to balance over time.

Start doing more exercises that maintain or improve your balance (as outlined in this chapter). Do some flexibility (Chapter 13) and resistance (Chapter 11) training, including core exercises, as well.

Improving Balance to Stay on Your Feet

Maintaining your balance is important during almost all physical activities. You can lose your balance easily enough when you're standing or walking, but most falls occur when you're moving, not just standing. Your head, trunk, and arms constitute two-thirds of your body weight, but with every step you take, that weight is carried and supported mainly by the hip muscles of your stationary leg.

Your balance during walking and other activities largely depends on how well you can balance on one leg at a time.

If your hip muscles are weak, you may tilt to the side. If you slip when you're already leaning, you're more likely to fall. Being strong and flexible is the only way you're able to counter tilting, slipping, leaning, and other imbalances without ending up on the ground.

Knowing which muscles to focus on

The most important muscles for balance are the ones that lift your legs to the side, lift your toes, and keep you moving forward — basically, the muscles that drive your hip, knee, and ankle strength. Strengthening muscles in those areas of your body and keeping them strong throughout your lifetime dramatically lowers your risk of falling at any age.

The primary muscle that lifts your legs to the side is one of the *gluteal* (buttocks) muscles, the *gluteus medius.* Your main toe lifter is the *tibialis anterior,* on the front of your shins. The *gastrocnemius* muscle on the outside back of your calves keeps you moving forward with its power and strength.

To strengthen the critical muscles in your legs that balance you, make sure to do side leg raises, toe raises, and calf raises.

Like a stork: Practicing standing on one leg

You can improve your balance with very basic exercises that are quite easy to do. Testing your balance by standing on one leg is the simplest move (refer to "Checking your own balance" earlier in this chapter). Now it's time to improve your ability to do it.

Bringing out your inner stork

Balance practice can be as simple as working at standing on one leg at a time. For best results, do this exercise two to three times a day, alternating legs.

Hold onto or brace your hand against a table, chair, wall, or another sturdy object when you first begin practicing this activity. You can find an illustrated version of this exercise in the later section "Working on Balance in Your Spare Time."

Taking it to the next level

As you become steadier on one leg, challenge yourself by using only one fingertip for support, followed by no support at all (but have something sturdy nearby to hold onto if necessary).

Using more advanced techniques as you feel able helps you boost your balance ability even further. When you're easily able to stand on one leg while holding on with both hands without getting too tired or losing your balance, try these progressive challenges:

1. Hold on with only one fingertip.

2. Don't hold on at all (see the "Single Leg Balance" exercise in Figure 12-1 later in this chapter).

3. If you're very steady, close your eyes (with or without holding on).

Supercharging Your Balance with Anytime Exercises and Activities

This section gives you lots of exercises that can help improve your balance, regardless of how young and steady you still are. You can do them almost anytime, in your home, and as often as you like with minimal or no equipment; just make sure you have something sturdy nearby to hold onto if needed.

The more of these exercises you do, the better your balance becomes. Doing even a few of them regularly improves your balance more than practicing your stork moves by themselves. (See the earlier section "Like a stork: Practicing standing on one leg" for this exercise.)

I've also included a chin-tuck exercise that helps improve your posture and remove or lessen an excessive bend in your upper back likely caused either by slumping or by getting older.

TIP

The exercises and activities in this section are critical for keeping the balance muscles in your legs strong. Practice them daily for best results.

Boost your glutes with side leg raises

Stand behind a sturdy chair with your feet slightly apart, holding on for balance. Slowly lift one leg out to the side with your toes facing forward. Lower your leg and repeat. Switch legs. *Note:* You can also do this exercise while lying on your side if you prefer.

Kick back with toe raises

Standing with your hand on the back of a chair or against a wall, straighten one leg so that your foot is off the floor in front of you and flex your ankle to point your toes up at the ceiling. Hold this position as long as you can. Relax and repeat until fully fatigued. Do these toe raises using the other leg as well.

Keep moving forward with calf raises

Stand with your toes on the edge of a step while holding something stable. Raise yourself up as high as you can and lower yourself slowly back down. Repeat ten times and then try doing it with the other leg. You can also work one calf at the same time. These are a more challenging version of the "Standing Calf Raises" resistance exercise shown in Chapter 11 because you do them with your toes on a step instead of standing on the floor (but still while holding on). *Note:* To make these raises even harder to do, hold a weighted object, like a dumbbell or full water bottle, in your free hand.

Grab a towel with your toes

Place a towel on the floor and practice grabbing it with the toes of each foot, alternately, while sitting. Repeat the exercise while standing.

Stand on a cushion

Find some cushions or pillows of varying firmness. Put them on the floor and stand on them with your legs alternately together and farther apart. Keep moving your position periodically to give your ankle muscles more practice at various odd angles.

Change the way you stand

Try various things that change how your body deals with standing still. Try standing with your eyes open or closed. Tilt your head to one side or keep it straight. Talk or keep silent. Keep your hands at your sides or move them out from your body.

Get up with sit-to-stand exercises

Practice standing up and sitting down from a stable chair that has no arms. Don't use your hands or arms for support or balance — only your legs. Lean forward slightly when attempting to stand up.

Walk heel-to-toe

Position your heel just in front of the toes of your opposite foot each time you take a step. Begin doing this exercise following along handrails or with a wall next to you, just in case you start to feel unsteady.

Travel backward

Try walking backward along a wall or a kitchen counter without looking back. Use the wall or counter to steady yourself as needed.

Practice posture by tucking your chin

You may not realize how much having poor posture is also affecting your balance, but it is. Over time, your body tends to bend forward, moving your center of balance the same direction, making your body unstable as you walk, and increasing your chances of falling. Good posture makes you feel better and is very important to preventing back and neck pain and maintaining better balance.

Here's how to practice this chin-tuck posture exercise:

1. Stand with your back to the wall with your heels 2 inches from it.

2. Hold your chin down onto your chest.

3. With your chin tucked in, try to touch the wall behind you with the back of your head.

REMEMBER

Don't despair if you can't do this posture activity right away or that well. Most people over 50 years old don't succeed in doing it. But it's still a good posture exercise to practice daily anyway.

Using Yoga or Tai Chi to Boost Flexibility, Strength, and Balance

As I note throughout the chapter, getting more flexible improves your balance and prevents falls. Yoga and tai chi both include movements that work on flexibility, strength, and balance at the same time. Working your joints and muscles with yoga, tai chi, or stretching to maintain and increase your range of motion around joints helps prevent injuries, along with keeping you on your feet.

TIP

Getting involved in tai chi or any form of martial arts training allows you to practice your balance while gaining lower body strength. Look for yoga and tai chi programs at your local Y or other health club, community center, or senior center.

TECHNICAL STUFF

If practiced in its true spirit, yoga can balance your body and mind, which enhances both your physical performance and mental well-being by counterbalancing the effects of your *sympathetic nervous system* (the fight-or-flight one). If you're mentally stressed, practicing such techniques can help you relax and calm down. Vigorous styles of yoga that are a workout in themselves aren't as good for relaxing and maximizing the effects of your *parasympathetic nervous system* activity, which works as the counterbalance to the sympathetic nervous system. Go for the kinder, gentler yoga moves for maximal relaxation.

Working on Balance in Your Spare Time

You have many options when it comes to practicing exercises to improve your balance. Some of the ones in this section are variations on ones you already discovered in earlier sections, and the rest are new ones to try.

Single leg balance

This exercise (Figure 12-1) also works on bringing out your inner stork, but it starts at the point where you're not holding on at all. If you need to hold on with one or both hands when you start out, certainly do so.

1. Stand with a chair in front of you to hold onto it for balance, if needed.

2. Bend your right knee and lift your right foot off the ground.

3. Hold that position for about 10 to 20 seconds.

4. Lower your right leg and raise your left foot for 10 to 20 seconds.

5. Repeat Steps 2 through 4 several times.

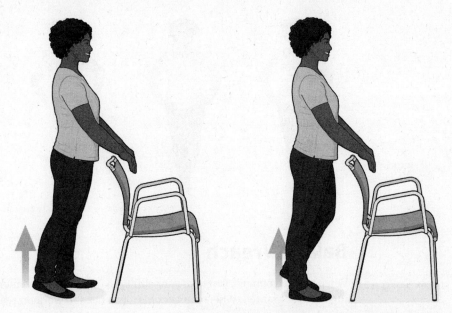

FIGURE 12-1:
Single leg
balance.

Illustration provided by the American Diabetes Association and David Priess.

Three-way leg swing

This leg swinging activity (Figure 12-2) is harder to do than you think, but it really benefits your balance if you practice it often. Start out cautiously with something nearby to steady yourself on until you get good at doing it.

1. Stand on one foot, hands on your hips (or hold onto a chair or the wall).

2. Swing your other foot forward and hold it in that position for 5 seconds before returning it to the starting position, and repeat this move ten times.

3. Next, lift that same leg out sideways ten times, holding for 5 seconds each time.

4. Finally, lift the leg backward ten times, holding for 5 seconds each time.

Stand on your other foot and follow Steps 2 through 4 to practice with both legs equally.

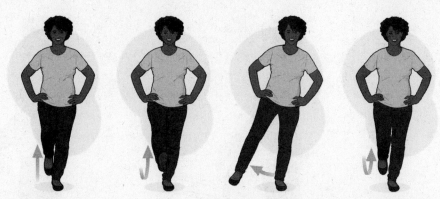

FIGURE 12-2:
Three-way leg
swing.

Illustration provided by the American Diabetes Association and David Priess.

Balance/reach

When you're younger, you take your ability to do a lot of movements without fall-ing over for granted. When you get older, you need to work on reaching for things while staying on your feet, as shown in Figure 12-3.

1. **Bend your knees and lower your body while reaching across your chest with your right arm; hold this position for 5 seconds.**

2. **Return your right arm to its starting position and then reach across with your left hand; hold this position for 5 seconds.**

3. **Repeat Steps 1 and 2 ten times.**

Forward lean

Even leaning forward can be harder to do well when your balance declines. Improve your ability by practicing this exercise (Figure 12-4).

1. **Stand on both feet with your hands on your hips.**

2. **Bend forward as if to touch your forehead to the wall.**

3. **Hold this position for 10 to 15 seconds.**

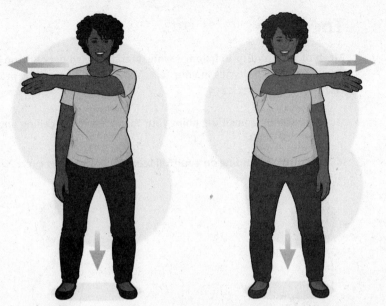

FIGURE 12-3:
Balance/reach.

Illustration provided by the American Diabetes Association and David Priess.

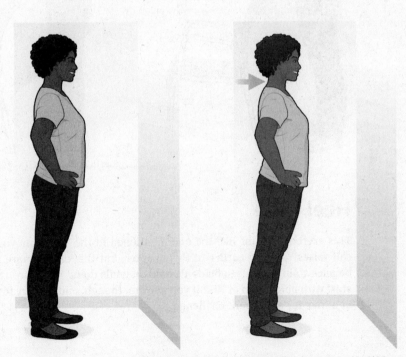

FIGURE 12-4:
Forward lean.

Illustration provided by the American Diabetes Association and David Priess.

Toe raise

Much of your ability to balance while standing also depends on the strength and flexibility of the muscles in your feet. Make them stronger by practicing the exercise shown in Figure 12-5.

1. **In a standing position, point your toes toward the ceiling and rock back on your heels.**

2. **Return to standing on your full feet, and repeat this cycle 20 times.**

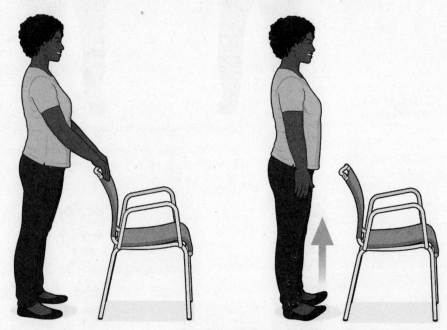

FIGURE 12-5:
Toe raise.

Illustration provided by the American Diabetes Association and David Priess.

Heel raise

This exercise is a lot like the one mentioned in the "Keep moving forward with calf raises" section earlier in this chapter, but this one is more focused just on balance ability because you don't hold on while doing it (Figure 12-6). It's fine to start with holding on at first if you need to, though, and also try it raising one heel at a time for a different challenge.

1. **Standing on both feet, rise on the balls of your feet, lifting your heels.**

2. **Repeat this movement 20 times.**

TIP

You can also try this exercise one leg at a time by raising one heel five times and then doing the same with the other heel.

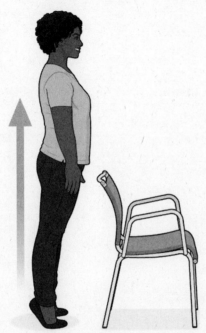

FIGURE 12-6:
Heel raise.

Illustration provided by the American Diabetes Association and David Priess.

IN THIS CHAPTER

» **Uncovering the flexibility benefits of static and dynamic stretching**

» **Getting some pointers on good stretching form and relaxation techniques**

» **Making sure you know flexibility stretches for all areas of your body**

» **Striking some yoga poses that help make you more flexible**

» **Trying out some basic stretches**

Chapter **13**

Focusing on Flexibility

O ne cornerstone physical activity that you must, must include in your fitness routine is flexibility training. It doesn't have to take a lot of your time, but including some stretches or flexibility exercises into your daily life makes a big difference in how well you age with diabetes — and how nimble you stay throughout your lifetime.

REMEMBER

The sad truth is that everyone gets less flexible with each passing year, but now is the time to fight back to combat this loss.

This chapter shows you why flexibility training improves your body's function, keeping you more limber and less likely to get injured. Basic stretches should flex all the major joints in your body regularly. Though you can do traditional (static) stretching or dynamic flexibility moves, the outcome of either type of activity is better movement. You can try some other activities like yoga, too, if you want to.

Breaking Down What Stretching Does for You

Doing stretching, yoga, or some other flexibility exercise at least several times a week is an important part of being active. Working on your flexibility keeps you doing all the activities you enjoy, along with improving your balance to keep you on your feet.

Stretching regularly can help you

>> Move and reach more fully

>> Relax stiff, sore, and tired muscles

>> Lower your risk of sports injuries

>> Prevent falls due to lack of flexibility

>> Combat the loss of flexibility from aging, inactivity, and diabetes

REMEMBER

Flexibility training is doubly important for anyone with diabetes. Everyone loses flexibility over time due to aging, but elevated blood glucose levels speed up this loss by binding to joint structures (like collagen) and making them more brittle and less flexible.

Figuring out why flexibility matters

Reduced flexibility leads to a smaller range of motion around your joints, which increases your chances of getting joint and muscle injuries. You're also more likely to develop joint-related problems often associated with diabetes, such as diabetic frozen shoulder, tendinitis, trigger finger, and carpal tunnel syndrome.

Having decreased motion around your joints increases the likelihood of getting injured, falling, and choosing to be inactive due to your fear of falling again. Regular stretching to keep full motion around each of your joints can help prevent all these problems.

REMEMBER

People with poorly managed and long-term diabetes are more prone to painful joint issues that can immobilize or limit movement.

Evaluating static versus dynamic stretching

You can choose to do either *static* (traditional) or *dynamic* (done during movement) types of stretching. Both increase your flexibility around joints.

You hold static stretches for at least 20 to 30 seconds; don't bounce to get into the position. Dynamic stretching involves slow, gentle movement to induce the stretch (but still no bouncing). For example, tai chi has many dynamic stretches in its forms, while yoga incorporates more static movements. (I discuss both of these practices and their flexibility benefits later in the chapter.)

Dynamic stretches are like static ones in that they often use the same body position, but they include some extra movement. For example, instead of holding a position to stretch your calves for 15 seconds or longer, a dynamic calf stretch includes walking on your toes forward and backward and then on your heels the same way. This stretch can progress to include a heel-to-toe walk or be done faster.

Studies have compared dynamic stretching to static stretching. Doing dynamic stretching right before running improves speed more than static stretching does. But static stretching increases how far your joints can move (their range of motion) more than dynamic movements can. Static stretching programs appear to increase flexibility in your *hamstrings* (muscles on the back of your thigh) more than dynamic movements do in most studies. Both dynamic and static stretching have their places in your flexibility routine.

REMEMBER

Static stretching is likely better for boosting your mobility, and you can use dynamic stretching to prepare for a sport and improve power. Choose what works best for you. Not every type of stretching is right for everyone.

Considering whether dynamic moves mean fewer injuries

Ever heard of someone pulling a hamstring after forgetting to stretch before playing a softball game? Maybe the lack of stretching wasn't what caused that to happen. Although stretching used to be recommended to prevent injuries during activities, its ability to lower your chances of getting injured has been a controversial topic of late. The issue may also depend on what type of stretching you do beforehand.

Doing a dynamic warm-up prior to an explosive athletic activity may reduce your risk of injury. Dynamic stretching allows your muscles to tolerate the stresses of a given sport with less strain by preparing your muscles to move in a coordinated way. Or it may reduce your risk by helping you practice moving a certain way that gets rid of awkward and inefficient movements that could get you injured. In any case, there's little or no evidence that doing static stretching before activities reduces your chances of getting injured.

TIP

Stick with dynamic stretches before an activity if you're trying to keep from pulling your hamstring or otherwise injury yourself.

Stretching Effectively

Ideally, stretching should be a part of every exercise session. When your muscles are cold, they're not very pliable and are more prone to injury. You're less likely to pull or injure a warmed muscle. The best time to stretch is likely at the end of your workout, when your muscles and joints are warm. You can also stretch after a light five-to-ten-minute warm-up or anytime during your workout if you want.

TIP

Some people benefit from doing gentle stretches after their initial warm-up and then deeper stretches at the end of the workout. See what works best for you.

Stretch the major muscle groups, including those in your calves, thighs, hips, lower back, shoulders, arms, and neck on both sides of your body. Sport-specific stretches are most beneficial, so focus on the muscles and joints that you have been or will be using during an activity. Make sure to stretch opposing muscle groups equally (like biceps and triceps in the upper arm). Activities that you should consider doing at least three days per week are dynamic or static stretching and balance training (refer to Chapter 12), as well as other activities that benefit flexibility like yoga and tai chi, which I cover later in the chapter.

To stretch safely, find the position where you can feel the stretch but not any pain. Pain indicates you need to decrease the stretch or change position to relieve it. Hold that position for at least 20 to 30 seconds to do static stretching, and repeat each stretch twice. You should never bounce when stretching; just hold your muscle in its lengthened position and relax while taking deep breaths. Remember to breathe throughout all stretching exercises. Head to the earlier section "Evaluating static versus dynamic stretching" for examples of dynamic stretching.

Reviewing Muscles and Basic Stretches

You have so many options to stretch your various muscles that you can't go wrong when picking some to do. Just make sure to warm up first and then stretch all the major muscle groups in your neck, shoulders, and upper body, along with those in your core and lower body. Do extra stretches for any areas that feel especially tight during any flexibility routine.

TIP

Some illustrated stretches are at the end of this chapter, but you can find many online on a variety of websites. Other examples appear in Table 13-1.

TABLE 13-1

Static Stretching Exercises by Body Part

Body Part	Area Stretched	Stretching Exercises
Upper body	Neck	Neck to side Neck to front and back
	Shoulder	Arm across chest Arm overhead (back scratch) Arm behind back
	Upper arm	Doorway Back scratch
	Wrists	Wrist flexion Wrist extension
Body core	Abdominals	Side trunk bend Cobra yoga pose Backbend
	Lower back	Lying knees to chest Spinal twist Cat yoga pose
Lower body	Hips	Forward lunge Sideways lunge IT band leg cross (bow) Seated butterfly Seated twist
	Quadriceps	Standing quad Lying quad Sideways lunge
	Hamstrings	Standing hamstring Modified hurdler Tip-over tuck Bridging with leg to chest
	Glutes	Forward lunge Lying knees to chest
	Calves	Standing calf Standing bent knee calf

Arms, neck, and shoulders

Your shoulder joint has three main parts to its primary muscle that you need to stretch (the front, middle, and back part of your *deltoids*). Also, get your *pectoralis* muscles (pecs) on the front and your *trapezius* on the back of your upper torso. Flex those areas by moving your arm from the shoulder joint in various directions. For your upper arm, stretch the *biceps* in the front and the *triceps* in the back. Your wrist muscles are optional, but you can stretch them by moving your wrist in all four directions. Don't forget to throw in a stretch for your neck that will limber up your upper back at the same time.

Core muscles

Use side stretches (alternately leaning and stretching to each side) to get some of your core muscles more flexible, including your abdominals (*rectus abdominus* and *obliques*). You can also use some yoga poses later in the chapter to stretch your abs (cobra pose) and back (cat pose) muscles.

FINDING THE RIGHT GEAR FOR STRETCHING

Clothing is probably the most important gear you need for flexibility activities. Look for comfortable workout clothes to stretch in. A T-shirt and a pair of shorts, yoga pants, or sweats work well; loose-fitting clothing is more comfortable, although anything that allows your free range of motion around all joints is acceptable.

Some people invest in mats that can be used for floor exercises during yoga, flexibility training, and other activities. If you don't have access to a mat, find the most comfortable surface that you can to do your stretching on (preferably not tile or wood flooring).

You may want to find or invest in some other equipment that you can use for stretching exercises. This extra gear includes a Styrofoam roller, which you can use to work out many areas of your back, upper back, neck, chest, and shoulders. You can find them online, and many gyms have them. Stretch bands and exercise balls can also help enhance your flexibility.

Legs, hips, and buttocks

Stretch out the front (*quadriceps*) and back (*hamstrings*) of your thighs using either standing or lying stretches. Stand upright and bend back at your knee to bring your foot to your buttocks to stretch the front (or do the same lying on your side). You can lie on your back and pull your knees up to your chest to stretch the backs of your thighs, along with your *gluteals* (glutes, or buttocks muscles). Also, stretch your *iliotibial band* (ITB), a band of tissue that runs along the outside of your hip, thigh, and knee, as well as other hip muscles (*flexors, extensors, adductors,* and *abductors*), by crossing your legs at the knee while standing and arch and lean to the side like a bow. Don't forget to stretch your calf muscles (*gastrocnemius* and *soleus*).

Practicing Some Yoga Poses

Yoga originated in India and stands for "union" in Sanskrit. Its practice is meant to connect the mind, body, and spirit by allowing you to hold physical poses while concentrating on being in the moment through your slowly measured breathing.

REMEMBER

Though it's a lower intensity activity, yoga can help your balance improve as well because it works on the endurance of muscles involved in your body core.

Practicing yoga helps you build strength and flexibility at the same time — and both are very important for everyone. Yoga also makes you more aware of your posture. Most of the standing poses are the foundation of more complex ones. Start with easy ones and work on using good form and aligning your body parts, all while keeping your balance.

TIP

Hold each yoga pose through two full breaths when you start, working up to four or five breaths as your strength and balance increase.

Basic and foundational poses

Start with these easy poses to build your foundation.

Mountain pose (Tadasana)

Standing: Essentially, this pose just practices standing up straight and tall:

1. **Stand as tall as possible, with your feet together and your arms straight down by your sides.**

2. **Make all parts of your feet touch the floor evenly, expand your ribs, straighten your spine, hold your head straight up, and fully extend your hands and fingers down toward the ground.**

3. **Hold this pose for five breaths while inhaling and exhaling through your nose (or your mouth, if using your nose is difficult for you).**

Easy pose (Sukhasana)

Sitting: For this pose, sit (eventually comfortably) cross-legged on the floor (use support cushions under the sides of your legs to start out if it's too uncomfortable):

1. **From a seated position, cross your shins parallel to the floor, bringing each foot beneath the opposite knee.**

   Each time you do this pose, alternate how your legs are crossed.

2. **Lengthen your spine, keeping the natural arches in the spine, and sit up straight while pulling your shoulder blades toward each other.**

3. **Place your hands on your lap or knees with palms up or down.**

Staff pose (Dandasana)

Sitting: This pose practices sitting on the floor with your legs straight out:

1. **Sit with your legs together and stretched out in front of you, your hands next to you on the floor.**

2. **Flex your feet, extending out through your heels.**

3. **Pull the tops of your thighs up toward your hips and down to the floor, using your abdominal strength to help you sit straight.**

4. **Draw your shoulders back and down along the spine, bringing the bottom of the shoulder blades toward each other.**

5. **Keep engaging your abdominal muscles to maintain this pose.**

As a variation, lift your arms straight up overhead, pointed toward the sky, and hold that position.

Cobra pose (Bhujangasana)

Lying: Done while lying on your stomach, this pose stretches out your abdominal muscles and arches your back in the opposite direction of sitting:

1. **Lie on your stomach, pointing your toes straight back, with your arms bent at the elbow and hands on the floor lined up with your shoulders.**

2. **Keep your elbows bent and close to your body while you inhale and lift up from your midback to raise your just chest up off the floor.**

3. **Lift your head and push up with your forearms to come up higher, all the way up to a point where it feels good to you.**

4. **Bring your ribs forward, draw your upper arm bones back, and lengthen your neck, allowing you to feel the bend through your entire spine.**

5. **Look up, but only if you maintain the length in the back of your neck.**

   To keep your neck safe, keep the back of your neck long at all times while you're doing this pose.

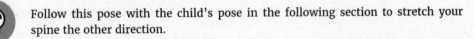

6. **Lower your body on an exhalation, rest, and repeat Steps 2 through 5.**

Follow this pose with the child's pose in the following section to stretch your spine the other direction.

Child's pose (Balasana)

On all fours: This resting pose curls your back opposite from the cobra pose in the preceding section:

1. **Kneeling on the floor, spread your knees to hip width, keeping your big toes together.**

2. **Exhale and rest your stomach between your thighs, lowering your buttocks toward your heels and lengthening your spine.**

3. **Put your arms on the floor alongside your torso, palms up, and release the fronts of your shoulders toward the floor, forehead on the floor.**

   You can also stretch your arms straight out in front of you if that feels more comfortable.

4. **Rest in this pose for 30 seconds to a few minutes, breathing deeply.**

More-advanced yoga poses

These poses are somewhat more advanced and build on the basic poses in the previous sections.

Cat pose (Majaryasana)

On all fours: This pose practices arching your back like a cat stretching and should be followed by the cow pose in the following section:

1. **Start on your hands and knees, looking down at the floor, with your fingers spread.**

2. **Exhale and round your spine toward the ceiling by pulling in your abdominal muscles and gently contracting your buttocks.**

   Try to keep your shoulders and knees in position and release your head toward the floor.

3. **Inhale and come back into the starting position.**

Cow pose (Bitilasana)

On all fours: This pose stretches your back opposite to the cat pose:

1. **Start on your hands and knees in a tabletop position.**

2. **Place your head in a neutral position, gazing toward the floor.**

3. **Inhale, open your chest, and allow your stomach to sink toward the floor.**

4. **Lift your head to look straight forward or look up (whatever is comfortable).**

5. **Hold this pose before you exhale and return to a neutral tabletop position.**

Downward-facing dog pose (Adho mukha svanasana)

On all fours: This pose forms an upside-down V out of your full body:

1. **Start on your hands and knees with your hands slightly forward of your shoulders.**

2. **Spread your fingers and imagine clawing into the ground to create a little suction cup of air in the middle of your palm.**

3. **While exhaling, lift your hips back and up to push yourself back into an upside-down V pose, keeping your knees initially bent.**

4. **If you can, straighten your legs while keeping the length in your spine.**

   Otherwise, skip to Step 5.

5. **Press your upper arms toward each other, keeping the space across the tops of your shoulders, and hold this position.**

Chair pose (Utkatasana)

Standing: This pose is done standing, making a chair out of your lap:

1. **Standing with your feet together, bend your knees 90 degrees (or as close as you can to that without pain) while keeping your back straight.**

2. **Reach your arms over your head, letting your hips move back a little toward your heels.**

3. **Hold this pose, keeping your focus straight.**

Tree pose (Vrksasana)

Standing: This pose makes you practice standing on one leg with the other foot propped against the leg you're standing on:

1. **Standing with your weight distributed equally on both feet and your hands in a prayer position in front of you, bend your right knee, bringing the sole of your right foot high onto your inner left thigh.**

   If you have trouble balancing when you first try this pose, bring your foot lower onto your left leg (just not directly on the inside of your knee).

2. **Keep both of your hips squared toward the front.**

3. **Repeat this move standing on your right foot.**

Half lord of the fishes pose (Ardha matsyendrasana)

Sitting: Starting from the staff pose earlier in the chapter, this position gently twists your spine:

1. **Sit with your legs outstretched in front of you in the staff pose.**

2. **Lift your right knee and place your right foot on the outside of your left leg at knee height.**

3. **If you can, bend your left leg and place your left foot on the outside of your right hip.**

   If that doesn't work for you, just keep your left leg extended as in Step 1.

4. **Place your right arm behind you, breathe in, and extend your left arm up to the ceiling.**

5. **Bend and hook your elbow behind the knee as you twist to the right.**

6. **With every breath in, try to lengthen your spine; on exhalation, move deeper into the twist.**

7. **On a final exhalation, come out of the twist by moving back into the staff pose, and then repeat the twist on your other side.**

FINDING YOUR WAY WITH TAI CHI

The ancient Chinese exercise form known as *tai chi* is excellent for improving balance, which isn't surprising given that it's the foundation of all martial arts forms. It also requires you to move many of your joints through a wider range, which increases your flexibility naturally. Getting involved in tai chi or any martial arts training allows you to practice your balance while gaining lower body strength and more flexibility around your joints. Lower-body resistance training also doubles as balance exercise, and this includes many of the movements involved in tai chi.

As an added benefit, tai chi participation can lower A1C levels in older adults with diabetes.

Trying a Whole-Body Approach to Relax

You can try a whole-body approach to increase your flexibility through yoga, meditation, or progressive muscle relaxation exercises. When you get stressed, a common physical reaction is to tense up the muscles in your shoulders, neck, and other areas of your body, which can limit your flexibility in those areas as well.

Exercise is an important tool to manage mental stress. Gentle, slow movement like yoga and stretching can be helpful for some people to feel more relaxed overall, while others prefer to destress with more vigorous activity such as walking, swimming, or other types of aerobic exercise. In either case, relaxing is important to your mental and physical health.

One way that exercise helps with stress is by making you take deeper breaths, which brings more oxygen to your muscles and can help them relax. This kind of deep breathing is also what happens naturally as your body shifts from being awake to sleeping. More blood flow into those areas helps your joints stay more limber as well.

Training your body and mind to destress

Each time you work out, you physically damage your muscles. But you ultimately end up stronger, faster, and better, and your body responds by releasing fewer stress hormones during workouts.

When you practice using relaxation techniques to control your stress levels, your mind learns to reduce your body's *sympathetic nervous system* (fight-or-flight) stimulation and keep your adrenaline and other hormone levels lower. The more consistently you practice relaxation, the more easily you can avoid eliciting a strong stress response the next time life happens. During recovery, your *parasympathetic nervous system* (the opposing one is the sympathetic nervous system) keeps your heart rate low and digestion high, so it's no wonder that a warm shower, a big meal, and a long nap after a workout make you feel more relaxed. You're in an *anabolic* (building and repairing) state then, and your muscle glycogen is being restored while your muscles are being repaired and strengthened.

Lower stress with deep breathing

The negative aspect of emotional stress is that it can greatly increase your release of the hormone *cortisol*, which increases insulin resistance and lowers your immunity to common colds and illnesses. Feeling stressed or catching a cold or the flu due to stress greatly impacts your insulin action and metabolic health.

Whenever you start to feel stressed, try this breathing exercise to relax:

1. **Place one hand on your chest and the other on your abdomen.**

2. **Take full, deep breaths in through your nose and out through your mouth, feeling your stomach push out and your chest rise.**

3. **Exhale slowly, feeling your stomach go in and your chest deflate.**

   Use your abdominal muscles to fully push the air out of your lungs.

4. **Take a series of these deep breaths to take time out and destress.**

Filling your lungs with air also improves the oxygenation of your blood, which is great for your body, brain, and mental state.

Checking out a positive, stress-releasing activity

If you can lie down, try this stress-releasing activity as well. If you don't have anywhere to lie down, or if you fall asleep easily, do this exercise sitting upright in a chair in a quiet place. Figure out what works best for you, and do it several times a day to see whether your stress levels start to go down:

1. **Lying down, close your eyes and take a few deep breaths.**

2. **Try to quiet your mind by erasing all thoughts of your day or problems.**

3. **Think about a pleasant place to be — on a beach, resting on the grass on a warm sunny day, or wherever you feel most at peace.**

4. Relax and visualize all the tension flowing out of your body, replacing it with calmness.

5. Feel good about yourself and create positive thoughts about the changes that are taking place in your body.

TIP

Your thoughts and beliefs about yourself affect the neural connections that allow you to change your habits, so try to keep your thoughts as positive as possible.

Using visualization to perform better

Sport psychologists recommend relaxation to enhance performance in athletic events. Relaxation techniques can help you control the stress of competition as well as the stress coming from other avenues of your life.

To relax, sit quietly and focus your mind, or even try relaxing while exercising. For example, try punching the air with your fists to release your anger or anxiety and consciously relaxing the tense muscles and joints in your body — all while you're working out.

Use your imagination to visualize more blood flowing to all the parts of your body that need it. Some studies have shown that people can enhance blood flow to their feet simply by visualizing it, verifying that a strong mind-body connection exists.

Also, take deep and steady breaths and release them slowly, particularly during your warm-up and cool-down periods when you're not working as hard. Whenever you start to feel winded during a workout, take deeper breaths to bring more oxygen into your lungs and body.

Working on Flexibility with Some Stretching Exercises

You can do many different static stretches to flex your joints. Here are a few simple ones to get you started.

Neck stretch

Your neck is one of the main places you tense up when you're stressed. Stretch it out as shown in Figure 13-1 to get more movement back.

1. Stand with your feet apart and your knees slightly bent (or sit in a chair with your back straight and your feet on the floor).

2. Relax your shoulders and bend your head toward your right shoulder.

3. Hold it there for 5 seconds and then tilt it to the left for 5 seconds.

4. Tip your head forward toward your chest.

5. Hold this position for 5 seconds and then tilt your face toward the ceiling for 5 seconds.

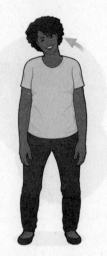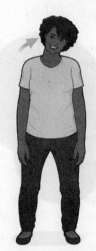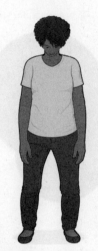

FIGURE 13-1:
Neck stretch.

Illustration provided by the American Diabetes Association and David Priess.

Shoulder/upper-back stretch

The upper shoulder is an area that most people lose flexibility in over time. Practice the stretch in Figure 13-2 to keep or get some mobility back in that area.

1. Stand with your feet a little apart.

2. Slightly bend your knees and tense your stomach muscles.

3. Relax your shoulders and pull your right arm across your chest by grabbing onto your elbow with your left hand; hold the stretch for 10 seconds.

4. Repeat Step 3 with your left arm.

You can also do this exercise while seated in a chair.

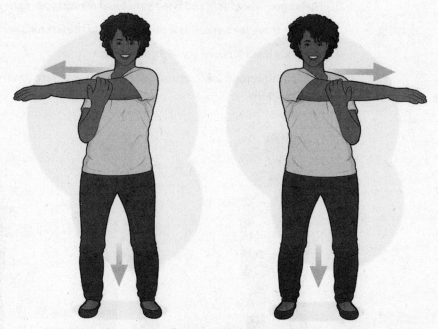

Illustration provided by the American Diabetes Association and David Priess.

FIGURE 13-2:
Shoulder/
upper-back
stretch.

Chest/shoulder stretch

You can do this stretch standing or seated. If standing, bend your knees slightly as shown in Figure 13-3; if seated, sit forward in your chair to fit your arms behind you.

1. Tense your stomach and relax your shoulders.

2. Try to clasp your hands behind your back, and then bring your shoulders back and push your chest forward.

3. Hold the stretch for about 10 seconds.

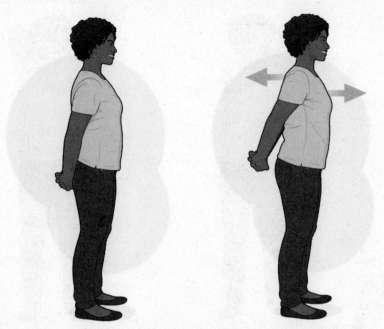

FIGURE 13-3:
Chest/shoulder
stretch.

Illustration provided by the American Diabetes Association and David Priess.

Upper-back/back of arm stretch

This stretch (shown in Figure 13-4) is another essential one to keep your shoulders flexible. It's also a good move if you like to scratch your own back.

1. Stand with your feet apart, your knees slightly bent, and your stomach tensed.

2. Relax your shoulders and bend your elbows while pulling your right arm straight up by pushing on the back of your right elbow with your left hand.

3. Hold the stretch for 10 seconds.

4. Repeat Steps 2 and 3 with your left and right arms reversed.

You can also do this exercise while seated in a chair.

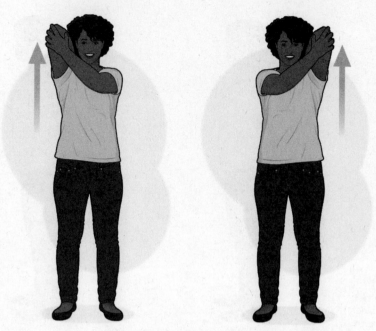

FIGURE 13-4:
Upper-back/back
of arm stretch.

Illustration provided by the American Diabetes Association and David Priess.

Back of upper-leg stretch

Most people get some tightness in the backs of their thighs that can get worse over time. Work on reversing it with the stretch shown in Figure 13-5.

1. **Stand behind a chair with your legs straight, holding the back of the chair with both hands.**

2. **Bend forward from your hips, not from your waist, keeping your back and shoulders straight.**

    Your upper body will be over the floor.

3. **Hold this position for 10 seconds, relax, and repeat Step 2.**

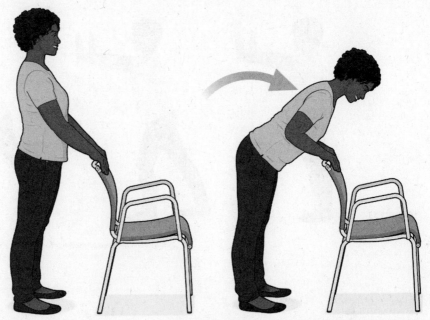

FIGURE 13-5:
Back of upper-leg stretch.

Calf stretch

Your calves are another area that can get too tight, especially if you ever wear shoes with heels. Work on getting your calves more flexible (Figure 13-6).

1. With straight arms, put your hands on the wall in front of you.

2. Place your feet shoulder-width apart.

3. Move your right foot back from the wall about 12 inches while bending your left knee.

4. Holding your back and your right knee straight, bend your elbows slightly; lean in a few inches toward the wall to stretch your right calf.

5. Hold the stretch for about 10 seconds and then repeat Steps 3 and 4 with the other leg, again holding for 10 seconds.

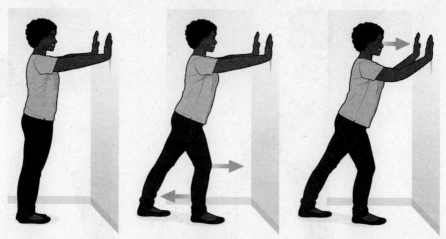

FIGURE 13-6:
Calf stretch.

Illustration provided by the American Diabetes Association and David Priess.

Chapter 14

Mixing It Up with Cross-Training

I f you're like a lot of other people, you may get bored doing the same physical activities day after day. More than 50 percent of people who start exercise training programs drop out in the first six months, so what you do to keep your workout fresh sometimes matters more for getting the most out of training and staying with it. Cross-training covers a lot of ground, including combining different types of activities (like cardio and resistance training) in one workout, doing both during the week, or including other types of training in your routine.

In this chapter, you discover the various advantages of cross-training, uncover the diabetes benefits of cross-training cardio and resistance, and examine the pros and cons of the cross-training approach called CrossFit.

Benefiting from Doing Cross-Training

You may want to do a variety of activities on a weekly basis, an approach known as *cross-training*. For example, you can walk on Monday, Wednesday, and Friday but swim on Tuesday and take dance classes on Saturday. Cross-training is good for you because it does the following:

>> Uses several different activities to help you reach your exercise goals

>> Adds variety by including activities like walking, cycling, rowing, swimming, arm bike, weight training, aerobic classes, tai chi, and yoga

>> Helps fight insulin resistance

>> Leads to lower doses of diabetes medications for many people

>> Gives you flexibility in your program (for example, substituting indoor machines for outdoor walking if it's raining outside)

>> Reduces injuries because you don't repeat the same movement all the time

>> Minimizes boredom because you're always changing up your exercises

>> Uses different muscles during various activities so more muscles get the benefit of exercise training

>> Makes your daily activities easier on your joints and body

>> Keeps your body challenged to adapt and improve in different ways

>> Allows you to rest some muscles so they can recover from workouts without stopping you from exercising altogether on other days

>> Helps you develop new exercise skills and proficiencies

The following sections explore a few of these benefits in more detail and give you some suggestions for practicing cross-training.

REMEMBER

What cross-training ensures above all else is the ability to continue being active and more motivated to move your body for the rest of your life.

Increasing blood glucose and glycogen use

In terms of managing insulin resistance (and blood glucose), this approach is also very effective. Usually, as your body becomes accustomed to doing an activity like walking or cycling, your blood sugar is less likely to drop while you are doing it. By participating in each activity less frequently, you tend to use more of your blood glucose and stored glycogen during each one — which is beneficial if you're using workouts to help raise your insulin action or lower your blood glucose.

Experiencing fewer injuries

Nothing is worse than getting sidelined from your regular training due to overuse or acute injuries caused by being active. (Refer to Chapter 9 for more on these types of injuries.) Constantly stressing your body in the same way can lead to tendinitis in joints, bursitis, tendon ruptures, muscle tears and pulls, and possibly acute injuries. Each activity you do stresses your muscles and joints differently, so doing a variety lowers your chances of getting an injury.

REMEMBER

Stick with moderation in all your exercise activities for the best results. For example, although the training approach called CrossFit can be an effective way to cross-train, it has been notorious for resulting in muscle and joint injuries for its participants because it relies on overtraining as a means of getting stronger and more fit. I discuss CrossFit in more detail later in the chapter.

Cross-training helps you deal with any activity-related injuries without losing all your conditioning while waiting for the injury to heal. If you have lower leg pain, you can still work out your upper body doing other activities and vice versa. Try to alternate weight-bearing activities like walking with non-weight-bearing ones (for example, swimming and stationary cycling) to avoid injuring another part of your body while waiting for an existing injury to get better.

REMEMBER

Always wear proper footwear, and you will be less likely to get injured. If you choose to wear worn out or poorly fitted shoes, you may make existing issues such as flat feet, high arches, wide feet, or joint problems worse. Shoes with more stability like cross-training athletic ones provide more arch support and reduce risk of injuries. Custom orthotics may also be beneficial for some people. Talk with your health care provider or a foot doctor to find out what may be the proper styles of shoes for your unique feet. In addition, many sporting goods or running specialty stores can help match you with the right athletic shoes.

Enjoying more variety

Cross-training adds variety to your exercise program when you include activities like walking, cycling, rowing, swimming, arm cycling, weight training, aerobic classes, yoga, and more. You have more flexibility to choose different options based on your time constraints, the weather, and other factors. Mixing up your activities also allows you to work a variety of muscles. Each activity recruits either different muscles altogether or the same ones in different patterns; regardless, you experience a wider use of the muscles in your whole body.

REMEMBER

Because you do each activity less frequently when you vary them, you won't experience as pronounced a training effect specific to each one.

Staving off boredom

For some people, *exercise* is a four-letter word; they'd rather excise it from their vocabularies and their lives. Even calling it "physical activity" instead isn't enough to keep them from getting bored with doing it.

However, people do find that when they engage in a variety of activities — some of them more enjoyable to them than others — they're more willing to put up with the ones they don't like just to be able to do the others on alternate days. So, in addition to making your workout routines more enjoyable, cross-training can help you fend off the boredom that's more likely to pop up when you really don't like doing activities you feel forced to do.

Taking the right approach to any type of cross-training

Engage in cross-training activities by following these tips:

>> Choose a variety of activities that you enjoy, and include them all in your exercise program instead of just having a single activity.

>> Improve your ability in a favorite activity by adding in others that use similar areas of the body. For example, if you like to walk, doing some cycling can make you stronger when you walk, so do some of both.

>> Substitute these other activities every second or third day you exercise, or do different activities with every session. For example, walk half the time and cycle or do resistance exercise the other half.

>> Substitute as many different exercise activities as you want to during a workout if you enjoy that approach more and it keeps you more engaged.

>> Keep changing your exercise activities — daily, weekly, monthly, or seasonally — to stay challenged and motivated.

Table 14-1 provides a sample plan for cross-training that includes all the activities recommended for people with diabetes (especially if you're 40 or older and need to do some balance training).

TABLE 14-1 **Example of Weekly Cross-Training Exercise Plan**

Day	Aerobic (include intervals and vary aerobic activities)	Resistance (exercises done can vary by day)	Flexibility (do when warmed up)	Balance (do any time of day)
1	15 minutes	30 to 45 minutes	5 minutes	5 minutes
2	30 to 60 minutes		5 minutes	
3	15 minutes	30 to 45 minutes	5 minutes	5 minutes
4	Daily activities		Yoga class	

Day	Aerobic (include intervals and vary aerobic activities)	Resistance (exercises done can vary by day)	Flexibility (do when warmed up)	Balance (do any time of day)
5	15 minutes	30 to 45 minutes	5 minutes	5 minutes
6	20 to 30 minutes		5 minutes	Tai chi class
7	60 minutes (long day)		5 minutes	5 minutes

Combining Cardio and Resistance Work to Combat Diabetes

The latest recommendations from the American Diabetes Association are that doing cross-training may give the greatest benefits for blood glucose and insulin sensitivity. Cardio and resistance training are likely the most common type of cross-training.

So, for example, in addition to walking, you may want to do some resistance training at least two nonconsecutive days per week (but preferably three). It can further improve your sensitivity to insulin and help you better manage your blood glucose; for older women with type 2 diabetes, the combination of aerobic and resistance training may also afford a more significant decrease in abdominal fat than aerobic training alone does, with increased muscle mass to boot. (Head to Chapter 10 for more info on cardio training and Chapter 11 for details on resistance.)

CrossFit Training with Diabetes

A concerned young man with type 1 diabetes asked whether it was safe for him to do CrossFit training, which is a strength and conditioning program consisting mainly of a mix of aerobic exercise, gymnastics (body weight exercises), and Olympic weight lifting. Its programming is decentralized, but its general methodology is used by thousands of private affiliated gyms, whose actual programs vary tremendously from site to site. The young man was already doing CrossFit training and wanted to continue, but a blog he'd read claimed that because intense training causes the liver to release excess glucose during training, people with type 1 diabetes may fare better with less-intense, lower-volume activities such as power lifting.

However, there's no reason why a young and healthy person with diabetes shouldn't be able to engage in CrossFit training without worrying excessively about the temporary rise in blood glucose levels that it may cause. To limit the rise in blood glucose, simply approach CrossFit training like any other intense workout, which can cause elevations in blood glucose even in people without diabetes. Insulin users just need to check their blood glucose frequently and adjust insulin doses and food intake to have adequate amounts in their bodies during and following workouts. (Flip to Chapters 3 and 7 for details on adapting insulin dosing and food consumption, respectively, for exercise.)

TIP

Doing some easy cardio exercise after an intense workout such as CrossFit can help lower blood glucose naturally in everyone. Also, exercisers experience a bigger blood glucose rise in the early morning compared to later in the day due to having more glucose-raising hormones and less insulin on board in the morning, pre-breakfast. If you opt for CrossFit, schedule it for the afternoon or evening to help minimize any blood glucose spike if that's a big issue for you. If you do CrossFit in the morning, you may need to take some insulin (if you use it) to cover the rise in your blood glucose.

REMEMBER

CrossFit isn't without hazards, though. Make sure you are using correct form to prevent injuries, as you should do with any sport. One concern is that CrossFit's online community enables athletes to follow the program without proper guidance, increasing the risk of improper form or technique that leads to injury. Some people have caused significant damage to the cartilage in their knees doing such training inappropriately. Undertaken correctly, CrossFit isn't inherently bad or ineffective, but beginning exercisers starting out shouldn't do too much. Besides, you can gain strength similarly from resistance exercise programs done correctly that don't cause undue muscle soreness, so getting really sore isn't necessary and can be harmful.

For example, a young woman who was a physical therapist and a regular CrossFit participant woke the morning after a particularly grueling session consisting of hundreds of reps of arm exercises and found she couldn't bend her elbows. She was shortly thereafter diagnosed in the ER with *rhabdomyolysis* (*rhabdo* for short), a condition in which damaged skeletal muscle tissue breaks down rapidly. Many other reports of rhabdo related to CrossFit have surfaced. Strenuous exercise is a known — albeit rare — cause of rhabdo, which can cause kidney failure when breakdown products (*myoglobin*) of damaged muscles end up in the blood.

WARNING

Severe symptoms like muscle pain, vomiting, and confusion are signs of significant muscle damage and possible kidney failure. Seek treatment right away if you have severe muscle pain and dark-colored urine.

4

Keeping Fit at Any Age or Any Stage

IN THIS PART . . .

Get more active, even if you're carrying some extra weight or dealing with health issues that may complicate exercise.

Uncover special considerations for active females with diabetes.

Ditch your age constraints, whether you're young or old, and get moving more.

Train your best as an athlete with diabetes.

IN THIS CHAPTER

» Understanding how your extra weight affects you

» Focusing on the right activities for your condition and joint health

» Dropping and maintaining your weight (and seeing how your medications impact it)

» Understanding the effects of certain types of weight loss

» Waking up to sleep's influence on weight loss

Chapter **15**

Training with Extra Body Weight

C arrying around a little extra body weight — like at least two-thirds of all Americans do — can change what types of activities may be best for you to get involved in. Getting started is as easy as getting up from your chair and moving more often. Keeping going means that you may need to focus on doing lower impact activities that put less stress on your lower limbs.

If you have arthritis in your hips or knees, that may also change what you choose to do. Rest assured that you can find some appropriate activities and find out more about being active in this chapter. You may even lose some weight as a result — and get tips on how to keep it off for good.

Limiting the Impact of Your Extra Weight Gain

You may have heard that gaining weight is what caused your prediabetes or type 2 diabetes. But it's just as likely or even more likely that your weight gain is just a symptom associated with insulin resistance, prediabetes, and diabetes rather than a direct cause. It's possible to become insulin sensitive without losing much or any weight. However, having excess body fat does have its downside. The following sections help you understand how that additional weight, particularly fat, can affect your health.

Aiming to be fit and thin (if possible)

As your body weight increases, so does your risk of dying from heart disease or developing type 2 diabetes. However, the more physically fit you are, the lower your risk of dying from any cause is — even if you're overweight.

REMEMBER

Although being fit and thin is still best for your health and life span, being fit and fat is healthier than being thin and unfit. In other words, you can gain extra fat and reduce your risk of developing health problems by being regularly active. Being overweight or obese and being physically unfit are stand-alone risk factors for heart disease, early death, and type 2 diabetes. So if you can't lose weight, then get fit.

Recognizing that where you store your fat matters

When you store fat just in fat cells (particularly just under the skin, as *subcutaneous fat*), you aren't likely to have as many health problems compared to when your body puts it in other places. If you store most of your fat in your hips (making you pear-shaped), you may be perfectly healthy, metabolically speaking. Being shaped more like an apple with fat around your middle, however, can be the indicator of many problems with your metabolism — and health issues in your future if you don't do what you can to prevent them with changes in your lifestyle.

Losing your belly fat if you can

Storing excess fat within your belly (as *visceral fat*) is undeniably bad for your health. Having a lot of visceral fat increases your risk for heart disease, high blood pressure, and even type 2 diabetes. The spillover of excess fat into organs like the liver or heart is what damages them. (Head to the later section "Storing less fat in your liver" for more on how fat affects the liver.) If you can put those excess calories as fat in your fat cells instead, you can actually prevent or delay these harmful effects.

Visceral fat stored deep within your abdomen is the worst type of body fat for managing blood glucose because it makes your insulin work less effectively.

Keeping the bad fat out of your muscles

Your muscles also store extra fat as you get heavier, and that can make your muscles more resistant to insulin. Because your muscles are responsible for most blood glucose use orchestrated by insulin in your blood, developing insulin-resistant muscles has a substantial negative impact on your blood glucose. And the only remedy appears to be exercising regularly.

Regular exercisers, paradoxically, can store more fat in their muscles without getting insulin resistant. Athletes have large amounts of fat stored inside their muscle fibers, and they're extremely insulin sensitive for the most part. That alone tells you that the total amount of fat stored there isn't as critical as whether you're staying active, although exercising may impact the types of fat packed away in muscles and how they're stored there.

Storing less fat in your liver

Storing extra fat in your liver may contribute to low-level inflammation throughout your body, and that inflammation is what is believed to lead to insulin resistance, type 2 diabetes, heart disease, and other metabolic health problems. So your liver (and whether it has excess fat in it) may prove to be a crucial link between weight gain and prediabetes or type 2 diabetes.

When packed with fat, your liver gets resistant to insulin, and that can lead your liver to release too much glucose into your blood overnight (among other bad effects). Having an insulin-resistant liver may cause elevated blood fats and cholesterol levels that contribute to the development of heart disease. You can compound the problem with dietary choices that contribute to your liver's insulin resistance, including foods that are highly processed, contain excess calories, or are consumed in large portions.

You have the power to lower your body's inflammation and improve your metabolic health, both of which are tied to the health of your liver. Being active and eating more fiber naturally through foods are the most important changes you can make to lower inflammation and prevent metabolic diseases by getting rid of at least some of the fat that may be stored in your liver.

Keeping Active to Manage Your Weight

Many people decide to be physically active to help them lose weight and improve their body shape. Regular physical activity makes a huge difference in whether you gain weight, keep the same weight, or lose more. The lifestyle behaviors that help you keep your weight down (like regular exercise) are likely to improve your diabetes management as an added benefit.

Preventing type 2 diabetes with activity

Regardless of how much weight you lose or don't lose by being active, being regularly active can prevent you from developing type 2 diabetes in the first place or reverse prediabetes. Losing weight can also help manage diabetes in people, regardless of what type they have.

The Diabetes Prevention Program (a lifestyle management program designed to prevent type 2 diabetes) study found that weight loss is most directly associated with lower risk of getting type 2. But in the study, participants' weight loss was predicted by how much exercise they did daily, and only the ones who continued to exercise around 60 minutes a day — most just by walking — after the study ended maintained their new, lower body weights. The rest who were sedentary gained most or all the weight back over time.

Choosing aerobic and resistance workouts

Remember, you can become more fit regardless of your body weight. You can also gain almost all the health benefits of having a higher fitness level without struggling to lose weight and keep it off. Both moderate aerobic exercise and resistance training help you lose belly (visceral) fat that dieting alone can't. (I discuss these kinds of exercises in Chapters 10 and 11, respectively.)

TECHNICAL
STUFF

Both aerobic and resistance training are more effective at helping you lose visceral fat than dieting alone. Research examined how improving lifestyle habits helped obese people with too much of this inside-the-belly fat. Though exercising helped them get rid of more of this bad fat, having a healthier diet also kept their insulin working better, showing that making both changes at once is beneficial. Another study showed that doing interval training while cutting back on carbohydrates and eating fewer calories for two weeks ensures that you lose the unhealthy visceral fat from inside your abdominal region while keeping more muscle.

TIP

Try to keep your muscle and gain more with resistance training to boost your metabolism, lower your blood glucose, and prevent gaining back the pounds you lost.

Giving your backside a break

How can you get more active when you're sedentary and overweight? Most activities are possible, but ease into being more active by taking small steps in that direction. It's not a race to the finish; you're just trying to establish a lifetime habit of being more active.

>> **Stand up whenever possible.** Burn calories by standing as much as you can every day. Stand up when talking on the phone at work or home. Have standing meetings at work. Get a standing desk. Encourage others to stand with you.

>> **Move more all day long.** Make a habit of moving as much as you can throughout the day. Even if you find it challenging to fit in regular workouts at a gym or prolonged and continuous walks or other activities, you can get more fit and lose weight by staying as active as you can every day doing any physical movement. That includes standing, fidgeting, taking more daily steps, stretching, pacing in your office, walking the dog, and much more.

>> **Break up sedentary time.** Even just getting up from a sitting activity at least once or twice an hour for a few minutes boosts your metabolism and prevents insulin resistance regardless of whether you have diabetes. Everyone needs to avoid sitting for long periods of time. What you do when you get up doesn't have to be strenuous or prolonged; it just needs to occur frequently. Stand up, walk around at any speed, do a few leg bends, or stretch for two to five minutes before sitting back down.

Starting out slowly but steadily

Getting active with extra body weight is all about starting out slowly and progressing slowly for the best results. You want to get fit and possibly lose some weight along the way. It's possible if you go about it the right way.

>> **Begin with lower impact activities.** Do activities that don't require you to carry around your full body weight, such as swimming, classes in a swimming pool, seated exercises, stationary cycling, stretching, and light resistance training. Extra fat stored under the skin acts to insulate you and keep you warmer in the pool, where you lose body heat faster than in air. Just walking or moving in the water is a good choice. Additionally, the water helps hide your figure, if that's a concern for you, and may lower your resistance to exercising in public. Seated exercises or stationary cycling also reduce stress on your lower limb joints.

>> **Work your way up to doing more.** One of the main reasons people drop out of exercise programs is that they start out working out too hard, which can cause injuries. Don't push yourself as hard as a cast member on *The Biggest Loser,* or you're likely to get sidelined by an injury or just lose interest. Do continue to move forward with what you're doing, though, and progress to other activities and to doing them at a higher level to get more fit.

Picking activities you enjoy

As with all things, if you enjoy doing something, you're more likely to continue doing it over time. This concept is critically important with physical activities and even more so if you're trying to manage your weight. If you hate doing an activity, eventually you come up with one excuse or another to stop. When you're packing some extra weight, doing any activity can feel harder than it might be when you've lost a few pounds.

REMEMBER

Most people quit before they start enjoying an activity. Nothing is quite as important to establishing an active lifestyle as choosing activities to do that you find to be enjoyable or fun.

TIP

Join others to do physical activities with you as well to make them social events to enhance your enjoyment. You can help them all get thinner, too.

Dealing with Arthritis and Other Joint Problems

Carrying extra body fat raises your chances of getting arthritis (osteoarthritis being the most common type that develops with aging) in your hips, knees, and ankles, which may limit your ability to exercise. Despite that, being active is an effective means of managing arthritis, including the more severe rheumatoid type (which is an autoimmune condition like type 1 diabetes), and its associated discomfort. Being active can make your pain and discomfort less over time instead of aggravating it.

Working out with arthritic joints

Start with basic range-of-motion exercises (including stretching) to increase your joint mobility. Later you can include specific resistance exercises that strengthen the muscles surrounding your affected joints. Doing so also helps you maintain your leg strength, which is critical to basic movements like getting up out of a chair, climbing stairs, and walking.

Doing moderate aerobic activity that is weight-bearing (like walking) can reduce arthritis pain in hips and knees. If you have arthritic knees or hips and don't enjoy walking because it's too uncomfortable or painful, you can choose to do non-weight-bearing activities instead.

If you have arthritis in your lower extremities, also consider the following options:

>> Easy or moderate workouts rather than vigorous ones

>> Varied activities from day to day to avoid overstressing joints in the same way each time

>> Warm-ups and cool-downs to keep joints more limber

>> Some weight loss to take stress off your painful joints

>> Activities that don't make you carry your weight, such as swimming, aquatic exercises, cycling, and seated workouts

You may also want to seek out a physical therapist, athletic trainer, personal trainer, or other fitness professional to help you design an exercise program specific to your needs.

TIP

Your buoyancy in water takes the strain off painful joints so you can move them more fluidly. Swimming and aquatic classes (like water aerobics) in either shallow or deep water are both appropriate and challenging activities to improve joint mobility, overall strength, and aerobic fitness. You may also want to try walking in a pool (with or without a flotation belt around your waist).

Managing discomfort or pain

After exercising, you may want to apply ice to your joints (particularly your knees) for 15 to 20 minutes to reduce swelling and help prevent undue soreness. In addition, consider taking nonsteroidal anti-inflammatory medications (NSAIDs) like aspirin or ibuprofen to lessen any residual discomfort, but avoid taking them if your kidneys are not working well. Check with your doctor if your arthritis pain becomes worse over time, and avoid activities that feel like they make your joints more painful.

Avoiding other joint issues

Having diabetes increases your risk of experiencing joint-related injuries and overuse problems like tendinitis. Choosing a more moderate exercise like walking rather than jogging or running may be prudent to reduce the potential for joint trauma.

Diabetic frozen shoulder, trigger finger, and other acute joint problems can also come on with no warning and for no apparent reason, even if you exercise regularly and moderately, and they may recur more easily as well. You may benefit from the expert help of a physical therapist if you develop any of these issues.

The best defense against injuries is good blood glucose control, along with flexibility exercises (see Chapter 13) and doing cross-training (Chapter 14).

REMEMBER

Losing Weight and Keeping It Off

To improve your health, you don't have to reach some unrealistically low body weight. In fact, losing just 10 pounds improves your insulin action, lowers your body's inflammation, raises your good cholesterol and lowers the bad, and improves your metabolic efficiency. And you can learn how to keep it off for good.

Losing some weight along the way

Going on a diet to lose weight isn't the best long-term solution to managing your body weight or reducing your diabetes risk. Even though you can lose weight on a diet, dieting doesn't work for most people. It becomes progressively harder to lose weight the longer you stay on a diet, which makes it harder for you to stay motivated to follow it. Consequently, many people give up after they've been on a diet for a while, and they fail to meet their target weight loss.

So how can you lose weight? The best way is slowly, over time, accomplished by doing physical activities *and* cutting back on your calories by a small amount. You won't even realize that you're "dieting" while you're doing it. Just don't diet or severely restrict your calories without being active, or you'll lose too much of your muscle and likely eventually end up fatter than you were before. Consider consulting with a registered dietitian to set up an individualized, weight-reducing meal plan for you.

If you must choose between dieting and exercising to lose weight, always choose being active, even if that makes you lose weight more slowly.

TIP

Keep in mind that what you normally weigh can change gradually over your lifetime. But your body has a preferred weight, and when you try to change that quickly by dieting, your body resists the effort to keep it off. If you do daily physical activity while you're losing weight and after, you'll be less likely to gain fat back later because you keep more muscle.

Keeping the weight off

The biggest problem with dieting without exercise is that even if you do lose some weight, you're not likely to keep off it. More than 90 percent of dieters who have successfully lost weight ultimately regain the pounds they struggled to lose. If you go back to eating the same foods that you ate prior to your weight loss, you are likely to return to your previous weight

Most people gain back even more than they lost, regardless of the diet they followed. And you may end up fatter than you started before you lose weight.

Regaining the weight is probably even worse for your health than never losing it in the first place. A greater percentage of the weight you gain back is fat (unless you're exercising a whole lot and gaining muscle). In most cases, you end up with more total body fat than if you had never lost any weight, even if your weight only goes back to your pre-diet level. In other words, you ultimately end up even fatter from dieting.

Being a successful "loser"

Keeping off the weight you lost for more than six months is very uncommon even among successful dieters. If you're one of those people, congratulations. If not, you can benefit from looking at how others have done it. If you lose weight rapidly, you are more likely to gain it back.

How can you become one of the success cases? Some people have figured it out. The National Weight Control Registry has tracked over 10,000 individuals who have lost at least 30 pounds and kept the weight off for at least a year. What method or weight loss plan people use to lose weight doesn't appear to matter; their food choices ranged from conventional lower-calorie, moderate-carbohydrate diets like Weight Watchers and Jenny Craig to low-carbohydrate ones like Atkins and South Beach. What matters more are the lifestyle habits that almost all of them adopt:

>> They're conscientious about eating more healthful foods in appropriate portions.

>> They exercise almost daily (expending about 2,000 calories a week).

>> They eat a healthy breakfast.

>> Most eat about 50 percent of calories as carbohydrates, 30 percent as fat, and 20 percent as protein.

>> Only 17 percent follow a low-carbohydrate diet going forward, regardless of what diet they followed to lose the weight.

Conversely, those who regain the most weight take in more calories, eat more fast foods and fat, and are less physically active.

Burning calories by moving more

Most people fail to prevent weight gain that typically comes with getting older. Also, the greater release of insulin you get from eating excessive amounts of carbohydrate may cause you to gain body fat. Carbohydrates are usually converted into and stored as fat when you're sedentary, but not so much so when you're active.

Remember, what matters more is whether you're fit. Simply get physically active and don't worry about maintaining a specific weight. Despite the hundreds of thousands of calories you typically eat each year, your body has the innate ability to match food intake with calorie intake and can maintain your body weight within a pound or two. Likely, the biggest contributor to weight gain is burning too few calories in daily movement.

Cutting back by 50 calories a day

You can prevent or reverse weight gain over time by making small changes in your daily habits. A pound of fat equals about 3,500 calories, so if you eat just 50 more calories than you use each day (the equivalent of less than a quarter cup of cooked rice), you can gain 5 pounds of body fat in a year from that alone. If you cut back by 50 calories instead — by leaving a few bites uneaten or skipping a small treat — and expend an extra 50 calories a day by doing some extra walking, stretching, or other easy activity, you can lose 10 pounds of body fat in a year instead. Choose to tip the scale in your favor.

Using more measurements than just the scale

Exercising causes you to retain and gain some muscle mass, which is what you want to have happen given that muscle is sensitive to insulin and is a storage place for carbohydrates and blood glucose. Muscle is denser than body fat and weighs more. When you lose fat while gaining muscle, your scale weight may change very little (or even rise slightly at first), even though your total fat percentage is getting lower.

REMEMBER

Be patient when waiting to see the positive changes on the scales if you're trying to lose weight while exercising. And don't use weight loss as the only measure of your success because fitness counts, too.

If you feel compelled to weigh yourself frequently after you start an exercise program, don't. Focus on your waist and hip measurements and how your clothes fit instead — the so-called clothes test. When you're starting your activity program, only weigh yourself once a week at the same time of day. Even if exercising regularly doesn't make you lose all the weight you want to, it can still help you lose your fat and keep your muscle.

SCALE WEIGHT WITH EXERCISE GOT YOU DOWN?

About the only thing that exercise can't do for you is to make your body weight go down faster than dieting alone does. This effect isn't bad, just frustrating. When you go on a diet, the weight you lose is a combination of body fat, muscle mass, and water weight. Exercising while dieting helps you retain and even gain some muscle mass, which is beneficial because muscle is sensitive to insulin and a good place to store your extra carbohydrates and glucose.

The downside of retaining or gaining muscle — if it can be considered a downside — is that muscle is denser than body fat and weighs more. When you lose fat while gaining muscle, your weight on the scale may change very little (or even rise slightly at first) even though your body composition is changing for the better.

Slow reductions in body weight don't mean that you aren't making any headway. Give it some time. You didn't gain all your weight overnight, and you're not going to lose it that way either. If you lose weight slowly by cutting calories while being more active or just by exercising, you're much more likely to keep it off compared to losing weight rapidly from starving yourself and not being active.

Avoiding Insulin Weight Gain and Using Diabetes Medications to Lose Weight

Taking insulin can potentially lead you into gaining weight if you don't manage its use well. You can adopt some strategies to keep weight gain from happening whether you have type 1 or type 2 diabetes. Some other diabetes medications can contribute to fat gains as well. Luckily, some newer medications can help you lose weight. You may want to talk with your doctor about using them and avoiding the ones that cause weight gain if you want to get thinner.

Dodging weight gain from insulin use

Why is using insulin sometimes associated with weight gain? On insulin, your blood glucose is (usually) in a tighter range, and you stop losing some calories as glucose in your urine. You may also gain weight from having to eat extra to treat any lows caused by using insulin.

REMEMBER

Lifestyle changes, such as cutting back on refined carbohydrates that require larger doses of insulin to cover them and exercising regularly, are likely your best bets to counteract any potential weight gain caused by insulin use.

Weight gain with type 1 and type 2 diabetes

Most people diagnosed with type 1 diabetes gain some weight as soon as they start using insulin. Many of them lost weight before diagnosis — some of it muscle — so not all the weight regain is necessarily bad.

However, you can gain excess weight from taking too much daily insulin and then needing extra carbohydrates to treat low blood glucose. You can also gain weight if you're taking the right dose of insulin to cover your food and you're simply eating too many calories. In any case, gaining fat weight from insulin can lead to "double diabetes," meaning that you can become more insulin resistant like many with type 2 diabetes and need larger insulin doses. People with type 1 may need lower insulin doses if they're active.

Readjusting the ratio of basal to meal-associated insulin — specifically, lowering your basal doses and raising your pre-meal insulin — without increasing your total daily insulin dose may prevent weight gain if you have type 1 diabetes.

REMEMBER

Many people with type 2 diabetes try to delay going on insulin as long as possible because they've heard horror stories about how much weight it can make them gain. (Or they just don't like shots.) Making lifestyle changes like including exercise as a part of your daily routine can help lower your insulin needs and offset weight gain with supplemental insulin use.

Keep your total insulin needs low

What else can you do to avoid weight gain with insulin? First of all, try to keep your insulin needs as low as possible because the more you take, the greater your potential for weight gain is. The best way to keep your insulin needs in check is to engage in regular physical activity. For example, some people with type 2 diabetes who were studied gained weight from insulin use while others didn't. The main difference between them was that the gainers were less physically active. Although taking insulin doses that effectively manage blood glucose can also lead to weight gain in type 1 diabetes, being more active can prevent it.

WARNING

Insulin treatment is often associated with weight gain and more frequent bouts of *hypoglycemia* (low blood glucose).

During any physical activity, your muscles can take up blood glucose and use it as a fuel without insulin. Following exercise, your insulin action is heightened for a few hours up to 72 hours. During that time, you need smaller doses of insulin to have the same effect.

TIP

If you have type 2 diabetes and start exercising regularly, you may lose fat weight and can lower your insulin doses more or get off insulin completely.

REMEMBER

Regular exercise is the best way to prevent insulin-induced weight gain. But you need to adjust your insulin doses downward to prevent lows that cause you to take in extra calories to treat them so you don't gain weight.

Try using different insulins

You may be able to avoid weight gain by looking at the type of insulins you're using. For example, once-daily Levemir used by people with type 2 diabetes causes less weight gain and less frequent hypoglycemia than N insulin, even combined with use of rapid-acting injections of meal insulin. The same is likely true when using Lantus, Basaglar, Toujeo, and Tresiba. In type 1 diabetes, individuals end up eating less when using Levemir compared to Lantus, leading them to gain less weight. (Chapter 3 has the lowdown on these and other insulins.)

Table 15-1 breaks down how common insulins can impact weight gain. You may be able to avoid weight gain from insulin taken for meals just by altering when you take it (before vs. after eating), as you can see in Table 15-1.

TABLE 15-1   **Insulin Effects on Weight Gain or Loss**

Type of Insulin	Insulin Use Causing Weight Gain	Weight-Friendly or More Weight-Neutral Insulin Use
Long-acting	Humulin N, Novolin N, Humulin R, Novolin R, Lantus, Basaglar, Toujeo	Levemir, Tresiba
Short-acting (for meals)/inhaled	NovoLog, Humalog, Apidra, Fiasp, Admelog, Afrezza (when taken before meals, so you have to eat to match your insulin and may eat more than desired)	NovoLog, Humalog, Apidra, Fiasp, Admelog, Afrezza (when taken after meals, so insulin taken to cover only as much food as you eat)

Both the type of insulins you use and the doses you take are important to consider in the overall management of your diabetes and your body weight. Making sure that your doses are regulated effectively helps prevent blood glucose lows and highs.

Adjusting other diabetes medications to lose weight

Even when you begin exercising more, your non-insulin medications may be working against your ability to lose weight. Focus on reducing diabetes medications that contribute to weight gain and replacing them (if needed) with ones that are *weight-friendly* — that is, they don't affect body weight, they help with weight loss, or they cause less weight gain. Table 15-2 shows both categories of medications; you can read more about each type of medication in Chapter 3.

WARNING

To change any of your medications to more weight-friendly ones, consult directly with your health care provider for help with making appropriate adjustments.

PRESCRIBING WEIGHT LOSS CAN DO MORE HARM THAN GOOD

When you found out about your type 2 diabetes from your doctor, he or she probably told you to lose weight, eat better, take your medications, and exercise more. Maybe the recommendations weren't exactly in that order, but if you are overweight, losing weight was probably near the top. Sometimes, it's the only thing people are told to do.

Unfortunately, because long-term dieting has such a high failure rate, a blanket prescription to lose weight can potentially harm you more than help you. Although some weight loss may boost your insulin action, losing large amounts of weight is unnecessary to achieve your blood glucose goals — not to mention unrealistic — and shouldn't be the primary focus.

Consider the case of one woman diagnosed with type 2 diabetes in her early 40s. At the time she weighed 270 pounds, which categorized her as morbidly obese, and her A1C was almost double the recommended levels at 14 percent. Over the next few months, she started eating better and exercising more, and her overall diabetes control vastly improved. Her A1C dropped to 8 and then to under 6 percent — reflective of an average blood glucose level within normal, nondiabetic limits. When she saw her doctor again, he expressed disappointment that she hadn't lost any weight. In fact, he told her that she obviously didn't care about her health because weight loss should be her main focus, and she failed to lose any.

This doctor's fixation on weight loss alone wasn't only misguided (he ignored her great overall blood glucose levels) but also emotionally counterproductive for the woman, failing to give her the encouragement and praise she deserved for so effectively managing her diabetes on her own. He didn't understand that starting a new program of regular exercise can make you gain weight rather than lose it in the short term, but you're still likely gaining muscle while losing fat.

Doctors would serve patients far better by monitoring short-term changes in their body fat levels rather than their scale weights. And they should reward patients for meeting their blood glucose goals, especially when they do it by adopting a healthier lifestyle.

Medications Causing Weight Gain	"Weight-Friendly" or Neutral Medications	
TABLE 15-2	**Diabetes Medication Effects on Weight Gain or Loss**	
Sulfonylureas: Amaryl, DiaBeta, Diabinese, Glynase, Glucotrol, Micronase	**Metformin:** Metformin (generic), Glucophage, Glucophage XR, Riomet, Glumetza	
Glinides (Meglitinides): Starlix, Prandin	**DPP-4 inhibitors:** Januvia, Onglyza, Nesina/Galvus, Tradjenta	
Thiazolidinediones (TZDs): Actos, Avandia	**GLP-1 receptor agonists:** Byetta, Victoza, Lyxumia, Bydureon, Trulicity, Ozempic, Eperzan, Adlyxin	
	SGLT-2 inhibitors: Invokana, Farxiga, Jardiance, Steglatro	
	Amylin analog: Symlin	
	Alpha-glucosidase inhibitors: Precose, Glyset	

Considering Other Weight Loss Issues

When you lose excess body fat, you can potentially let loose a lifetime of accumulated toxins stored in your fat, like PCBs and DDEs from insecticides. These substances can lead to nerve damage and are the main reason why losing weight when you're older may not be that good for you. Another reason is the increased risk of fracturing a hip, getting frail, and being admitted to a nursing home because you no longer have the strength to care for yourself. This scenario can happen if you lose too much of your muscle and strength from dieting when you're older.

Along with toxins, any medications stored in fat are released during weight loss. Unless your doctor lowers the dose of fat-soluble medications you're on when you're losing weight, you may end up with higher than normal or advisable amounts in your bloodstream.

If you've done the yo-yo dieting thing (cycling between losing and gaining weight), you can end up losing so much of your muscle that you're too weak to move your own body weight. That makes you "fat frail" (known as *sarcopenic obesity* in the medical world). Having too little strength can greatly lower your quality of life. What's more, losing too much muscle lowers how many calories you need daily, making it easier to gain weight even when eating the same number of calories as you used to. It's a vicious cycle.

WARNING

Losing weight unexpectedly without trying to could be a sign that you're ill. If you find your weight dropping without dieting or exercise, you may need to see your doctor to rule out disease as a potential cause, especially if you can catch problems while they're easier to treat.

TIP

Don't let these statistics on significant and later-in-life weight loss scare you away from trying to get fit. Do start moving more to improve your muscle mass and your overall health.

Keeping Diabetes from Making You Blue

Many people with diabetes or prediabetes who have body weight issues are more prone to suffering from emotional disorders like depression and anxiety, along with body image issues. True clinical depression is much different from the occasional bout of "the blues." Depression lasts much longer, often going on for months without any lasting relief.

When depressed, you may feel sad and hopeless and lose interest in things you normally enjoy. Other symptoms include eating or sleeping unusual amounts (whether that's more or less), feeling low in energy, having trouble concentrating, and having negative feelings about yourself.

Having diabetes makes you more than twice as likely to suffer from the most serious form of depression, *major depressive disorder*. Almost half of all people with diabetes have some level of depression, and it's even more likely if you have heart disease, arthritis, or other health issues. Feeling blue can sabotage your usual diabetes care because you may not feel like being active or making healthful food choices, and it may even lead you to binge eat, gain more weight, and feel even worse about yourself. If you haven't had a reason to smile today, try to find one.

REMEMBER

Depression itself may contribute to the development of diabetes rather than the other way around, which is why you should focus on managing your mental health as well as your physical state.

Getting Enough Sleep to Get Thinner

Getting adequate sleep each night helps you burn fat and lose weight. Too little sleep increases levels of the hormone *cortisol,* which contributes to belly fat, insulin resistance, and type 2 diabetes. And losing sleep can even keep you from losing weight when you're dieting.

In a study, middle-aged adults who slept 8.5 hours per night lost about 3 pounds in two weeks, but those sleeping only 5.5 hours per night lost less than half that much. On top of that, sleeping less lowered the proportion of fat weight lost by 55 percent. The sleep-deprived adults felt hungrier, and their bodies used less energy during the day to compensate for lack of sleep.

Unfortunately, sleeping well isn't as easy as it sounds. Aging causes you to sleep less deeply and more fitfully. The normal aches and pains of aging can keep you awake at night, or you may have medical conditions that make it harder to get enough deep sleep. Many people with diabetes suffer with *sleep apnea*, which can result in greatly disturbed sleep patterns.

Aging also leads to lower levels of a natural body hormone called *melatonin*, which is related to falling and staying asleep. Melatonin comes from the pineal gland in the brain and controls your sleep and wake cycles. These naturally decreased levels lead to greater insulin resistance. Taking over-the-counter melatonin supplements 30 minutes before you go to bed may help you sleep better and lower your morning blood glucose as well.

IN THIS CHAPTER

» **Grasping how diabetes combined with other conditions can impact your workout needs**

» **Working around central or peripheral nerve damage**

» **Choosing activities to exercise with cardiovascular disease**

» **Staying active in spite of diabetic retinopathy**

» **Deciding how to be active with kidney issues**

Chapter **16**

Exercising with Health Complications

So you know you need to be more physically active, but you have [*insert your health issue here*] to worry about, which makes you choose to stay on the couch instead. Is it loss of sensation in your feet that makes you more unstable while walking? A diagnosis or symptoms of heart disease? Some early changes in your eyes or your vision that you see as a barrier to exercise?

Certain health complications or other physical conditions can impact your ability to exercise safely and effectively. Though not usually entirely limiting, some diabetes-related health complications require adaptations in your physical activity choices.

Regardless of the health issue or issues you may be dealing with, this chapter shows you that you can find a way to be more active, both safely and effectively. It's just a matter of making some adjustments or taking some precautions to make sure that you don't injure yourself or cause your condition to get worse. You've got this.

Dealing with Health Complications

Although 85 percent of older adults over 65 have a health problem that they may view as a deterrent, anyone with a chronic health problem or two generally responds well to exercise training. But having diabetes does carry some additional risks.

As you may already know, diabetes is associated with a number of short-term and long-term health complications that require you to understand them to exercise safely. The leading cause of death in all Americans is heart disease, regardless of whether you have diabetes. You are at greater risk for developing complications like stroke, high blood pressure, vision loss, kidney disease, joint problems, nerve damage, foot ulcers, and lower-extremity amputations that may affect your choice of activities or how you approach them.

REMEMBER

Keeping your blood glucose as close to normal as possible is the best way to prevent many, if not all, of these potential health problems. That's where regular exercise, a healthful diet, effective use of diabetes medications, and a blood glucose meter come in handy.

TIP

If you're just getting started, you may want to consult with your health care team or an exercise professional to help you develop a physical activity plan that factors in your diabetes management, complications, heart disease risk, other health problems, personal goals, and exercise preferences. If you choose to go it alone, simply follow the exercise guidelines published by the American Diabetes Association (accessible online at `http://care.diabetesjournals.org/content/39/11/2065`) and respect your potential limitations while staying as physically active as possible.

Exercising Safely with Nerve Damage

Loss of sensation or pain in your feet (or hands) is called *peripheral neuropathy,* and it increases your risk of damaging your feet or lower limbs during exercise. If you have damage to other nerves in your body (*autonomic neuropathy,* affecting nerves in the spinal cord), you can experience different issues related to this condition. In this section, I explain why being active may help and how to exercise safely if you have either of these issues.

Working around damaged feet and legs

When you're missing the usual symptoms of pain or discomfort from impact on your feet or friction and pressure from footwear, you're much more likely to get an irritated area on your foot without being aware of it. In some cases, a simple blister can progress into a full-blown infected abscess or ulcer and ultimately result in an amputation if not detected and treated in time.

Even if you haven't lost much sensation in your feet that you know of, developing a foot ulcer on the bottom (*plantar*) surface or sides of your feet may be a sign you have some peripheral neuropathy already. Your doctor can check for signs of this condition or refer you to a specialist if necessary.

When staying active, inspect your feet daily for sores, blisters, irritation, cuts, or other injuries that can develop into ulcers. If you can't easily pull your feet up to look at the bottoms, place a mirror on the floor and hold your feet over it to inspect them yourself or ask someone else to check them for you.

Have a doctor look at any unusual changes in the skin of your feet sooner rather than later. You can avoid the possibility of gangrene and possible amputation of your toes or your foot if you get problem areas treated early.

Picking the right socks and shoes

If you've lost sensation in your feet, use shoes with silica gel or air midsoles (the middle section of the shoe that provides the most stability and shock absorption). Also, wear polyester or cotton-polyester blend socks to prevent blisters and keep your feet dry during physical activities.

Pure cotton socks aren't recommended for exercise because they tend to get and stay wet, which can lead to irritation and injury of your feet.

Choosing appropriate activities

Although being regularly active can't fully reverse nerve damage in your feet, exercise can slow its progression and prevent your getting more out of shape from sitting around all the time. Exercise may improve circulation in your lower legs and feet and help prevent ulcers.

If you've lost most or all of the sensation in your feet, you may need to switch to doing more activities that minimize potential trauma to your lower extremities. Aquatic activities like swimming, pool walking, and water aerobics are good choices, but they're not an option if you have any open sores. You can also do rowing, upper body cycling (using an arm crank), chair exercises, stationary cycling, yoga, seated resistance training, and abdominal work.

Work on improving your flexibility and balance to prevent falls, which are more common if you lose sensation in your feet. Chapters 12 and 13 offer balance and flexibility exercises, respectively.

WARNING

If you have unhealed ulcers, minimize walking or weight-bearing activities until they've fully healed. While they're healing, keep your feet clean and dry, avoid swimming, stay off your feet, and inspect them daily.

You don't need to avoid all activities done on your feet if you've lost sensation, but not doing them daily (cross-training) helps. Combined resistance and interval exercise training are both good to do occasionally. All these activities — both the ones that make you carry your weight and those that don't — can improve your fitness, muscle tone, balance, and awareness of your lower extremities.

If your peripheral nerve damage causes dull, shooting, or throbbing pain in your extremities after you go for a walk or do other weight-bearing activities, switch to others that don't cause you lasting pain or discomfort. If the pain is constant, you may need to seek treatment for painful diabetic neuropathy or be tested for peripheral artery disease (more on this condition later in this chapter).

Staying on top of central nerve issues

If you have damage to your central nervous system (*autonomic neuropathy*), it can manifest in a variety of ways, almost all of which may impact your ability to be active safely and effectively. For example, you may be more likely to experience *silent ischemia* (reduced heart blood that doesn't have any other symptoms), which can result in a "silent" or symptomless and undetected heart attack. Your chances of dying suddenly during exercise are higher after your heart has become unresponsive to nerve impulses (a central nerve condition known as *cardiac autonomic neuropathy*, which is discussed more below), particularly if you have some underlying heart disease present.

Here are some possible conditions that result from central nerve damage and guidelines on what you should do to stay safe during exercise:

>> **Cardiac autonomic neuropathy:** This is the most concerning of all the central nervous system damage that can occur when your blood glucose stays elevated over time. If you have this condition, you may have an elevated heart rate at rest (for example, 100 beats per minute or higher rather than the normal 72), and it may keep your heart from beating as fast as normal during exercise. Keep the following points in mind:

- If you have cardiac autonomic nerve damage, take a conservative approach to exercise and physical activities.

- Have your doctor test your heart's responses before you start an exercise program so you know how exercise affects your heart rate.

- Warm up for at least ten minutes and cool down longer than normal, particularly when you're doing strenuous activities.

- Don't use heart rate to monitor your exercise intensity because it may be lower than expected during activities; instead, use a subjective rating (such as "somewhat hard" for moderate) or the talk test (which I cover in Chapter 4).

» **Orthostatic hypotension:** When you change your body position rapidly during an activity, your blood pressure may drop (a condition called *orthostatic hypotension*) and make you feel lightheaded or dizzy, or you may faint.

- Avoid activities with rapid postural changes (like racquetball) because your blood pressure may not respond fast enough and you can faint.

- Try to stay fully hydrated during exercise to remove the potential for dehydration to add to these symptoms.

» **Impaired thermoregulation:** Your body is less able to move blood around to help you cool down, making you more likely to overheat and get dehydrated during exercise.

- Don't exercise in extreme hot or cold environments because you may not be able to regulate your body temperature well at either end of the spectrum.

- Stay fully hydrated by drinking fluids during exercise, especially when you're exercising in hot and humid conditions.

» **Gastroparesis:** If your ability to digest food has been affected, any carbohydrate you use to treat low blood glucose during exercise may take longer to work, and your low may get more severe. Consider the following:

- Eat only small portions and avoid eating a large meal before exercise; the latter may delay the emptying of food from your stomach.

- Check your blood glucose before and after exercise because you're more likely to develop low blood glucose.

- To treat a low, take glucose tablets before your blood glucose goes down to 100 mg/dL to prevent severe hypoglycemia.

Being Active with Vessel Disease

If you have diabetes or prediabetes, you may also already have the beginnings of cardiovascular disease, which can cause heart attack, stroke, lowered blood flow to your heart, or reduced leg blood flow. When stable, none of these conditions should prevent you from exercising, but you may need to change up what you're doing or take other precautions to avoid problems.

Individuals with diabetes in supervised "cardiac rehab" exercise programs engage in various activities. You may choose to join such a program if you know you have cardiovascular disease, or you may exercise on your own or with others.

Regular exercise helps improve blood flow through your body and reduce the severity of cardiovascular changes you may already be experiencing.

REMEMBER

Heart disease

Heart disease — which is caused by plaque formation in the coronary arteries and reduced blood flow to the heart muscle — has been associated with insulin resistance and inflammation. But it may not be as directly related to how well your blood glucose is managed. If you have any symptoms related to heart disease you need to take precautions to exercise safely.

Dealing with reduced blood flow to your heart

If you experience *angina* (chest pain) due to reduced blood flow to your heart muscle (a condition known as *ischemia*) during an aerobic activity like walking, you may want to do a different activity.

You probably won't have the same problem during resistance workouts. Lifting a heavy weight 10 to 12 times may increase your blood pressure more than aerobic exercise does, but it doesn't raise your heart rate as much. Your blood pressure rises more and sends more blood to your heart muscle during this type of workout than an aerobic one.

If you have some coronary artery blockage from plaque buildup, moderate weight training may be a safer activity for you than most higher intensity aerobic ones, and resistance training is recommended nowadays for almost everyone to increase strength and preserve muscle mass.

REMEMBER

If you prefer walking or another aerobic activity but experience angina when active, keep your heart rate about ten beats per minute lower than the point at which you start to experience pain or tightness in your chest during the activity. For example, work no harder than 120 beats per minute if you have symptoms that start at 130 beats.

WARNING

Recognizing that you're having a heart attack

Exercising only slightly increases your risk of having a cardiovascular event like a heart attack (*myocardial infarction*) while you're doing it. But training regularly lowers your chances, so being active is still always better than being a couch potato.

That said, know the usual warning signs of heart attack:

>> **Chest discomfort:** This discomfort in the center of the chest may feel like bad indigestion, uncomfortable pressure, squeezing, fullness, or acute and stabbing pain. It may last or be intermittent.

>> **Discomfort elsewhere:** The pain or discomfort may be localized somewhere other than your chest. Pain radiating down one or both arms or the back, neck, jaw, or stomach is known as *referred pain* because it originates in your heart due to lack of oxygen but is felt elsewhere.

>> **Shortness of breath:** This warning sign can occur with or without chest discomfort and is symptomatic when it's unusual or unexpected.

>> **Other symptoms:** Sudden sweating, nausea and vomiting, lightheadedness, and undue, unexplained fatigue are all signals you may be having a heart attack.

WARNING

If you experience a sudden, unexplained change in your ability to exercise (such as extreme fatigue that comes on quickly), without any other symptoms, immediately stop exercising and consult with your physician as soon as you can to rule out silent ischemia.

WARNING

Don't delay in calling 911 or seeking other immediate medical attention if you're experiencing any of the signs or symptoms of a heart attack. Treatment in the first few minutes is critical for surviving a major cardiac event with minimal lasting problems.

High blood pressure and stroke

Being regularly active doing aerobic exercise lowers the potential impact of most other cardiovascular risk factors, including high blood pressure, regardless of what type of diabetes you have.

High blood pressure, or *hypertension,* is associated with elevated levels of insulin in your body, which are common with insulin resistance. Getting up off the couch and exercising regularly can lower your blood pressure and reduce how much insulin is in your bloodstream — both of which are very good for your overall health.

Exercising safely with high blood pressure

If you have high blood pressure, you may need to avoid high-intensity or heavy resistance exercises that can cause your blood pressure to rise dangerously high and bring on heart attack or stroke. Limit your involvement in heavy weight training; near-maximal exercise; activities that require intense, sustained contractions of the upper body, such as water-skiing or windsurfing; or any exercise that involves holding your breath.

TIP

Appropriate blood pressure medications should help keep your pressures lower during activities, so take them as prescribed.

Recognizing that you're having a stroke

Watch out for stroke warning signs, which all have a sudden onset in common. Go to the emergency room right away for life- and brain-saving treatment within a couple of hours for the best possible outcomes if you do have any of the symptoms of a stroke.

Stroke warning signs and symptoms include sudden

>> Numbness or weakness, especially on one side of the body (for example, legs, arms, face)

>> Confusion

>> Trouble with normal speaking or understanding

>> Loss of vision in one or both eyes

>> Trouble with walking, loss of balance, or lack of physical coordination

>> Severe headache and dizziness

>> Symptoms like sweating, nausea and vomiting, lightheadedness, or undue, unexplained fatigue

WARNING

To lower your risk of stroke, if your *systolic blood pressure* (the higher number) is above 200 mmHg or your *diastolic blood pressure* (the lower one) is above 110 mmHg, avoid exercising until they're lower.

Peripheral artery disease (PAD)

Another form of cardiovascular disease, *peripheral artery disease* (PAD), is a common circulatory problem that limits blood flow to your legs and arms. Plaque can form in any artery, not just the ones feeding the heart and brain, and PAD usually occurs in peripheral arteries in the legs.

Knowing whether you have PAD

Pain in your lower legs while standing or walking is a common symptom of PAD. Measuring the blood pressure in your leg or ankle compared to in your arm is how doctors diagnose PAD. If it's higher in your leg, you may have blockage there that is raising the pressure.

If you experience symptoms in your legs during or after physical activity and you haven't yet been diagnosed with PAD, see your doctor to get a definite diagnosis before proceeding with your exercise program. You want to know for sure because having PAD may mean that you have widespread plaque formation in other arteries around your body.

WARNING

If plaque in your leg arteries ruptures, it can block blood flow and cause pain, changes in skin color, sores or ulcers, difficulty walking, and even gangrene. See your doctor right away if you have any of these symptoms.

Luckily, PAD is treatable. Certain prescribed medications that lower your blood pressure can dilate your leg arteries and relieve symptoms. Surgery can also improve blood flow to your legs by bypassing blockages.

Exercising with PAD

You can get your PAD under control and maintain your normal activities. In fact, walking or other daily exercise helps you maintain optimal circulation in your legs. It may improve the blood flow to your feet, especially when combined with eating a more healthful diet and quitting smoking.

Using pain as your guide, engage in easy or moderate walking and take rest periods as needed. You may have to choose activities that don't cause pain. If walking hurts too much, try doing seated exercises, water workouts, upper body resistance training, or stationary cycling.

Eyeing Ways to Exercise with Retinopathy

Individuals who have diabetes can develop up to eight different eye complications over time, including cataracts, macular edema, and retinopathy. You can lower your risk of getting any of these with better overall blood glucose management and limiting your post-meal spikes. All eye diseases have the potential to obscure vision and make participation in certain activities (such as outdoor cycling) more dangerous. But, luckily, they're not usually a complete barrier to exercise. The following sections address one of the more common issues, *diabetic retinopathy* (caused by abnormal growth of blood vessels inside the eye back on the retina that can bleed when severe).

WARNING

If you notice sudden, dramatic changes in your sight while exercising, stop all activity immediately and check with your eye doctor for further guidance.

Mild or moderate retinopathy

If you have diabetic retinopathy that is only mild or moderate, with no active bleeds, some precautions are necessary. Avoid activities that dramatically increase the blood pressure inside your eyes, such as heavy resistance training, breath-holding during exercise, or doing activities with your head lower than your heart.

Severe (proliferative) retinopathy

If you have severe, or *proliferative*, retinopathy (that is, you have growth of abnormal vessels in the back of your eyes that can hemorrhage or detach your retina), you can do exercises like swimming, walking, low-impact aerobics, stationary cycling, and other endurance exercises at a low to moderate level as long as your eyes aren't actively bleeding internally. You should be able to see when such hemorrhages occur (if your vision isn't already totally blocked by prior bleeds that haven't fully cleared out).

However, you must avoid certain activities until the condition has stabilized over time with treatment. Although exercise doesn't make this eye disease worse overall, it can make hemorrhaging worse (by increasing pressure inside your eyes) or contribute to a retinal tear or retinal detachment.

WARNING

Avoid doing these activities with unstable proliferative diabetic retinopathy:

>> Heavy resistance training

>> Running or jogging

>> Most racquet sports

>> Boxing

>> Competitive contact sports (such as basketball and football)

>> High-impact aerobics

>> Activities where you keep your head down or lower than your heart

>> Jumping

>> Jarring activities

>> Any activity that elevates blood pressure a lot

WARNING

Never engage in moderate or vigorous exercise with an ongoing eye hemorrhage. Doing so may cause extra bleeding into your eye and further block your vision. Wait until the hemorrhage has stopped and then see your eye doctor for guidance before doing any more intense exercise.

MANAGING SEVERE PROLIFERATIVE RETINOPATHY

More severe forms of eye disease like proliferative diabetic retinopathy can cause your eyes to form weak, abnormal blood vessels in the back of the eye (the retina). These vessels can break, tear, or bleed into the vitreous fluid in the center of your eye, filling it with blood that can obscure vision temporarily or permanently.

Ideally, you should have a dilated eye exam by an ophthalmologist at least once a year and close to when you start any new vigorous exercise. A recent exam isn't necessary prior to doing easy or moderate activities.

If you have severe or unstable eye disease, you need to change your exercise regimen to prevent bleeding into your eye and loss of vision. Let your eye doctor know about your planned exercise routine to find out if you should modify it based on the results of your latest eye exam.

Staying Active with Kidney Disease

Regular exercise training is recommended for anyone with diabetes-related kidney disease, regardless of how severe it is. Exercise doesn't worsen diabetes-related kidney problems (such as nephropathy). In fact, being active may help keep such problems from progressing as fast. Letting yourself get deconditioned when you have kidney problems only adds to your level of fatigue.

What should you do to be active?

>> With kidney disease at any stage, you may have a reduced capacity to exercise. Start out with low to moderate activities rather than anything too hard and progress slowly.

>> Try to exercise daily, even if you just do easy exercise on days that you're feeling more tired.

>> You can even exercise *during* dialysis sessions if you have the chance. Only avoid exercising during dialysis if certain substances in your blood (hematocrit or total red blood cell count, calcium, or potassium) become unbalanced or if you get extremely fatigued immediately afterward.

>> If you have a kidney transplant, you can safely start exercising six to eight weeks after surgery, when you're stable and free of signs of rejection of the new kidney.

Exercise increases the excretion of protein and microalbumin in your urine, both of which are used as lab indicators of kidney problems. Abstain from exercising hard on a day that you're collecting your urine to be tested. Otherwise, your results may be skewed and misinterpreted as evidence of kidney damage or disease progression when your kidneys are healthy.

Managing Exercise with Health Issues

Be prepared for the type of exercise you're doing. For example, invest in the right shoes for the activity and dress in layers so that you can add or remove clothing if you need to. Avoiding activities that cause you any pain or that aggravate any preexisting health problems you may have is also important.

If you've been mostly sedentary, the best advice is to start with mild or moderate exercise and progress slowly to prevent potential problems with any health complications. Brisk walking and other mild and moderate activities are generally safe to start on your own, but if you want to do vigorous activities, see your health care provider first to get checked for complications that certain activities may worsen.

Precautions for exercising with diabetes in addition to any health complications include the following:

>> Carry a blood glucose meter to check your blood glucose level before, possibly during, and/or after exercise, or if you have any symptoms of a low.

>> Immediately treat low blood glucose during or following exercise with easily absorbed carbohydrates like glucose tablets or regular soft drinks (see Chapter 5).

>> Inform your exercise partners about your diabetes, and show them how to administer glucose or another carbohydrate to you should you need assistance.

>> Stay properly hydrated with frequent sips of cool water. Chapter 7 has details on hydration.

>> Consult with your physician prior to exercising with any of the following conditions:

- High blood pressure

- Neuropathy (nerve damage), either peripheral or autonomic

- Foot injuries (including ulcers)

- Proliferative retinopathy or current hemorrhaging

- Kidney disease

- Serious illness or infection

>> Seek immediate medical attention for chest pain or any pain or discomfort that radiates down your arm, jaw, or neck.

>> If you have high blood pressure, avoid activities that cause large increases in your blood pressure, such as heavy resistance work, head-down exercises, and anything that forces you to hold your breath.

>> Wear proper footwear, and check your feet daily for signs of trauma such as blisters, redness, or other irritation.

>> Stop exercising immediately if you experience bleeding into your eyes related to unstable proliferative retinopathy.

>> Wear a diabetes medic alert bracelet or necklace with emergency contact information.

>> Carry a cellphone with you when you exercise outdoors or alone.

No matter what you choose to do to be physically active, the most important thing is that you're doing it. So many health complications associated with having diabetes long-term are preventable with healthful lifestyle changes — including regular physical activity. Even if you're already suffering from some of these long-term issues, you really don't have any excuses left for not getting moving to improve your health while you're alive.

REMEMBER

The best advice is to use having diabetes as *an excuse to exercise,* not as a reason to remain sedentary.

Chapter **17**

Being Active and Female

Females of all ages face special challenges to blood glucose management that are directly related to changes in their hormones. Adolescent girls have raging hormones as their bodies mature that make them more insulin resistant. Women of childbearing age must manage the effects of fluctuating hormones related to monthly cycles, contraceptive use, and pregnancy. Older women deal with hormonal changes when going through menopause and lose the protective effects of estrogen on heart health.

This chapter takes you through how these changes can impact you and your body's responses to physical activity and how to best navigate your way through them all. Knowing more about how to deal with these issues helps you get the most out of your daily movement while still managing your blood glucose effectively.

Understanding How Female Hormones Affect Insulin and Exercise

After going through puberty and before reaching menopause, females continually must factor in the effects of fluctuations in their hormones, including *estrogen* and *progesterone*. These two are the most important hormones made by the ovaries and are considered female sex hormones, but the ovaries also produce some of the more typically male hormone, *testosterone*. Not only do these hormonal swings affect mood and mental state (think PMS), but they can also lead to physical changes (not all of them pleasant or desirable).

Hormonal swings and insulin action

The hardest part for anyone dealing with diabetes is that female hormones influence how effectively insulin works. Changes in their levels can make blood glucose more challenging to manage during certain times of the month.

REMEMBER

Changes in hormonal levels during a woman's normal monthly menstrual cycle can have a large impact on insulin action and blood glucose responses. This monthly cycle has two distinct phases dictated by hormone levels:

>> *Follicular,* which goes from the start of *menses* or *menstruation* (the "period") up to *ovulation* (when eggs are released) at mid-cycle

>> *Luteal,* spanning the time from ovulation to just before the start of the next period

Women are more insulin resistant during the luteal phase (second half of the cycle, the time after ovulation) because of the greater release of estrogen and progesterone during that time. Many women find that their blood glucose levels start to increase gradually seven to ten days before menses and then instantly decrease the day their monthly bleeding begins. If you take insulin you may have to increase your basal doses and/or your total insulin dosing to compensate for greater insulin resistance leading up to your period.

TECHNICAL STUFF

The normal menstrual cycle can last anywhere from 21 to 35 days in adult females, although the average cycle is 28 days long. It's more variable in young teens, lasting from 21 to 45 days. Menstruation also varies from 2 to 7 days (or lasts even longer in some cases). Some women's periods are as regular as clockwork, while others differ in timing from one month to the next.

Not all females are affected equally, with differences related to the actual increases in your female hormone levels. The higher they go, the greater the potential rise in your blood glucose when you have diabetes.

Use of oral contraceptives can alter hormonal fluctuations in women as well. Most of these contraceptive pills, injections, or patches deliver low-dose estrogen and progestin. Although this combination of hormones prevents a woman from ovulating (and getting pregnant), it may also cause her insulin action to be somewhat reduced. But at least insulin action remains more balanced over the monthly cycle with fewer swings, leading to greater predictability and easier glucose management if you use contraceptives.

AVOIDING EXCESSIVE INSULIN RESTRICTION

Insulin promotes the storage of body fat. Because of that fat, some people deliberately take less insulin than they need or skip it altogether — known as *voluntary insulin restriction* — to lose weight or prevent gaining more. Most people who engage in this practice are younger females with type 1 diabetes, although anyone who takes insulin may potentially do so. It's not good for your health, though, and can lead to complications both in the short-term and down the road.

Needing lower doses of insulin overall normally promotes better health, but restricting it purposefully or skipping doses is a completely different situation. Restricting necessary insulin can raise your blood glucose, starve your cells, and lead to the serious condition *diabetic ketoacidosis,* or DKA. Taking too little insulin can also have dire long-term health consequences related to poor diabetes management.

Another interesting fact is that after you go through menopause, you may be more insulin resistant overall (even though your female hormones are greatly diminished). But the levels are relatively stable all the time and not changing from one day or week to the next.

Exercise responses with hormonal changes

Hormonal changes can also affect female athletes who are trying to manage their blood glucose while competing in sports and athletic events. Although very little research has looked at how menstrual cycles can affect sports performance, it appears that monthly cycles may not have much of an impact.

Women may have a higher risk of tissue injuries, especially tears of the anterior cruciate ligament (ACL) in the knee, at certain points in their menstrual cycles. According to limited research, women appear to be more likely to experience such an injury in the first half of their menstrual cycle, especially as they approach ovulation. Although more research is needed to confirm this finding, it's potentially concerning for women athletes.

Staying Active During Pregnancy

Pregnancy typically lasts for 40 weeks, which is slightly more than nine months. Staying physically active throughout your pregnancy, if you can, is so important. Whether you had diabetes before you got pregnant or you develop it while you're expecting, being active can lead to a better pregnancy and a healthier baby.

Keeping your blood glucose in check ensures fewer problems with your pregnancy, childbirth, and the baby.

Being active does not increase the risk of having a low-birth-weight baby, a preterm delivery, or a miscarriage. On the contrary, regular exercise likely reduces your risk of having pregnancy complications, such as *preeclampsia* (elevations in blood pressure that require bed rest) and gestational diabetes.

Keeping insulin lower and fitness higher

During pregnancy, your higher levels of hormones spare your blood glucose for your developing baby (fetus). To do so, they make you very insulin resistant, which can make your insulin needs go up dramatically. Even if you're regularly active, the release of the same hormones during pregnancy as during the luteal phase (second half) of your menstrual cycle ensures that your insulin requirements rise to new highs while you're expecting.

Staying physically active will keep you from having to raise your insulin doses as much, even during the last few months of your pregnancy, and keep you from getting out of shape. You're likely to have a shorter time in labor if you're fit, and who doesn't want a faster delivery?

REMEMBER

Being pregnant isn't a reason to sit around and de-train for nine months. It should be your excuse to prioritize being active above all else in your daily routines — to better your health and the health of your unborn child.

If you have to stop exercising during your pregnancy for any reason, expect your insulin needs to go up dramatically, due to the combination of hormones and decreased insulin action from being inactive.

Avoiding excess weight gain by exercising

Regular exercise also keeps you from gaining too much pregnancy weight. Normal pregnancy weight gain is 25 to 35 pounds. If you're underweight to start, you may need to gain 28 to 40 pounds during pregnancy, and if you're overweight, only 15 to 25 pounds.

Almost half of American moms reportedly gain more than the recommended amount of weight during pregnancy, putting themselves and their babies at risk for health problems. These can include issues like elevations in blood pressure (which can lead to preeclampsia and eclampsia) during pregnancy and complications with labor and delivery (particularly when babies weigh more than 9 pounds). After pregnancy, the mother's extra weight can make her more insulin resistant and lead to problems with lactation.

REMEMBER

Beyond recommended amounts of weight gain, the excess is just extra body fat that you'll have to work extra hard to take off later. Why not just prevent gaining too much in the first place by being active while pregnant? Doing so can mean having fewer stretch marks on your belly, too.

Pregnancy also increases the energy costs of doing any activity. That means you burn more calories during all your activities for nine months, particularly the weight-bearing ones. That's like getting two workouts for the price of one when it comes to using up excess calories.

Exercising throughout pregnancy

Although being active before you get pregnant is a good idea, it's not too late to get started if you're already with child. In fact, all pregnant women are highly recommended to get in 30 minutes of moderate-intensity physical activity on most, if not all, days of the week.

Choosing the right activities

You have a lot of physical activities to choose from when you are pregnant and only a limited number that are better left until after your baby is born (see the following section). If you've been sedentary and are new to exercise when you're pregnant, be more cautious and slowly work up to doing the recommended amounts. If you're already active, you can generally keep doing what you've been doing, although you may need to lower your intensity of some of your workouts later during your pregnancy.

Physical activity recommendations for women during pregnancy include the following:

>> **Overall (duration, intensity, type, and frequency):** 30 minutes of moderate-intensity activity (either aerobic or resistance) at least most days

>> **Aerobic:** Walking, stationary cycling, swimming, aquatic activities, conditioning machines, prenatal exercise classes, prenatal yoga, seated exercises, and possibly jogging or running (if you've been highly active before pregnancy)

>> **Resistance:** Light or moderate resistance exercises (see Chapter 11)

>> **Progression:** If just starting out, increase the duration of moderate exercise slowly; if already more active, maintain or lower intensity during pregnancy instead of attempting to progress to higher levels

TIP

During the third trimester, consider substituting non-weight-bearing activities like aquatics and stationary cycling for running or doing excessive amounts of walking. That will be easier on your back and your leg joints.

You can continue doing both aerobic and resistance training safely. But your exercise intensity will likely need to go down, particularly in the later stages of your pregnancy.

Avoiding the wrong activities

You should avoid certain activities when pregnant — such as contact sports, sports with lots of directional changes (like racquetball), skiing (downhill or water), cycling outdoors (when balance becomes an issue), horseback riding, and scuba diving. But you can continue doing most other ones.

Don't do any exercises lying flat on your back past the second trimester because doing so can reduce blood flow to your developing baby.

Other activities to avoid include the following:

>> Any activities that increase the risk of falling or abdominal trauma

>> Activities done in environmental extremes (too hot, too cold, or at high altitude)

Managing gestational diabetes

Gestational diabetes — or diabetes that develops and lasts during pregnancy only — affects as many as one in seven pregnancies. It's diagnosed when an expecting mother's blood glucose rises too high (usually the third trimester). It's usually discovered with an oral glucose tolerance test (see Chapter 1 for details) at 24 to 28 weeks of pregnancy, although pregnant women who are at high risk for it may need to be tested sooner.

If you're regularly active before becoming pregnant or start early into it, you're less likely to experience a rise in your blood glucose during your pregnancy. You'll also lower your risk of developing type 2 diabetes later in life if you can avoid developing gestational diabetes.

If you're at high risk for gestational diabetes, you may be able to prevent it with lifestyle changes during pregnancy. If you do develop it, you may be able to manage it with just dietary improvements and regular physical activity, although insulin and/or oral medications may be necessary to achieve optimal blood glucose levels in some women.

IN THIS CHAPTER

» **Understanding why kids become inactive**

» **Finding activities to keep the youngest and oldest active**

» **Discovering more about how being physically inactive impacts seniors**

» **Seeing how physical activity helps brain function and mental health**

» **Tracking your biological age through specific markers**

Chapter **18**

Taking Special Considerations for Kids and Seniors

aving a sedentary lifestyle can impact you whether you're young or old, from being a toddler all the way to living more than a hundred years. It's estimated that one in three Americans will have diabetes by the year 2050. The current generation of Americans may be the first to die before their parents due to health conditions that can often be managed or prevented with a healthier lifestyle that includes being more physically active.

This chapter leads you through the unique metabolic challenges related to physical inactivity at both ends of the age spectrum. "Youth" includes all kids under the age of 18, although infants, toddlers, children (ages 5 to 11), and adolescents (ages 12 to 17) may respond differently in some cases. The goal for everyone at any age should be optimal health and mobility, and being regularly active can help you achieve this. Nurture your innate ability to be independent (whether you're young or old) by staying active no matter your age.

Getting at the Root of Physical Inactivity of Today's Youth

Do you ever find yourself telling your kids to go do something active and then sitting around yourself? If so, you aren't alone; more than 60 percent of all American adults (parents included) aren't regularly active, creating a poor model for the next generation.

A lack of physical activity — particularly vigorous exercise — is a consistent contributor to weight gain in youth. The amount of TV watched during childhood and adolescence is associated with a greater chance for type 2 diabetes, poor fitness, high cholesterol, smoking, and obesity in adulthood. The removal of physical education from many schools and the decline in the numbers of kids participating in after-school sports and other physically active extracurricular pursuits contribute to inactivity as well.

REMEMBER

Many pediatricians are now recommending that all youth be restricted to one to two hours a day using TVs and computers combined (although extra time on computers may be allowed for homework).

TIP

Sitting quietly for extended periods is so foreign to kids' natures that it's almost physically impossible for them to do for long. The next time you get ready to put your child into a stroller or chair simply for convenience, consider whether trapping them in a sedentary state is necessary.

KIDS AREN'T JUST MINI-ADULTS

Kids aren't like adults, and not just because kids are smaller. As far as physiology goes, children's bodies respond differently to exercise than adults' bodies do. Children (ages 5 to 11 years) and even adolescents (ages 12 to 17 years) face some unique issues related to physical activity.

Until children go through their final growth spurt and reach puberty, they aren't physically mature. Their bones still need to calcify. Their nervous systems and muscles are immature. How they make ATP from muscle glycogen stores is different and more limited. They have a harder time managing their body heat during exercise because they have a limited ability to heat and cool themselves.

Adults are like the tortoise in the tortoise and the hare scenario, plodding along at one slow pace, while the kids sprint ahead like jack rabbits but then frequently stop and wait for the adults to catch up. Exercise programs for youth should accommodate these distinctions and match the unique physiology of their growing, maturing bodies.

Encouraging Kids to Be Active

You want to start your kids off young learning a healthier way to live, which includes being physically active. For youth of any age with diabetes, exercise can have a positive impact on blood glucose and body weight. You need to keep in mind that they may react differently to activities than adults do, so make sure to keep them exercising safely.

REMEMBER

No matter what you do, don't make being physically active a punishment or negative consequence for your kids. Check out the nearby sidebar "Avoiding making exercise a punishment" for details on this topic.

Examining the effects of exercise on blood glucose

Heavier youth with type 2 diabetes often have a harder time achieving optimal diabetes management, although regular exercise almost invariably improves it. Youth with type 1 diabetes who are active may not necessarily improve their blood glucose, but they will require less insulin and achieve the same long-term health benefits. Being sedentary still leads to worse blood glucose than being active for kids with any type of diabetes.

REMEMBER

If managed effectively, kids with type 1 diabetes can improve their blood glucose with exercise. Youth who exercise more than twice weekly have better A1C levels, particularly if active for 60 minutes at a time or more.

Resistance training lowers insulin resistance in kids of any age, although muscle mass doesn't increase much before they hit puberty. Regular resistance exercise and aerobic training reduce the total daily dose of insulin due to improved insulin action and can promote a healthy weight and help prevent complications.

Keeping kids safe during activities

Here are some facts you need to know about kids and exercise to keep them safe:

>> Their bones, nerves, and muscles are immature before puberty, so resistance training doesn't boost strength or muscle size before puberty.

>> Lifting heavy weights can injure the growth plates in the long bones, which can stunt their growth.

>> Overusing joints like the shoulder (such as by repeatedly throwing a ball) can damage the rotator cuff muscles and surrounding joint structures.

» Injuries can be avoided with a modified training schedule, especially for youth that participate in sports year-round.

» Excessive endurance training can negatively affect bone maturation and health by causing loss of calcium from bones before puberty.

» Youth can only effectively use ATP and creatine phosphate stored in muscle for energy. Longer activities are harder because their lactic acid energy systems (lasting 30 seconds to 2 minutes) are limited by smaller muscle glycogen stores. (Chapter 4 has more on these energy systems.)

» Prepubescent youth use more blood glucose and less muscle glycogen during moderate exercise.

» Carbohydrate drinks may be necessary during extended activities (such as running, soccer, and swimming) for kids to participate at full tilt.

» Immature sweat glands limit kids' ability to sweat to cool down, so give them cool fluids and frequent rest (in shade) during exercise in the heat.

» Keep children warm during outdoor activities in the cold because they can't heat up as well, especially when bench-sitting during sporting events.

As a parent, you should establish some controls and limits to keep your kids safe and injury-free. But youth can make some age-appropriate decisions for themselves, such as which activity to do on a given day.

Nurturing kids' innate love of movement

According to the guidelines, all youth should engage in at least 60 minutes of daily activity, including aerobic, muscle-strengthening, and bone-strengthening activities. Encourage both children and adolescents to be physically active daily as part of play, games, sports, transportation, recreation, physical education, or planned exercise. They can do these activities with their families, at school, and out in the community (for example, through volunteering or employment). Even *exergaming* (playing video games that provide exercise) can be an effective way to get them more active.

For sedentary youth, even participating in physical activity at less than recommended levels can give them some health benefits. If they're currently not doing any activities, they can start with smaller amounts and gradually increase duration, frequency, and intensity to meet the guidelines.

Here are some ideas for younger kids to get active:

» Take your dog out for a walk.

» Start up a playground kickball game or play tag.

>> Join an after-school sports team.

>> Go to the park and play with a buddy.

>> Help out doing chores around the house or with yardwork.

>> Ride your bike to school or to a friend's house.

>> Walk to the store with your parent.

>> See how many jumping jacks or push-ups you can do.

>> Race a friend to the end of the block and back.

Additional ideas for getting teenagers more active include the following:

>> Mow your lawn with a push mower.

>> Go for a walk around the neighborhood or in a nearby park.

>> Take the stairs rather than an elevator or escalator.

>> Bike, inline skate, or skateboard when going to work, running errands, or visiting friends.

>> Walk with a friend during lunch at school, or take family walks.

>> Get an active part-time job for after school or on weekends.

>> Volunteer to become a coach or referee.

>> Get involved in community activities that are physically active.

>> Sign up for a group exercise class or tennis lessons.

>> Use your parents' exercise equipment at home.

>> Take PE classes at school, even in your later years of high school.

>> Join an after-school sports league.

Making movement a family affair

When you see most children outdoors, they're trying to run around, play, and just have fun being active. Why not bring some of that joy that comes from moving your body back not just to sedentary kids but to the whole family?

TIP

Make being physically active fun for everyone with family bike rides, backyard games, hiking trips, or just dancing around the living room. Make sure to set an example for your kids by being active yourself.

Peeling those couch potatoes off the cushions

You may run into some additional challenges if your kid is the ultimate couch potato. If you need some help getting them moving, use other strategies to help motivate the most sedentary kids:

>> Have your kids get up and move around during ads on TV, even if they just walk in place, bounce up and down, or dance during them.

>> Set time limits for all sedentary activities. Have kids do 3 to 5 minutes of physical activity after every 30 minutes of sedentary activity (even reading or doing homework).

>> Turn the TV and all electronic devices off for a specified period of time every day to limit their screen time (no matter how much they protest).

>> Take TVs out of your kids' bedrooms.

>> Use active outings (like bowling or roller skating) as rewards for accomplishments.

>> Buy your kids things that get them active (like skates or a bike) rather than ones that make them sit or be inactive.

>> Ask your kids to do at least one physically active chore around the house or yard daily like sweeping, vacuuming, or raking leaves.

>> Make up a weekly physical activity chart for your kids to record their physical activities, and give them non-food rewards.

>> Do whatever you can to be an active role model, especially doing activities that your kids may think are fun.

>> Help them learn to spend time doing active playing rather than just forcing them to exercise.

>> Teach your kids some flexibility and warm-up exercises to do every day.

>> Use some sidewalk chalk to play hopscotch with your younger kids.

>> Play hide-and-seek with your kids, indoors or outdoors.

>> Plant and tend a garden together with your kids and grow some vegetables that they can eat.

>> Have your kids throw a ball in the yard for a dog.

>> Send your kids to summer camp (daily or overnight).

>> If their school isn't too far away, take the time to walk your kids to school instead of driving or busing them there.

AVOIDING MAKING EXERCISE A PUNISHMENT

You never want kids to associate their negative behaviors with exercise, even when they break a rule, stretch the truth, or otherwise behave as youngsters often do.

There's nothing wrong with being firm when you're trying to get your kids more active, and you do have the right to move their TVs out of their bedrooms. But if you're being senselessly rigid or appear to be punishing them in ways that force being active, your kids are going to react negatively. Remember to make being active as fun as it has the potential to be, and you'll even end up wanting to do it yourself alongside your kids.

>> Involve your kids in a fund-raising walk for charity and collect donations for how far they walk.

>> Adopt an elderly neighbor or relative who can use your kids' help with some chores around the house and yard.

>> Whenever you need to have a serious talk with your kids, take them out for a walk to do it.

>> When they're old enough for part-time jobs, help your teens find active ones (such as lawn care, waiter or busboy, grocery store stocker, and so on).

Looking at Aging and Health in Seniors

As they say, getting old is not for the faint of heart. In fact, aging has few benefits, except that it beats the alternative (dying early). Living a long time but not being healthy for many of your later years isn't desirable either, so you should set your sights on living long *and* well.

REMEMBER

How well you age is largely up to you and the lifestyle choices you make, especially when you have diabetes or prediabetes.

Getting older with diabetes has its own set of potential health complications. For example, whether you have type 1 or type 2 diabetes, you have an increased risk of bone fractures, likely related to elevations in your blood glucose over time. Preventing falls is important for lowering your risk of suffering a fracture or an injury.

Being aware of bodily changes over time

Aging causes bodily changes, many of which are independent of disease, even if you remain physically active throughout your lifetime. The aging process involves a gradual decline in the physiological function of your body's systems. From your mid-20s on, you can expect a number of changes to happen to your body and your mind. You experience slow changes in your various bodily systems, including your heart, lungs, muscles, nervous system, bones, and more. These changes are natural with aging and unavoidable.

REMEMBER

Being active can prevent disability from many chronic illnesses that you can avoid, but physiological aging is natural and not entirely preventable. Expect a slow decrease in your maximal heart rate, the amount of blood pumped by your heart, your lung capacity, and your maximal aerobic capacity over time.

Here's some of what to expect from these bodily changes as you age:

>> **Strength and endurance:** You have lower overall strength and endurance the older you get, particularly as you start to lose both muscle strength and mass.

- Your muscles selectively lose the fast-twitch fibers used for power and speed (used during heavy resistance or interval training).

- Doing training can't help you get these fibers back, but being active can delay or prevent their loss in the first place.

>> **Bone density:** Losing calcium and other minerals from your bones accelerates with age, particularly for women after they hit menopause, making your bones easier to fracture from falls or just in general.

>> **Body composition:** You have more fat and less muscle, even if your weight stays the same, which can make it harder for you to move your weight around.

>> **Metabolic rate:** A drop in your metabolism reflects how much muscle you've lost, but doing resistance training can offset this decline somewhat.

REMEMBER

Older adults face unique challenges to staying active, including joint injuries, arthritis, osteoporosis and fracture risk, instability, falls, and frailty.

Slowing the effects of time

Exercise is the best medicine to combat aging and preventable diseases because it can prevent, slow, or reverse at least some of the bodily changes listed in the preceding section. For instance, exercise can keep breathing muscles trained and strong, enabling you to take deeper breaths during exercise. You can fight the loss of faster muscle fibers by using them when you exercise through resistance training and pushing yourself to do harder weights or resistance. Likewise, doing balance exercises can help you improve your stability and prevent falls in the first place.

TECHNICAL STUFF

Although your body's maximal ability to use oxygen during exercise typically declines a steady 1.5 percent per year, older athletes who are highly trained have a slower decline more in the range of 0.5 percent per year. However, the decline is still steady even if it's slower. Master (older) athletes have the same insulin sensitivity as younger ones, making an increase in insulin resistance (and type 2 diabetes risk) largely preventable as you age. You can also keep your bones healthier: You can reduce the rate of mineral loss through regular exercise, particularly resistance training and weight-bearing activities like walking.

Recognizing whether decline is due to aging or inactivity

Though many people view getting chronic diseases like obesity or diabetes as inseparable from aging, such conditions aren't all inevitable as you get older. That said, you can hasten your ultimate demise by having an inactive lifestyle.

Regardless of whether you have diabetes, preventing an early death or lasting impairment from treatable health issues is worthwhile. Regular training can slow declines in muscle mass (at least to a point) and help you stay stronger. If you have diabetes, an added benefit is that having more insulin-sensitive muscle mass (where glucose is stored) helps to keep your blood glucose lower, and that adds greatly to your well-being if you can avoid health complications from diabetes. To live long and well, be vigilant about all aspects of your health.

Many of the usual declines in insulin action associated with aging, however, may be caused more by obesity and lack of physical activity than aging itself. Regular physical activity is critical to managing most of these conditions, and in many cases may actually prevent or possibly reverse them.

Being active raises insulin action

If you're physically trained, you already know that you generally have a heightened sensitivity to insulin. The reason apparently varies with the type of training you do.

Both aerobic and resistance training may improve insulin action, but apparently by different mechanisms. Resistance training increases your muscle mass, which lets you store more glucose in your muscles as *glycogen*. Aerobic endurance training doesn't make you gain as much muscle, but it does make your muscles take up more glucose — without needing much insulin — for 2 to 72 hours after you exercise. Sedentary, insulin-resistant, middle-aged adults doing 30 minutes of moderate walking three to seven days per week for six months reversed their prediabetes just by being active, even without changing their diets or losing any weight. Similarly, older adults who walked on mini-trampolines for 20 to 40 minutes four days per week for four months increased their blood glucose use for the same insulin release without any weight loss.

No matter your age, exercise training can improve your insulin action within just one week of training without weight loss or a true training adaptation in your muscles. Add in some resistance training, and then you're good to go.

Avoiding muscle wasting and fat gain

You may be focused on trying to get down to a slimmer you, but as you get older, losing weight can be a mixed bag (see Chapter 15 for a fuller discussion of this topic). In short, losing weight is usually beneficial to your health if you only lose body fat, but it can also be bad if what you're losing is your muscle mass. *Sarcopenia*, or muscle wasting, can vastly decrease your quality of life and speed up the aging process.

BEWARE OF POLYPHARMACY

Many older adults take multiple prescription medications for their various health problems. Some of these medications can result in side effects that require another medication to treat. Taking four or more medications per day (known as *polypharmacy*) is very common in older adults who have diabetes. Though not all medications negatively impact your ability to be active, some of them can make exercising more difficult.

One of the best examples is statins, a class of medications prescribed to adults to lower their cholesterol levels. Their use in people with diabetes is widespread. Statins, unfortunately, double your risk of having a muscle-related problem that can force you to be sedentary, and they increase your risk of acute injuries like Achilles tendon ruptures during activity. Certain diuretic medications ("water pills") you may take to lower your blood pressure can also reduce your exercise tolerance, give you low blood pressure, or cause you to fall due to dehydration.

If you take four or more medications daily, talk to your doctor about whether you may be able to change what you take or get by with fewer medications as you age — especially if any of them are keeping you from being as active. Exercising improves your cholesterol profile and lowers your blood pressure, so you may be able to solve some of your health problems without medication just by keeping physically fit and active, or at least use less medication to achieve the same results

Some research on overweight adults reported that sarcopenia is associated with insulin resistance in all individuals, regardless of how much body fat they have. If they're obese, they're even more likely to have elevations in their blood glucose. That study concluded that sarcopenia, independent of obesity, is associated with adverse blood glucose metabolism, especially in adults who are less than 60 years old. Having less muscle when you're younger than 60 may be an early predictor of possibly getting type 2 diabetes in such cases.

Losing weight without exercising regularly can cause you to lose muscle rather than fat and is a recipe for disaster when it comes to your long-term metabolic health.

A huge problem with losing a lot of weight after you reach middle age is that your loss will be at best about 75 percent fat and 25 percent muscle for the typical dieter. But when you gain weight back afterward (which is extremely common within six months to a year), up to 85 percent of what you gain back is pure body fat. Ending up with less muscle after dieting makes you burn fewer calories daily, which makes gaining weight easier even when you're eating the same number of calories after your diet as you did before. If you're one of those people who frequently cycles between losing weight and gaining it back, you'll likely end up with so little muscle that you may have trouble carrying around your extra weight.

When losing weight, you must regularly exercise to maintain your muscle mass. Being active is likely more important than how many calories you eat when it comes to maintaining a good body weight and your health. Dieters who fail to exercise lose more muscle mass. Exercising when you're cutting back on your calories stimulates your body to keep the muscle, which also keeps metabolism operating at a higher level.

What's the best long-term advice for managing your body weight and your muscle health? Lose the diets, keep yourself regularly active (including doing resistance training), and eat a healthful diet.

Getting Seniors Up and Moving

Exercise recommendations for seniors aren't that different from those for the general population. In fact, physical activity and exercise guidelines for adults who are 18 to 64 years old and generally healthy apply to older adults (ages 65 and older), with a few modifications. Chapter 9 covers the types and amounts of recommended activities (cardio and interval, resistance and core, balance, and flexibility training).

But some additional physical activity recommendations are specific to adults 65 and older. Many also apply to adults less than 65 with a chronic disease or other health issues that may limit their ability to exercise.

Cardio training and intervals

When you're older, factoring in how fit you are (or aren't) when you start an exercise program is important, especially if you've been living a mostly sedentary lifestyle. If you can't meet the recommendation of 150 minutes of moderate-intensity aerobic exercise weekly, be as physically active as your abilities and health allow. If you have an ongoing health issue, learn more about how it may affect your ability to do regular physical activity safely, and then get more active however you can.

In addition to being active by doing some moderate-intensity aerobic and muscle-strengthening activities, aim to be more active overall in your daily life.

As far as interval training goes, adding in short periods of working out faster or harder is possible. Doing some of the trendy workouts like high-intensity interval training isn't recommended — at least as a starting point — for most older adults. (See more about this type of interval training in Chapter 10.)

Doing workouts with vigorous interval training is likely not the best thing for you if you're currently sedentary and obese or have health issues that may get worse due to a high-intensity workout.

Resistance and core training

Doing resistance training at least twice a week is recommended for all adults, but it's absolutely critical for older adults who want to age well. It's the only way to reverse your loss of muscle mass and to keep from losing more as you age. Aim for three resistance workouts a week, on nonconsecutive days, to best prevent additional losses associated with aging and being inactive.

Resistance training that focuses on your core body muscles — your abdominal, low-back, and hips regions — is also essential for older adults. If you can keep your core muscles strong, you prevent low-back pain, improve your ability to walk and do other everyday activities, and decrease your chances of falling during activities.

Include core exercises in your resistance workouts two to three days a week for optimal strength and health as you age.

Balance training

Your biggest worry as you age should be injuring yourself in a fall; head injuries in particular can be lethal. Falling is one of the biggest concerns facing the aging population.

REMEMBER

For many older people, breaking a hip from a fall increases the risk of a quick decline in health and can lead to dying within a year or two. Do everything in your power to stay on your feet and avoid falls and potential injuries that can limit your health and vitality and cut your life short.

If you're forced to spend weeks or months off your feet healing broken hips or other bones, you lose muscle mass, strength, bone density, balance ability, and more — things that are even harder to get back the older you get. The best thing you can do is practice keeping your balance by doing daily exercises. Fitting them into your schedule doesn't take much time, and the payback from doing them regularly is so worth the effort. (See Chapter 12 for exercises you can practice to improve your balance.)

Flexibility training

Staying flexible is also important because being limber keeps you from falling as well (see the preceding section). Doing everything in life is easier if your joints are working well and let you move them through their full range of motion. As I discuss in Chapter 13, everyone loses flexibility with aging, and having elevated blood glucose can accelerate the process.

Fit in some stretching as many days per week as you can. Certainly, you should stretch anything that feels tight after your workouts, and always remember to warm up your joints and muscles first before trying to stretch them. You can stretch statically or during movement (dynamically), but static stretches are likely to increase your range of motion around joints more over time than dynamic stretching.

TIP

Check out a yoga or tai chi class to work on your flexibility, balance, and strength at the same time.

Breaking up sedentary time

The latest research confirms that interspersing your sedentary time with any type of movement improves your physical function, and it may preserve your ability to take care of yourself on a daily basis as you age. When you have diabetes, it can help lower your blood glucose as well.

TIP

Get up after every 30 minutes of a sedentary activity and move around for a few minutes. As long as you do something active, the specific activity doesn't seem to matter.

Moving more all day long

Many older adults with multiple health issues think that they can't exercise regularly, but they usually can. The people who are the most sedentary can get the greatest health benefits from simply moving more however they can. If you're in this boat, grab an oar (figuratively) and start paddling to get healthier.

Even if you have some limits on your activities due to your health, joint issues, medical treatments, or something else, being as active as you can be still pays dividends. Any muscles you're not using lose strength and mass over time. Bones become less dense and more likely to fracture when you don't walk or pick things up with your arms.

Brisk walking, gardening, yardwork, and housework are good examples of spontaneous or unstructured activities that boost your physical function, build strength, and expend calories. Even home-based interventions and tai chi programs may be effective in reducing your fear of falling and lead you to being more active overall. (Refer to Chapter 9 for more ideas on how to increase your daily activity.)

Having a disability that limits your mobility or puts you in a wheelchair doesn't mean that you can't be regularly active. Working just your upper body can increase your mobility as you gain enhanced upper-body strength, endurance, and flexibility. Any type of activity can also give you health benefits, even if you do it sitting in a chair or wheelchair.

Working Out for Your Mental Health and Function

Exercising has payoffs for your mind, too; it can improve feelings of overall well-being, along with reducing stress and depression. Just getting up from your desk at work when you're stressed out and going for a short walk can clear your mind, improve your mood, and enhance your productivity. Exercise is an effective remedy for mild to moderate depression.

KEEP YOUR ARTHRITIC JOINTS PAIN-FREE FOR LIFE

Living with the daily pain of arthritic joints can make you feel a lot less youthful. The most common type is *osteoarthritis,* caused by degeneration of bony joint surfaces, usually in the knees, hips, spine, hands, and toes. This "wear and tear" arthritis is more common in joints that have been previously injured, particularly traumatically (through contact sports injuries).

Arthritis can cause pain in affected joints after repeated use, especially later in the day. Or you may experience swelling, pain, and stiffness after long periods of inactivity (for example, after sleep or sitting long periods), and you feel better after moving around some. The pain doesn't come from the joint cartilage surfaces (they contain no nerve endings) but rather from the irritated nerves in adjacent inflamed areas. Pain can be continuous when almost all the cartilage surfaces of joints have been eroded, at which point your arthritis is quite advanced.

To prevent painful flare-ups, avoid doing intense activities that can further injure your joint's bony surfaces. Moderate aerobic exercise is okay as long as you do it at an intensity that doesn't make it worse (for example, don't do vigorous running if you have bad knees).

Focus on strengthening surrounding muscles that will support and protect your painful joints. For your knees, strengthen both groups of muscles in your thighs that affect knee movement including your quadriceps in the front and hamstrings in the back. Try non-weight-bearing activities like stationary cycling, aquatics, and light to moderate resistance work to lower stress on joints. See Chapter 15 for more recommended activities.

Physical activity also has the power to lower your risk of Alzheimer's disease and other forms of dementia that occur in adults of all ages. Even in younger individuals, being a couch potato leads to brain *atrophy* (shrinkage), and just six months of regular aerobic training reduces rates of brain shrinkage. All physical activities increase blood flow and oxygen delivery to your brain and boost the part of your brain called the *hippocampus,* the region associated with memory and spatial navigation.

REMEMBER

Being active not only can delay or prevent dementia but also may be able to restore some of what you've lost mentally. Just as daily exercise strengthens certain muscle groups, mental exercise strengthens and enhances your ability to think, reason, and remember things.

Try doing any and all of these mental exercises to stimulate all your senses, logical thinking, and mental reasoning:

>> Memorize any list and recall as many of the items as you can later.

>> Listen to or read the news and later write a summary of all that you heard.

>> Read challenging articles and books of all types.

>> Think of a word and then of as many others as you can that begin with the same two letters.

>> Take a sentence from something you're reading and try to make other sentences using the same words in a different order.

>> Play online or video games, particularly ones that require quick responses and even some physical activity. (Don't use your new gaming habit as an excuse to be sedentary, though!)

>> Play card or board games that require mental reasoning, such as pinochle, bridge, chess, checkers, or Othello.

>> Do crossword puzzles, anagrams, Sudoku, or other reasoning games.

>> Practice doing math problems in your head, particularly ones that you personally find challenging.

>> Learn a new language, either on your own or by taking a class.

>> Sign up for other courses that are challenging and fun for you.

>> Look at and then draw an object a day to stimulate short-term memory. To work long-term memory, once a week draw all seven objects from the past week without first looking to see what they were.

>> Draw a plan or map of any place you visit that was new to you.

>> When eating, try to identify the individual ingredients based on taste.

>> Use smell and touch to identify objects with your eyes closed.

>> Vary the route that you take home to see if you can figure out a slightly different way to arrive at the same place.

>> Use your creativity to think up new ways to exercise your mind daily.

Assessing How Well You're Aging, Really

Not every organ or tissue in your body ages at the same rate. If you can enhance their function, you may be able to slow down the biological changes that make you feel your age. Taking a look at select biomarkers may give you a better feel of how well you're really aging, biologically speaking, compared to your actual chronological age.

Some areas to look at are your blood pressure, blood glucose and cholesterol levels, maximal aerobic capacity, breathing capacity, and bone density. The younger you appear on these measures, the longer you're likely to live well (no matter how long that ends up being). Feeling well while they're alive is more important to most people than simply living a long time — especially if they're unwell or aging poorly. You can check out how well you're aging through the measures that follow.

>> **Cardiovascular function:** This aging biomarker is indicated by your blood pressure. It's easily measured as *systolic* (recorded as the first number, such as "130" for a reading of "130 over 85") and *diastolic* blood pressure. If it's normal, your top (systolic) number will never be over about 120. But it goes up in many people as they age and their blood vessels become stiffer. If you want to lower yours, exercise regularly, lose some weight (especially around your middle), cut back on your salt intake, eat more fish, and take medications to control it.

>> **Breathing capacity:** This measurement represents how strong your breathing *(ventilatory)* muscles are and how expandable your lungs remain. A health care provider can measure both the total amount of air you can force out of your lungs quickly and how much air you breathe in and out. Having emphysema can severely limit your breathing ability and increase your aging, so if you smoke, consider stopping now to slow down your lungs' rapid aging.

>> **Metabolic activity:** Lab work you get at your checkups should include your fasting blood glucose and cholesterol. After an overnight fast, your blood glucose should be between 70 and 99 mg/dL — the lower the better. If yours is between 100 and 125 mg/dL, you're in a prediabetic range, and over 125 mg/dL is a diagnosis of diabetes. Any elevation in your glucose levels above normal can make your blood vessels age more rapidly.

For your cholesterol, lower totals are better for avoiding heart disease. Have your cholesterol subfractions measured (like HDL and LDL) because they're not all equally bad, and some are actually beneficial. Fluffy LDL-cholesterol is likely harmless.

>> **Bone mineral density:** You can get a bone mineral density scan to find markers of aging like thinner bones, arthritis, and bone spurs. If your bone density is low for your age, you may be able to raise it with exercise training (especially weight-bearing and resistance workouts), hormone therapy (estrogen in women), calcium, and vitamin D.

>> **Systemic inflammation:** Your doctor can test your blood for various blood markers that indicate whether your blood vessels are inflamed. When certain compounds in blood are present, your blood vessels may not work as well and get injured over time, which can cause plaque to form and lead to heart attacks or strokes. Physical activity is known to have anti-inflammatory effects on the body, so getting more active lowers inflammatory markers in blood and lessens potential damage to slow down aging of blood vessels.

>> **Maximal aerobic capacity:** You may not need a maximal exercise stress test to test your heart disease risk, but you can do one just to find out your fitness level. This testing reflects your biological age by looking at the coordination and function of your heart, lungs, blood vessels, and muscles all together. The higher your maximal aerobic capacity, the younger your biological age. You can improve your aerobic capacity on your own with an exercise training program to a certain extent, but the rest of your maximum is determined by your genes.

>> **Muscular strength:** An easy way to get a snapshot of your muscle strength is to measure your hand grip strength with a special device called a *hand dynamometer.* When your strength starts to go on this test, it reflects how much muscle you're losing in the rest of your body — a marker of declining biological age. Doing resistance training can boost muscle strength through-out your body, slowing or preventing aging associated with loss of muscle.

>> **Reaction time:** Special testing equipment can measure how quickly you can react to stimuli, but it's hard to find. In general, your ability to react quickly reflects how well your nerves conduct messages to your brain and back to your muscles. The faster they go, the younger you likely are, biologically speaking. It's hard to improve your reaction time much with physical training, but it never hurts to get stronger to compensate for slower reaction times.

>> **Mental function:** Testing by your doctor or another health care professional can detect mild cognitive changes and dementia. How well your mind works often reflects the state of your body. See the preceding section for more on how physical activity can help with mental function and well-being.

>> **Skin elasticity:** You can do this easy skin elasticity test on yourself. Pinch up the skin on the back of one hand between the thumb and forefinger of your other hand. Let go and watch how quickly your skin returns to its normal shape. Compare your response to that of your kids or grandkids, and you can easily see that they're biologically younger when their skin snaps back into place more quickly than yours. You can't do much about how fast your skin ages other than eating healthful foods, staying out of the sun as much as possible, wearing sunscreen, and keeping yourself hydrated (because dehydrated skin stays pinched up longer, regardless of your age).

Chapter **19**

Managing Diabetes as an Athlete

An athlete lives in everyone, even if you don't consider yourself one. Being athletic is more a state of mind than anything else. That said, some people with diabetes are actual competitive athletes, taking part in professional sports, the Olympics, and collegiate and high school competitions.

This chapter is geared toward helping you if you're a competitive athlete, but it's relevant even if you're just a more serious recreational one. Many different factors can impact your exercise performance — which can be gauged by how well you do and how good you feel while doing it — and now just may the time for you to get a performance tune-up.

Taking Your Activity to the Next Level

Most of what you need to know about how to effectively progress your exercise training you can find in earlier chapters. How fast you progress should be an individual choice, but it does take time to establish an exercise habit and to increase your fitness level.

When your training has lapsed (or you're just starting an exercise program), you benefit from an initial conditioning phase lasting four to six weeks. After that, you move on to an improvement phase for four to five months and then to a maintenance phase from six months on. If you already have a higher level of fitness, you may be able to shorten or skip the initial conditioning altogether.

Bumping up your training intensity

When you already have a fitness base, additional gains happen if you work out more at the higher end of your intensity range. You can do short, harder intervals or sustained higher-intensity training. Intervals are equally effective, usually more motivating, and better for avoiding overuse injuries. (Discover more about interval training in Chapter 10.)

The *overload principle* of training states that you must keep challenging your body to have any further fitness improvements or gains in muscle strength, or else you just reach a plateau. Increasing your intensity works both during the improvement phase and after you reach the maintenance stage. At that point, your progress slows unless you continue to overload yourself by increasing your exercise intensity, duration, frequency, or a combination of these factors. If you're as fit as you want to get, just work on staying that way.

REMEMBER

Interval training during aerobic workouts is a viable way to boost your fitness, especially if you don't like doing sustained harder workouts.

Pumping it up until fatigue sets in

In resistance workouts, you maximize your strength gains by doing 8 to 12 repetitions of each exercise (usually 8 to 10 different exercises) until you're feeling fatigued. If you're a novice at resistance work, you can start out with lighter weights or more-flexible resistance bands that enable you to complete one or two sets of 12 to 15 repetitions on each exercise, but use enough weight or resistance to feel at least somewhat fatigued by the end of the last set.

If you want to get a lot stronger, your goal should be to ultimately move a greater resistance fewer times (maybe 6 to 10 repetitions). Doing hard work produces more of an overload on the muscle fibers and brings you greater gains in muscular strength and mass.

REMEMBER

After you gain muscle mass, you burn more calories overall, your resting metabolism increases, and your insulin sensitivity improves.

The current resistance training recommendations don't tell you how many sets of repetitions you should do on each exercise. It has been proven that you can gain strength by doing only one set — that is, you can get stronger doing just one maximal repetition one time a week — but you're likely to gain more strength by performing two or three sets of each.

When doing more than one set per exercise, you can increase the weight or resistance on each successive set, slightly decreasing the number of reps each time the load increases (for example, doing 15 reps on the first set and only 10 on the second, harder set). You can also do it in reverse and decrease the weight while upping the reps on the second or third set. The idea is just to fatigue the muscles you're using for any given exercise, and there are many ways to arrive at that goal.

TIP

If you have time for only one set, make it an intense, nearly maximal set that fully fatigues your muscles by the time you reach the last repetition.

Knowing why your training state matters

When it comes to managing diabetes, how well trained you are definitely matters. How hard you're working out affects what fuels your body is using. How long your activity lasts also makes a difference because some athletic events are so short that only the first and second energy systems come into play (see more on those in Chapter 4). They can be trained, but they don't change as much with training as the aerobic energy system that relies heavily on carbohydrates and fat for fuel.

Here's where your training state has the biggest impact. Being aerobically trained doing a specific activity can increase how much fat your body uses when you're working out or competing. Most energy is supplied by carbohydrates when you do an activity at a somewhat-hard to hard intensity level. You use up a lot of stored glycogen from active muscles but also use some blood glucose.

REMEMBER

The amount of fat you can use as an alternate fuel during aerobic activities depends on your training state, how hard you're working out, and how long you stay active.

After you're more trained, if you're working out at the same absolute intensity or pace, your muscles bump up their fat use. If you keep the relative exercise intensity the same by increasing your pace after you're trained, then fat use increases only slightly.

All this information matters to how well you can keep your blood glucose stable and near-normal during exercise. You want to be able to use more fat and spare your body's carbohydrate supply to do well in prolonged athletic events or endeavors. You want to avoid hypoglycemia that makes you slow down or stop so you can excel at your sport or any activity you choose to do with diabetes.

Take your training to the next level to get as fit as you can doing each activity that you participate in.

To a certain extent, you have to start the process over with each new activity you do, although being trained for one sport or activity does convey a higher starting level because your heart, lungs, and blood vessels may already be trained to operate at a higher level from your other types of training.

Carb Loading Effectively for the Athlete

Almost all serious exercisers benefit from carbohydrate (carb) loading before long-distance events and carb reloading afterwards. Having an adequate intake of carbs at both times enables you to begin exercise with fully restored or even over-full stores of *muscle glycogen* (glucose stored in muscle and used during exercise).

The original carb-loading protocol before events was three to seven days of eating a high-carb diet (8 to 10 grams of carbs per kilogram of body weight). This diet was combined with a day or two of complete rest or a reduced exercise volume known as *tapering*.

But even a single day with a higher carb intake and rest or tapering can effectively maximize carb stores. Carb loading has been blown out of proportion and misapplied to all sorts of sporting events (like 5K walks) during which you have no risk of running out of muscle glycogen. You don't need to spend a week, or even three days, over-consuming carbs and potentially lowering your insulin sensitivity and raising your blood glucose by doing so.

If you eat enough calories and rest the day *before* your event, you'll have enough muscle glycogen stored to make it through most athletic endeavors. However, you need to effectively manage your blood glucose that day for full glycogen storage.

Most athletes make sure to take in plenty of carbs after their event or workout as well to restore glycogen in muscles as soon as possible. It can be different for people with diabetes, though, because it takes having enough insulin in your blood to restore glycogen effectively.

Not taking enough carbs after exercise can make it hard to do your next workout, but some people purposefully don't eat enough to keep their insulin action higher for longer after workouts or sporting events. Insulin action stays higher until the glycogen in your muscles is fully restored. That usually takes one to two days when you eat a normal diet — but it can take much longer if you're eating low-carb (head to the following section).

TIP

Consider your event and your normal training schedule when deciding how many carbs to eat and when to eat them. If you need some extra help, consider meeting with a sports dietitian, especially one that is a certified diabetes educator if you can find one, to help design a food and carbohydrate plan to maximize your ability to train and compete.

REMEMBER

If you eat enough calories and at least 40 percent of them come from carbs, your intake likely is adequate for refilling of muscle glycogen stores *after* workouts as well.

Training Well with Low-Carb Eating

Even though your body improves its ability to use fat and ketones as a fuel for exercise when you're on a low-carb regimen, fat is never your body's first choice of fuels during moderate and intense workouts lasting more than a couple of minutes. If your body can get carbs, it uses them rather than fat, particularly as your workout gets more intense. It happens simply because using carbs is more *fuel efficient* — that is, you get more energy out of carbs for a given quantity of oxygen.

REMEMBER

Carbs are like using a higher-octane fuel, resulting in more bang for the buck. If you want to exercise intensely and you eat a very low-carb diet, you likely won't be able to perform at your highest potential level.

If you're eating enough calories to cover what your body needs on a daily basis (including what you use during exercise), you can get by with consuming 40 percent or less of your calories from carbs. Eating more than that doesn't necessarily benefit exercise because it's not a case of "some is good, so more is better." Most people who are training overeat carbs, given the limited amount and intensity of training that they do. (See the preceding section for more on proper carb loading before an event.)

Scrutinizing whether low-carb eating hurts performance

Fully restoring muscle glycogen if you deplete any during exercise takes 24 to 48 hours, assuming you're eating adequate amounts of carbs. If you're on a low-carb regimen, the process takes longer, and you may be trying to do your next workout with less muscle and liver glycogen on board.

REMEMBER

If you can do less intense exercise as well as you want to while eating low-carb and performing optimally at the highest level doesn't matter to you as much as just finishing your events with a respectable time, then an active low-carb lifestyle may work just fine for you.

Despite what you may think, running low on carbs doesn't automatically bump up your fat use during exercise. As everyone says in the exercise world, "Fat burns in a carbohydrate flame." What that means is that if you don't have carbs left in your muscles, you can't use fat as a fuel very well either. Without glycogen, your fat use is compromised, and you have to slow down your pace to a level where you just don't need much carbohydrate.

Do you need to restrict carbs so severely if you're exercising regularly? Probably not. Even people with type 2 diabetes can handle carbs better when doing regular physical activity that depletes some muscle glycogen. You feel less tired and more energetic when eating some carbs during and after exercise to speed up muscle glycogen repletion.

REMEMBER

On days off from exercise, a lower-carb diet may help keep your insulin sensitivity heightened for longer.

Anyone with type 1 diabetes needs to keep blood glucose as near to normal as possible to get optimal glycogen into muscle and liver storage depots. It won't be effectively restored if your blood glucose is running on the high side.

Using the window of opportunity for carbs

Taking in some carbs post-exercise is likely the most important time — particularly during that window of opportunity from 30 minutes to 2 hours after a workout when glycogen repletion rates are highest. That period is also when you need the least insulin to cover any carbs you eat.

REMEMBER

Your carb intake doesn't have to be a lot. Start with 15 to 30 grams, depending on how long and hard you worked out.

Troubleshooting Exercise Blood Glucose for Competitive and Serious Recreational Athletes

Many different factors can impact your blood glucose responses, and the more you know about them, the better equipped you are to figure out what works best for you in almost every situation. This process always takes some trial and error.

Sometimes it's still difficult to figure out what is causing the blood glucose or other exercise responses you're having. Try these strategies if you're experiencing any of these issues with being active with diabetes.

Managing hypoglycemia

Getting low blood glucose during physical activity not only is annoying but also can compromise your ability to complete your event or competition. No one likes to get low during exercise.

If you've been experiencing any exercise–related lows, consider taking some of these actions or precautions to avoid it, especially if you use insulin:

>> Check your blood glucose more often if you've had a bad low or exercised hard in the 24 hours prior to your latest workout.

>> Keep in mind that doing new or unaccustomed exercise is more likely to result in lows, both during and following the activity.

>> Exercise when your blood levels of insulin are lower (like before meals or first thing in the morning before taking any meal insulin).

>> Take in extra carbohydrates before, during, and after activity (the amount dependent on the intensity, duration, starting blood glucose levels, and so on).

>> Consume some protein and/or fat after exercise and also at bedtime to counteract lows later on (and overnight).

>> If possible, choose pre-exercise foods that allow you to take the smallest doses of insulin to cover them to keep circulating insulin levels lower.

>> Prior to doing longer duration exercise, lower your insulin levels during exercise by lowering your closest pre-exercise dose(s).

>> Lower pre-exercise insulin you take within two to three hours before doing an activity (or set a lower basal rate if you use an insulin pump).

>> Remember that how quickly insulin is absorbed depends on the size of the dose: Smaller doses (one to three units) are absorbed more rapidly than larger doses (five or more units), which linger for longer.

>> If using an insulin pump, you can lower your basal rate prior to the start of exercise for one to two hours as well as during (and after) the activity.

>> If giving basal insulin (like Lantus/Basaglar or Levemir), consider splitting the dose (although not necessarily evenly) to give it twice daily to allow for easier dose reductions pre- and post-activity.

>> If low following exercise, reduce your dose of rapid-acting insulin given after any activity, or lower basal insulin for 4 to 12 hours.

>> Your insulin needs are lower when you're regularly active, and you may need permanently lower basal (and mealtime) insulin doses.

>> Doing an all-out sprint for 10 to 30 seconds helps counteract most lows during exercise, but only if your insulin levels aren't too high.

>> Avoid massaging the area where you just gave some insulin (because massaging it can speed up its absorption).

>> Getting in a hot tub or other prolonged heat exposure can speed up the absorption of any insulin taken (causing lows first, then highs later).

Handling hyperglycemia

If you've been experiencing high blood glucose related to being active, consider these possible ways to troubleshoot and correct your levels:

>> If your pre-exercise blood glucose is over 250 mg/dL and has been for more than a few hours, consider giving some insulin and waiting for the level to decrease (particularly if you have moderate or higher ketones).

>> If your blood glucose is over 300 mg/dL with no ketones, exercising is okay, but use caution because you can dehydrate more easily.

>> For early morning exercise (before breakfast), you may need a small dose of insulin (less than normal) and/or a small snack to break your fast to reduce your glucose-raising hormones like cortisol.

>> Eating a full meal within an hour of exercising can slow digestion and result in high blood glucose an hour or two afterward, particularly when you consume lower glycemic index foods and drinks. (Chapter 6 has more on the glycemic index.)

>> Stay hydrated during activities because dehydration can make blood glucose seem higher and cause you to give too much insulin later.

>> After you've trained for a few weeks doing a certain activity, you likely need fewer carbohydrates or smaller insulin reductions than before.

>> When you've participated in an activity that makes you get very sore (peaking two to three days afterward), you may be more insulin resistant because you can't restore muscle glycogen until your muscle damage from the activity is repaired.

>> For blood glucose elevations right after exercise, cut back on your carb intake during exercise, reduce your insulin less, or take some insulin after exercise (but make it a smaller amount than normal).

>> If the stress or intensity of competitions raises your blood glucose, keep basal insulin higher during the activity and only give 50 percent or less of your usual correction dose to lower glucose during or afterward.

>> If you carb load before events, take enough insulin to cover your carb intake; otherwise, it can raise your blood glucose and limit glycogen storage. Check out the earlier section "Carb Loading Effectively for the Athlete" for details on this training approach.

>> If you disconnect your pump during activities and your blood glucose starts to rise over time, reconnect at least once an hour and supplement with at least a portion of your missed basal dose to cover it.

>> Consider an untethered pump regimen where you give some of your insulin a long-acting insulin injection (Lantus, Basaglar, Levemir, Toujeo, or Tresiba) and the remainder as a reduced basal rate through the pump. Then if you disconnect, you still are receiving some background insulin and are less likely to have hyperglycemia post-exercise.

>> Keep insulin from getting too hot or too cold, or its action may diminish and cause usual doses to not cover your insulin needs.

>> Injected or pumped insulin is absorbed faster in smaller doses, so after a larger dose, you may end up too high first and then too low later on.

>> Smaller doses of basal insulin are absorbed more rapidly than larger ones (think 5 units versus 20) and often don't last as long as they're supposed to (24 hours for Lantus/Basaglar, closer to 12 hours for Levemir).

Avoiding early-onset or excessive fatigue

Did you ever DNF ("did not finish") a race or a competition? Certainly, that can happen if you twist your ankle, cramp up, or otherwise get injured. But sometimes your performance is affected when you get tired too soon during an event or if the fatigue is so bad you simply can't go on.

Here are actions you can take to prevent fatigue that comes on early or is bad enough to make you stop before you reach your athletic goals:

>> Prevent both hypoglycemia and hyperglycemia (see the preceding sections) to delay or prevent fatigue when you're physically active.

>> Keep your blood glucose as close to normal as possible for a day or two beforehand so your body can store optimal amounts of carbohydrate in muscle and liver (as glycogen).

>> Consume carbohydrates during exercise to provide an alternate source of blood glucose (other than the limited amount your liver can release).

» Avoid hyperglycemia by having adequate insulin in your blood to counterbalance the release of glucose-raising hormones during exercise.

» Try out new food or insulin strategies during practices, not events or competitions.

» Keep yourself adequately hydrated before and during motion, especially if your blood glucose levels have been running above normal levels.

» If muscle cramps are causing you to stop early, consider supplementing with magnesium and possibly a B vitamin complex. Also have your blood iron levels checked because anemia can cause fatigue, particularly during exercise. The following section has more on these deficiencies.

Considering other performance variables

Has your exercise performance been less than you'd hoped recently? Many different things can cause poor performance or unusual fatigue, but here are some potential causes (and solutions) to consider when you have diabetes and are athletically inclined.

Inadequate rest time

If you're doing well with your workouts, but not with your races and events, you may simply not be resting long enough to restore glycogen, repair muscle damage (caused by every workout), and fully recover. Cutting back on your workouts (tapering) for at least one to two days before a big event is critical. During that time, keep your blood glucose as close to normal as possible so your glycogen levels are as full as possible for your race or event day.

Blood glucose and glycogen stores

Restoring your muscle glycogen between workouts takes eating enough carbohydrates and having insulin in your body that works adequately. Doing longer and harder workouts can deplete glycogen stores, and you may not be fully replenishing them fast enough because you're either not eating enough carbs or not keeping your blood glucose in check. You must have an adequate amount of insulin available to restore the glycogen in your liver and muscles.

Iron levels

Having low iron body stores can cause you to feel tired all the time, colder than normal, and just generally lackluster. You can be iron deficient without having full-blown anemia. A simple blood test can check your *hemoglobin* (iron in red blood cells) and your overall iron status *(serum ferritins)*. If your body's iron levels are low for any reason (such as having dialysis), taking iron supplements can help; so can eating more red meat, which has the most absorbable form of iron.

Magnesium status

Most adults with diabetes are magnesium deficient, especially when their blood glucose levels are higher than optimal, which causes more loss of magnesium through your urine. About 50 percent of the body's magnesium supply is found in the bone; nearly another 50 percent is inside body tissue cells and organs, and less than 1 percent is in the blood. It's a critical mineral because it impacts over 300 enzyme-controlled steps in metabolism, including protein synthesis, muscle and nerve function, immune function, blood pressure regulation, and blood glucose management.

Symptoms of low magnesium levels include agitation and anxiety, restless leg syndrome, sleep disorders, irritability, nausea and vomiting, abnormal heart rhythms, low blood pressure, confusion, muscle spasm and weakness, hyperventilation, insomnia, poor nail growth, and even seizures. Having a magnesium deficiency likely compromises your blood glucose and exercise, and you may even experience some muscle cramping (unrelated to dehydration). Low magnesium can also lead to potassium imbalances.

Refining and overprocessing foods causes a loss of almost all the magnesium found in those foods originally, and the abundance of these foods leads to a widespread magnesium deficiency even in people without diabetes. You can eat more foods with magnesium in them naturally — such as nuts and seeds (especially almonds), dark leafy greens, legumes (like black beans), soymilk, yogurt, oats, avocados, fish, and even dark chocolate. However, taking a supplement may also help correct deficiencies in your diet. (Magnesium in the aspartate, citrate, lactate, and chloride forms is absorbed better than magnesium oxide and sulfate.)

B vitamin deficiencies

With diabetes, thiamin (vitamin B1) deficiency is also a likely culprit affecting your athletic performance, particularly if you're not eating a healthful diet. The eight vitamins in the B family are integrally involved in metabolism and even red blood cell formation. People who take metformin to control diabetes may end up deficient in vitamins B6 and B12, both of which are essential for proper nerve function and muscle contractions. Thiamin (B1) is depleted by alcohol intake, birth control pill use, and more. Taking a generic B complex vitamin daily can help you avoid these issues, and excesses of most B vitamins are harmless (and simply peed out).

Insulin delivery

Insulin pumps can help manage blood glucose and deliver rapid-acting insulin analogs like Humalog, Novolog, Apidra, and Fiasp. The body metabolizes these altered insulins differently than it does long-acting Lantus/Basaglar.

The rapid-acting insulins have little to no insulin-like growth factor (IGF) affinity, and most adults are reliant on IGF rather than human growth hormone (which is only higher in youth) to stimulate muscle growth and repair. Lantus and Basaglar stimulate IGF activity, so you may want to talk with your doctor about combining insulin pump use (for meal boluses) with basal insulin injections to get more IGF activity to promote muscle repair between workouts.

TIP

Choose Lantus/Basaglar or Toujeo for your basal insulin needs because Levemir (another basal insulin) is less effective at raising levels of bioactive IGF.

Thyroid issues

Many people with diabetes also have thyroid hormone imbalances. Having lower levels of functioning T3 and T4 hormones can cause early fatigue and poor exercise performance, among other things. However, just checking your main thyroid hormones (TSH, T3, and T4) may not be enough. You may also want to consider getting your thyroid antibodies checked if your thyroid hormones levels are normal and nothing else is helping your exercise training. Specifically check for antibodies to thyroid peroxidase, especially if you have diagnosed celiac disease.

Moving forward when you're still stumped

REMEMBER

With diabetes as an added variable to consider in exercise training, the answer to what is affecting your performance isn't always simple and clear-cut.

If you've been through all the confounding factors in the preceding sections and had everything check out okay, consider other possible issues. The fix may be as simple as monitoring your hydration status (and staying better hydrated, especially when your blood glucose runs higher). Or you may need to bump up your daily carbohydrate intake; adding even just 50 grams per day to your diet may help. Check for other possible vitamin and mineral deficiencies (vitamin D, potassium, and so on). If you use statins to lower your cholesterol, be aware that some statins cause unexplained muscle fatigue, so you may need to talk with your doctor about trying a different one. Your performance can also be impacted by frequent hypoglycemia or hypoglycemia-associated autonomic failure (see Chapter 4 for a discussion of that issue).

DIFFERENTIATING BETWEEN INSULIN BODYBUILDING AND BODYBUILDING ON INSULIN

A well-known track and field athlete approached a diabetic endurance athlete to see whether he could get some of her Lantus insulin. He wanted it because insulin is an anabolic hormone, meaning it promotes uptake and storage of fuels from the blood, including not only glucose (into muscle or liver glycogen stores) but also fatty acids (into fat cells) and *amino acids* (the building blocks of protein used for muscle growth and rebuilding). Lantus/Basaglar in particular is known for its ability to release IGF, which stimulates muscle growth and repair.

In people without diabetes, *insulin bodybuilding* is the practice of injecting insulin they wouldn't release themselves to enhance nutrient uptake — specifically, amino acids into muscle to make muscles bigger. In other words, nondiabetic bodybuilders are using a natural hormone as a potential aid to give them a boost beyond what they'd get normally from effective training and nutrient intake. They've tried the same thing before with growth hormone and testosterone, but those substances are banned in most sports, leading the way for the entry of insulin abuse.

Insulin bodybuilding is potentially dangerous because it can cause severe hypoglycemia. Many of these athletes also consume excess carbohydrates to prevent hypoglycemia after dosing with insulin, so they can also gain excess fat.

However, you can approach bodybuilding safely with diabetes if you normally take insulin. To be effective at this sport, keep your blood glucose levels tightly managed to effectively refuel after workouts by using just enough insulin to avoid getting too low. Taking in a bit more protein before and/or after heavy workouts can promote muscle building, although others show no benefit beyond what you'd get with proper refueling.

Training athletes don't have to eat much extra protein or take creatine as a supplement, but they do need at least 1.4 to 1.6 grams of protein per kilogram of body weight (1 kilogram equals 2.2 pounds) daily to rebuild muscle. Protein requires some insulin (usually within three to four hours of consuming it, but not right away unless eaten with carbohydrates), so check your blood glucose levels a few hours after exercise and protein intake and dose with insulin (if you use it) if your blood glucose starts to rise to ensure those amino acids get into your muscles. Some researchers now recommend taking in at least 30 to 40 grams of protein at each meal to enhance maximum protein uptake.

5

The Part of Tens

Discover the best ways to ramp up your health through exercise.

Build a strong core at home using easy exercises.

Use easy strategies to motivate yourself to be active.

Chapter 20

Ten Tips to Boost Your Overall Health

Your exercise (and any other lifestyle changes, like choosing more healthful foods) should be as uncomplicated as possible and geared toward your unique health needs, beliefs, and goals and the types of activities you most enjoy. One of the general tips for getting people more active is usually to get a dog to walk, but this approach doesn't work for everyone for obvious reasons. Other avenues involve making your physical activity more social by involving your friends, family, and even coworkers. If you can make your physical activity more like a flash mob (where everyone participates willingly), just think how much fun and motivating it will be for you.

Regardless of how you get your activity, being active can improve your health beyond diabetes. Use the tips in this chapter to benefit the health of everyone you know.

Get Emotionally Fit with Activity

Emotional fitness can be loosely defined as "having a positive attitude and outlook." To boost your mood, try to focus on keeping your emotions positive; positive emotions include feelings like happiness, pride, confidence, and high *self-esteem* (satisfaction in yourself). Honestly, a positive, healthy emotional outlook is key to success in all aspects of your life.

Here's where physical activity comes in. It's well established that doing physical activity gives your mood at least a short-term boost. When you adopt an active lifestyle day after day for a lifetime, you set yourself up to experience that mood lift day after day for a lifetime. In turn, improving your mood, and therefore your emotional fitness, through physical activity will help you stay active from this day forward.

Go for the Endorphin Release

One of the greatest emotional benefits of exercise comes from the release of brain hormones called *endorphins*. These mood-enhancing hormones bind to natural receptors in your brain and lead to feelings of euphoria and a lesser perception of pain, and your body can release them during exercise. This release usually happens after you've been exercising for a while and gives you a second wind. Some people are positively addicted to this release of endorphins and need to get their daily fix.

As far as your diabetes goes, endorphins can boost how well your insulin works and lower your body's insulin resistance. Endorphin release is one of the main players in enhancing your insulin action through physical activity.

TIP

Try to get maximal endorphin release from doing daily exercise. You feel less depressed and anxious, maintain a better mood, and improve your health.

Enjoy Higher Dopamine Levels

Another hormone called *dopamine* activates the pleasure centers of the brain. Basically, it's the brain hormone that allows you to have feelings of bliss, pleasure, euphoria, drive, motivation, focus, and concentration — and who doesn't want to experience all those on a daily basis?

Many things you do release dopamine, but most of them — such as drinking caffeine or using cocaine — are bad for both your body and your diabetes. However, physical activity also leads to dopamine release.

It's believed that brain dopamine release activating pleasurable feelings is the primary reaction that leads to addictions (see the nearby sidebar "The power of endorphins and brain hormones").

THE POWER OF ENDORPHINS AND BRAIN HORMONES

Endorphins — all 40 types of them — are stress hormones with receptors throughout the brain and body that calm the brain and relieve muscle pain during intense exercise. Endorphins produced in the brain contribute to the feeling of well-being that usually arises from exercise. Exercise positively influences the same brain hormones (that is, endorphins, serotonin, dopamine, and norepinephrine) as antidepressants do, but it may be even more effective than drugs for treating depression. Each workout boosts your mood, at least for a little while.

As for addictions, they all involve an out-of-control reward system in the brain. All the things people become addicted to — caffeine, nicotine, carbohydrates, drugs, living on the edge, and so on — boost dopamine in your brain's reward center. Though dopamine in the reward center creates the initial interest in a substance or activity, structural changes in the brain that ensue can make an addiction hard-wired into the brain. Each time the brain connections link, the behavior comes closer to being a habit. Normally, connections stabilize and dopamine levels drop off over time, but with addictions, dopamine floods the system with each use. Addicts don't make bad choices as much as they fail to inhibit behavior that has become reflexive.

If you continually subject your brain to an overload of dopamine, the number of receptors dwindles over time. The more dopamine you get, the more you need to elicit the same rush. As a treatment, exercise works by forcing you to adapt to a new stimulus, which allows you to learn and engage in healthier activities.

One final neurological benefit of exercise is the release of two brain endocannabinoids, a class of neurotransmitters that dull pain. Marijuana and chocolate activate these receptors in the brain as well.

Serotonin release, which also occurs during physical activity, is associated with short-term improvements in mood as well. Aim to release endorphins, serotonin, dopamine, and other mood-enhancing brain hormones daily through activity to manage your blood glucose and improve your outlook simultaneously.

REMEMBER

Brain dopamine release during exercise is key to adopting an active lifestyle. When you release dopamine during exercise, you associate being active with an elevated sense of delight. That makes your brain recall pleasant feelings associated with training, which makes you more likely to want to continue doing that activity to get your boost of feel-good hormones.

TIP

Blood (and potentially brain) dopamine levels are apparently low in the morning in people with type 2 diabetes and are associated with lower insulin action. Getting active that time of day may boost dopamine and help lower any residual insulin resistance you have from fasting overnight, so get moving as soon as your feet hit the floor in the morning.

Drop Those Cortisol Levels

Another hormonal benefit of physical activity relates to levels of *cortisol*, which your body releases in reaction to stress. It responds to both physical and mental stress, going up when your blood glucose is high or you're sick or have an infection but also when you have any mental stress, anxiety, or depression.

It's a vicious cycle. If you're sick or stressed out, your cortisol goes up. Having higher cortisol in your body increases insulin resistance, and your blood glucose management can worsen over time, leading to even higher cortisol. Check out the sidebar "Is an excess of cortisol the root of your problems?" in this chapter for more on the effects of cortisol.

TIP

The best way to reverse this cycle of excess cortisol release is to exercise regularly but moderately. Exercise improves your energy levels and your physical health, and feeling better physically helps you get rid of your depressive thought patterns. Exercising reduces your level of stress, anxiety, and depression, which also lowers your cortisol. But don't overtrain because that can cause physical stress and raise cortisol on its own.

Boost Your Bodily Satisfaction

Being dissatisfied with your body size, shape, or weight can lead to having lower self-esteem and self-respect. If you perceive yourself as fat and out of shape, you're particularly vulnerable to a negative self-image. More women than men have negative feelings about their bodies. Exercising more frequently makes you feel better about your body, regardless of how much you weigh or how you look. Being active can improve muscle tone, which can also raise your self-esteem and improve your self-image.

IS AN EXCESS OF CORTISOL THE ROOT OF YOUR PROBLEMS?

The one thing that links insulin resistance, type 2 diabetes, and depression is having too much cortisol, which your body releases in response to any type of physical or emotional stress. Elevations of this natural hormone not only cause you to become more insulin resistant but also can weaken your immune system, making you more likely to get sick.

Having too much cortisol in your body is at least partially responsible for low-level systemic inflammation, which may be the link between depression and developing type 2 diabetes. Some researchers believe that depression itself may be contributing to the development of diabetes, rather than the other way around — another overwhelming reason to manage not just diabetes but also depression.

Your cortisol levels can also rise when your blood glucose is running too high, which makes your insulin action worse. Then the insulin that you take or that your body makes is less effective. If you're still making your own insulin, elevated cortisol causes your pancreatic *beta* (insulin-making) cells to work overtime to make more insulin.

Listen to Your Body

You'll have days when you want to forget about your diabetes or prediabetes and chuck your lifestyle changes out the window. When everything else in your life feels like a struggle, the last thing you need to do is add to it with physical activity that stresses you out mentally or physically. But that doesn't mean you should always skip your workout then, either. The best thing to do on those days is to pay attention to your physical and emotional cues:

>> Know when to take time off from exercise to avoid injuries.

>> Don't try to push yourself more than you need to on any given day.

>> Exercise at a moderate intensity some days, not intensely all the time.

>> Work out harder on some days and easier on others to stay motivated and injury-free.

>> Record your exercise, along with blood glucose responses and how you felt, what worked, and what didn't.

>> Figure out what to try next time to get the most from your activities.

Don't Use Poor Health or Age as an Excuse Not to Exercise

Poor health and increasing age are often major barriers to getting more active, but luckily you can overcome them in most cases.

Everyone is aging and losing some muscle mass as time marches on. Most of the diseases that people assume are inevitable with aging are caused by living a sedentary lifestyle, not advancing age. But you can fight and slow the decline by being physically active. Just making sure you can stay steady on your feet is important if you're dealing with health issues and getting weaker by being inactive. The chapters in Part 3 offer a variety of activities older or ailing folks can easily incorporate into their days.

The creation of new brain connections slows down dramatically with age. Starting at about age 40, you start to lose about 5 percent of your overall brain volume per decade until you reach 70 years old, when any number of conditions can accelerate the decline. Staying active and involved can slow the degeneration. Exercise slows down the natural decline in handling stress and helps maintain blood flow and blood supply to the brain, so use your poor health or advancing age as an excuse to exercise.

TIP

If you find structured exercise too overwhelming, focus on practicing doing the basic activities of daily living to maintain your function as you age. That approach may be even more effective for increasing your ability to take care of yourself than doing a structured resistance exercise program.

Tackle Health Problems Early On

Aging itself causes bodily changes, many of which are independent of disease. Such changes occur even if you stay active throughout your life, but being active can slow them down.

The aging process involves a gradual decline in the physiological function of your body's systems. The highest your heart rate can reach declines with time, your energy systems work less efficiently, and your reflexes get slower — even if you're working out all the time. But you'll have a higher maximal heart rate and better reflexes if you stay active compared with being a couch potato.

Human cells apparently can split and reproduce only a limited number of times before dying. After your cells get to the point that they're not turning over and renewing as fast, the aging process picks up speed. Things like weight gain around your middle (the so-called middle age spread) are often viewed as inseparable from aging, but they aren't inevitable as you get older — if you exercise regularly.

REMEMBER

Even if humans could find a way to prevent all diseases, hospitals and nursing homes would be full of people dying of just old age. If you stay active until you reach that point, at least you'll have a much higher quality of life while you are alive.

Prevention of early death or impairment from treatable problems is an essential part of longevity with and without diabetes. For example, physical activity can offset declining muscle mass (at least to a point) and keep you stronger to deal with daily living activities. And having more insulin-sensitive muscle mass where carbohydrates you eat can be stored helps to keep your blood glucose lower overall.

TIP

To live long and well, be vigilant about all aspects of your health and get problems treated earlier rather than later. Follow these guidelines to stay on top of your health:

>> Never assume that your health will be static.

>> Do what you can to prevent problems in the first place.

>> Do regular preventive care, like having mammograms (women) and prostate gland checks (men).

>> Get the recommended annual tests for people with diabetes, such as a dilated eye exam from an ophthalmologist and a foot check from a podiatrist.

>> Don't hesitate to seek out additional doctors and specialists you need to stay healthy.

>> Use the new monitoring tools and medications to better manage the peaks and valleys in your blood glucose.

>> Address your mental health as well; the stress of diabetes and life in general can affect your care and your blood glucose.

Plan Ahead for Exercise Success

One thing that can help you achieve your exercise goals is planning ahead. Look at your calendar, see exactly what your schedule looks like and how you can fit exercise into it, and then schedule it in. So maybe Monday you'll exercise in the morning but Tuesday in the evening. Treat it like any other appointment or meeting that you have to keep in your calendar, and you have an easier time staying on track and being consistent.

REMEMBER

If you take insulin, planning ahead is even more helpful in case you need to cut back on your doses to avoid low blood glucose. Plan exactly when you're going to exercise and what you're going to do, and have a backup activity plan in case something keeps you from doing your scheduled one.

After a short break from your routine because of a vacation, illness, or athletic injury, start scheduling your physical activity back in again. During any break — whether it's long or short — try to keep up all your movement during the day even if you can't do anything taxing. Just staying in motion helps keep your fitness level higher and makes getting back into regular exercise as quickly as possible easier.

Know It's Never Too Late to Start Being Active

Whether you've been a couch potato or just recently slipped out of your exercise habit, it's not too late to change course. Even if you haven't had much success with managing your blood glucose up to this point, it's not too late to reap some of the health benefits now. You can still improve your health and your fitness by starting to be more active and by making other healthful lifestyle changes.

REMEMBER

Even if you haven't been on top of your diabetes recently, you may be able to slow the progression of some of your complications or reverse them with a little more diligence — starting with being more active now.

Chapter **21**

Ten Easy Exercises to Build a Strong Core without Leaving the House

Many people who are stuck at home for one reason or another think they can't work on staying fit, but the truth is that you can get a stronger core and stay fitter without leaving home. You'd be amazed at how easy it is to get fit.

REMEMBER

Your body core — the muscles around your trunk and pelvis — is particularly important to keep strong so that you can go about your normal daily activities and prevent falls and injuries, particularly as you age. Having a strong body core makes you better able to handle your daily life, even if that's just doing grocery shopping or playing a round of golf.

Core exercises are an important part of a well-rounded fitness program, and they're easy to do at home on your own. To get started on your body core workout, you don't need to purchase anything. (Some of the advanced variations do call for equipment like a gym ball or dumbbells.)

TIP

Include all 10 of these easy core exercises in your workouts, doing at least one set of 15 repetitions of each one to start (for all that are done as reps). Work up to doing two to three sets of each per workout, or even more repetitions if you can. For best results, do these exercises at least two or three nonconsecutive days per week; muscles need a day or two off to fully recover and get stronger. Just don't do them right before you do another physical activity (because a fatigued core increases your risk of injury).

#1: Abdominal Squeezes

This exercise (Figure 21-1) is great for working your abdominals and getting your body core as strong as possible. If you're female and have gone through a pregnancy, getting these muscles in shape doing these squeezes is a must.

1. **Put one of your hands against your upper stomach and the other facing the other direction below your belly button.**

2. **Inhale to expand your stomach.**

3. **Exhale and try to pull your abdominal muscles halfway toward your spine.**

   This is your starting position.

4. **Contract your abdominal muscles more deeply in toward your spine while counting to two.**

5. **Return to the starting position from Step 3 for another count of two.**

Work up to doing 100 repetitions per workout session.

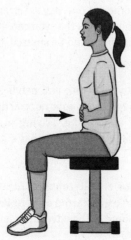

FIGURE 21-1:
Abdominal
squeezes.

© John Wiley & Sons, Inc.

#2: Plank or Modified Plank

Nobody likes doing planks, but they get the job done when it comes to boosting the strength of your core. Both planks and modified planks (Figure 21-2) work multiple areas, including your abdominals, lower back, and shoulders.

1. **Start on the floor on your stomach and bend your elbows 90 degrees, resting your weight on your forearms.**

2. **Place your elbows directly beneath your shoulders and form a straight line from your head to your feet.**

3. **Hold this position as long as you can.**

Repeat this exercise as many times as possible during each workout.

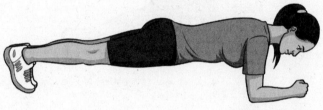

FIGURE 21-2: Plank.

© John Wiley & Sons, Inc.

TIP

If a regular plank is too hard when you start doing it, do a modified plank by bending your knees and resting on them instead.

WARNING

Avoid this exercise if you have shoulder or elbow problems or if you have diabetic *proliferative retinopathy* (bleeding inside your eyes; I discuss this condition in Chapter 16).

#3: Side Planks

A modification of regular planks, this side plank exercise (Figure 21-3) works some of the same and some slightly different muscles that include your abdominals, oblique abdominal muscles, sides of hips, gluteals, and shoulders. Try doing some of both types for the best results.

1. **Start out on the floor on your side with your feet together and one forearm directly below your shoulder.**

2. **Contract your core muscles and raise your hips until your body is in a straight line from head to feet.**

3. **Hold this position without letting your hips drop for as long as you can.**

4. **Repeat Steps 1 through 3 on the other side.**

Switch back and forth between sides as many times as you can.

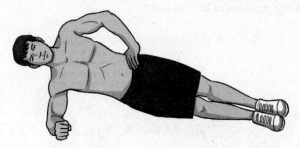

FIGURE 21-3:
Side plank.

TIP

Try these plank variations to mix things up a bit:

» **Raised side plank:** Lifting both your top arm and your leg upward brings other muscles into play and makes your core work harder to maintain balance, but don't let your hips sag.

» **Gym ball side plank:** Resting your supporting arm on a gym ball, use your core muscles to control the wobble to further strengthen your side muscles.

» **Side plank with lateral raise:** While holding the side plank position, slowly raise and lower a light dumbbell or other weight with your top arm to improve your coordination and strength.

» **Side plank pulse:** From the side plank position, add a vertical hip drive by lowering your hips until they're just off the floor and then driving them up as far as you can with each repetition of this move.

#4: Bridging

If you work on your abdominal strength, you also need to build the strength in your lower back to keep things balanced. Bridging (Figure 21-4) is a good exercise to do that because it works your buttocks (including gluteals), low back, and hip extensors. Remember to breathe in and out throughout this exercise.

1. **Keeping your shoulders on the floor, slowly raise your buttocks from the floor with your stomach tight and your lower back straight.**

2. **Gently lower your back to the ground.**

3. **Repeat Steps 1 and 2.**

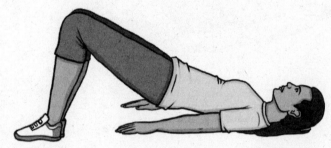

FIGURE 21-4:
Bridging.

© John Wiley & Sons, Inc.

TIP

Try the bridging with straight leg raise variation: With your legs bent, lift your buttocks up off the floor. Slowly extend your left knee, keeping your stomach tight. Repeat with the other leg. Do as many repetitions as possible.

#5: Pelvic Tilt

An easy exercise to do, the pelvic tilt (Figure 21-5) works your lower back and lower part of your abdominals.

1. **Lie on your back on the floor with your knees bent and feet flat on the floor.**

2. **Place your hands either by your sides or supporting your head.**

3. **Tighten your bottom, forcing your lower back flat against the floor, and then relax.**

4. **Repeat Steps 2 and 3 as many times as you can.**

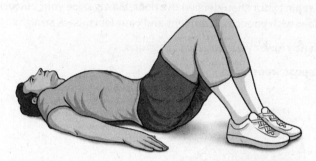

FIGURE 21-5:
Pelvic tilt.

© John Wiley & Sons, Inc.

#6: Superhero Pose

Whether you want to leap tall buildings with a single bound or not, try doing this superhero pose exercise (Figure 21-6) to get a stronger core. It works many areas, including your lower back, upper back, back of shoulders, and gluteals.

1. **Lie on your stomach with your arms straight out in front of your head on the floor.**

2. **Rest your chin on the floor between your arms.**

3. **Keeping your arms and legs straight, simultaneously lift your feet and your hands as high off the floor as you can.**

   Aim for at least 3 inches.

4. **Hold that position (sort of a superhero flying position) for 10 seconds if possible, and then relax your arms and legs back onto the floor.**

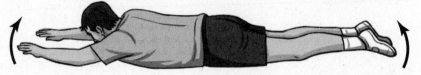

FIGURE 21-6:
Superhero pose.

© John Wiley & Sons, Inc.

If this exercise is too difficult, try lifting just your legs or arms off the floor separately — or even just one limb at a time.

#7: Knee Push-Ups

Push-ups are hard to do if you haven't built up the strength in your shoulders yet, so this knee version (Figure 21-7) is an easier way to start for most people. This exercise works your chest, front of shoulders, and back of upper arms.

1. Get on your hands and knees on the floor or a mat.

2. Place your hands shoulder-width apart on the floor.

3. Tighten your abdominal muscles to straighten your lower back and lower yourself down toward the floor as far as you can without touching.

4. Push yourself back up until your arms are extended, but don't lock your elbows.

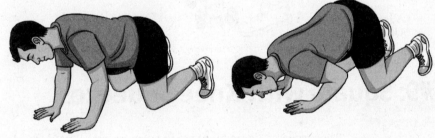

FIGURE 21-7:
Knee push-ups.

© John Wiley & Sons, Inc.

If knee push-ups are too hard for you, try doing wall push-ups to start instead. Stand facing a wall at an arm's length and place your palms against it at shoulder height and with your feet about a foot apart. Do your push-ups off the wall.

#8: Suitcase Lift

This exercise (Figure 21-8) is the proper way to lift items from the floor. Before you begin, place dumbbells or household items slightly forward and between your feet on the floor. You work the same muscles used in doing squats (lower back and lower body) with this activity.

1. **Stand in an upright position with your back and arms straight, with your hands in front of your abdomen.**

2. **Bending only your knees, reach down to pick up the dumbbells.**

3. **Grab the dumbbells or items in both hands and then push up with your legs and stand upright, keeping your back straight.**

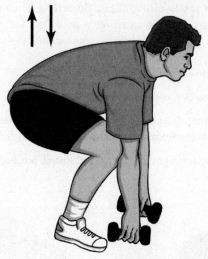

FIGURE 21-8: Suitcase lift.

© John Wiley & Sons, Inc.

#9: Squats with Knee Squeezes

These squats (Figure 21-9) are not your normal squats. They're more like a combination of squatting and wall sitting with a twist. You work the front and back of thighs, inner thighs (adductors), hip flexors, and extensors all with this one exercise.

1. **Stand with your back against the wall, with your feet aligned with your knees and straight out in front of you.**

2. **Place a ball or pillow between your knees and hold it there with your legs.**

3. **Inhale to expand your stomach and then exhale and contract your abdominal muscles.**

4. **Bend your knees and lower yourself into a squat.**

To avoid injuring your knees, don't bend them more than 90 degrees.

5. **Squeeze the ball with your thighs, drawing your stomach muscles more deeply toward your spine.**

6. **Do as many squeezes as you can up to 20 and then return to the starting position.**

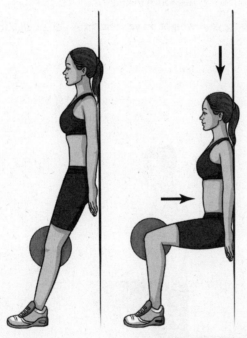

FIGURE 21-9: Squats with knee squeezes.

© John Wiley & Sons, Inc.

#10: Lunges

Lunges (Figure 21-10) are a common activity to work on the front and back of thighs, hip flexors and extensors, abdominals, and lower back all with one exercise. Do them with proper form to avoid aggravating your knees, though.

1. **Keep your upper body straight, with your shoulders back and relaxed and chin up.**

2. **Pick a point to stare at in front of you so you don't keep looking down, and engage your core.**

3. **Step forward with one leg, lowering your hips until both knees are bent at about a 90-degree angle.**

   Make sure your front knee is directly above your ankle, not pushed out too far, and don't let your back knee touch the floor.

4. **Focus on keeping your weight on your heels as you push back up to the starting position.**

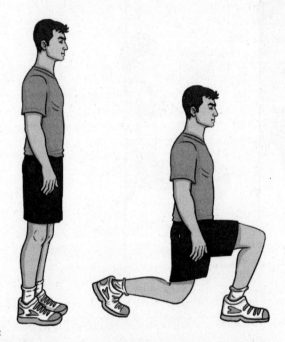

FIGURE 21-10:
Lunges.

© John Wiley & Sons, Inc.

TIP

To prevent injuries, if you feel any pain in your knees or hips when you do a lunge, do the following instead:

» Take smaller steps out with your front leg.

» Slowly increase your lunge distance as your pain gets better.

» Try doing a reverse lunge (stepping backward rather than forward) to help reduce knee strain.

Chapter **22**

Ten Ways to Get Motivated to Exercise (When You're Not)

Diabetes is a complex metabolic condition, and your blood glucose levels can impact you not only physically but also emotionally and mentally. Often, feeling depressed or anxious about diabetes management can be demotivating for taking better care of yourself. Whether that care involves getting more physically active or making more healthful food choices, getting and staying more motivated can only benefit you and your blood glucose.

REMEMBER

Exercise can lessen your feelings of stress, anxiety, and depression, among other mental benefits. In many cases, treating anxiety or mild to moderate depression with regular exercise is at least as effective as, if not more effective than, using medications to treat these symptoms; even just five minutes of aerobic exercise can stimulate anti-anxiety effects. And the side effects from being regularly active are much more positive. Being active can also positively affect your self-confidence, body image, and self-esteem.

But some days knowing all those benefits may not be enough to get you going. This chapter has you covered. Check out the following sections for ideas for those days where you just can't seem to get moving.

Check Your Blood Glucose

When you start a new exercise, checking your blood glucose before, during (if you're active more than an hour), and after your workout pays off. A reading that changes — especially in the direction that you want it to — can be very rewarding and motivating. If you don't check, you may never realize what a positive impact you can have on your diabetes simply by being active.

For example, say your blood glucose is a little high after you eat a meal, and you want it to go lower without taking (or releasing) any more insulin. You can exercise after your meal and bring your blood glucose down within two hours after eating and taking insulin, or you can avoid or lower post-meal spikes in your blood glucose. You wouldn't know the extent of the effect you can have without using your blood glucose meter or continuous glucose monitor to check.

Start with Easier Activities

Start slowly with easier activities and progress cautiously to working out harder. Exercising too hard right out of the gate is likely to make you end up discouraged or injured, especially if you haven't exercised in a while.

REMEMBER If you often complain about being too tired to exercise, your lack of physical activity is likely what's making you feel sluggish. After you begin doing even light or moderate activities, your energy levels rise along with your fitness, and your physical (and mental) health improves.

Pick Activities You Enjoy

Most adults need exercise to be fun, or they lose their motivation to do it over time. It's human nature to avoid doing the things you really don't like to do, so try to pick activities you truly enjoy, such as salsa dancing or golfing (as long as you walk and carry your own clubs). Having fun with your activities lets you more easily make them a permanent and integral part of your diabetes management. If you haven't found any that you enjoy much yet, choose some new ones to take out for a test run (so to speak).

TIP Choose an exercise that suits your physical condition and overcomes or works around your limitations.

Spice It Up

An essential motivator involves mixing your workouts up with different activities. People commonly complain about exercise being boring. Feelings of boredom with your program can be the result of repeating the same exercises each day. To make it more exciting, try different physical activities for varying durations and at different intensities. Knowing that you don't have to do the same workout day after day is motivating by itself. (For more tips on mixing up your workouts through cross-training, head to Chapter 14.)

Have a Plan B

Always have a backup plan that includes other activities you can do in case of inclement weather or other barriers to your planned exercise. For example, if a sudden snowstorm traps you at home on a day you planned to swim laps at the pool, be ready to walk on the treadmill or substitute some of the resistance activities from Chapter 11. You can always distract yourself during your second-choice exercise to make the time pass more pleasantly. Read a book or magazine, watch your favorite TV program, listen to music or a book on tape, or talk with a friend on the phone while you're working out.

Get an Exercise Buddy (or Several)

You don't need to go it alone when being active. Having a regular (and reliable) exercise buddy increases your likelihood of participating, and it also makes your activities more social and fun. Get your spouse, family members, friends, and co-workers to join in your physical activities, regardless of what time of day you do them. Having a good social network to support your new or renewed exercise habit helps you adhere to it over the long run.

REMEMBER

Your community may be a good place to look for other exercise options. To become more involved in structured exercise programs, find out what exercise programs are in your workplace or community. You can often find groups of health-conscious people walking together during lunch breaks, or you may be able to join a low-impact aerobics or other exercise class offered at your workplace, community center, or recreation center.

Take the time to find out what's available in your area. The more you can get involved in making your lifestyle changes as part of a larger community, the more likely you are to be successful in making them a lifelong habit.

TIP

If you can't find a human exercise buddy, borrow or adopt a dog that needs to be walked regularly.

Schedule It

Put your planned exercise down on your calendar or to-do list like you would other appointments. You show up for your doctor appointments, so why should scheduling your physical activity be any different? Never make the mistake of assuming it'll happen just because you claim that you want to do it a certain number of days per week or month. It takes some planning ahead and the commitment to make it a priority.

Set Goals and Reward Yourself

Setting goals helps keep your interest up. For instance, if you walk for exercise, you may want to get a pedometer and set a goal of adding in 2,000 more steps each day. Break your larger goals into smaller, realistic stepping-stones (such as daily and weekly physical activity goals) for all your active lifestyle changes, and use SMART goals (refer to Chapter 8). Trackers, activity logs, and other motivational tools are also widely available online.

TIP

Reward yourself when you reach your exercise goals (but preferably not with food). Who says that sticker charts and non-food treats are just for kids? Maybe you can promise yourself an outing to somewhere special, the purchase of a coveted item, or anything else that is reasonable and effectively motivates you to exercise.

If you miss one of your goals, try to make the rest of them happen anyway. Then reward yourself when you meet any of your goals, even if you don't make them all happen.

Take Advantage of Opportunities for Spontaneous Physical Activity

You don't have to do activities at a high intensity for them to be effective for diabetes and weight management. You can also add physical movement all day long doing anything you want to, including gardening, housework, and many other spontaneous physical activities, as I discuss in Chapter 9.

For instance, if you have a sedentary desk job, take the stairs rather than the elevator whenever you can. Walk to someone else's office or the neighbor's house to deliver a message instead of relying on the phone or email. Or park your car at the far end of the parking lot and walk the extra distance. Guess what? You've just gotten yourself more active without giving it much thought.

Take Small Steps

If you get out of your normal activity routine and are having trouble getting restarted, simply take small steps in that direction. You may need to start back at a lower intensity by using lighter weights, less resistance, or a slower walking speed. Starting out slowly with small steps helps you avoid burnout, muscle soreness, and injury.

For example, if you don't want to exercise on a given day, make a deal with yourself that you'll do it for a short time to get started (which is often the hardest part). Even doing only 5 to 10 minutes at a time (rather than 30 or more) is fine. After you're up and moving, you may feel good enough to exceed the time you planned on doing in the first place. The key is to begin through any means possible.

REMEMBER

You're in this for the long term, so even taking just small steps in the right direction will eventually allow you to reach your fitness goals and reclaim your good health.

Index

A

A1C (glycated hemoglobin)
  to average glucose equivalent, 36
  recommended goal for, 35
  test for, 16
abdominal squeezes, 348
abductors, 245
ACE inhibitors, 58–59
achilles tendinitis, 175
activity/activities. *See also specific exercises*
  about, 63, 141, 161
  aerobic, 194–201
  for athletes, 323–326
  avoiding certain, 173–174
  balance, 168–169, 225–237
  barriers to, 151–156
  blood glucose and, 83–84, 307
  bodily concerns, 81
  carbohydrates as fuel during, 70–71, 126–130
  cardio training, 181–201
  choosing, 358
  choosing for resistance training, 215
  choosing training types, 164–170
  cooling down, 171, 184
  core, 347–356
  cross-training, 259–264
  diabetes and, 22–23
  effect of female hormones on, 299–301
  emotional fitness through, 144
  encouraging in kids, 307–311
  energy systems, 66–70
  environment, 80
  equipment, 144–146
  errors in, as a common cause of injury, 177
  excuses not to, 344
  exercise myths, 157–160
  fat as fuel during, 70–71, 133–134
  finding, 141–144

  flexibility, 239–258
  glucose and, 65–66
  glucose response, 71–72
  health complications and, 285–297
  high blood pressure and, 291–292
  hormonal changes and, 301
  hormones, 64–66
  how it affects your body, 26–29
  hydration during, 136–137
  hypoglycemia-associated autonomic failure (HAAF), 82
  improving balance with, 229–231
  injuries, 174–180
  insulin action and, 313–314
  insulin needs for, 56
  insulin regimen changes, 80
  interactions with insulin, 53–54
  Kegel exercises, 170
  kidney disease and, 295–296
  in kids, 306
  managing with health complications, 296–297
  medications and, 46–49
  for mental health/function, 318–320
  motivation for, 146–150, 357–361
  myths about, 157–160
  with nerve damage, 286–289
  peripheral artery disease (PAD) and, 293
  planning, 345–346, 359
  positive, stress-releasing, 251–252
  during pregnancy, 301–304, 303–304
  preventing hypoglycemia after, 93
  preventing type 2 diabetes with, 270
  as a punishment, 311
  for resistance (strength) training, 203–224
  retinopathy and, 293–295
  routine for, 171–173
  scheduling, 360
  seniors and, 315–318
  spontaneity of, 98

activity/activities *(continued)*

spontaneous physical activity (SPA), 161–164, 360–361

starting with easier, 358

stretching, 252–258

timing of, 346

training effects, 79–80

travel backward, 231

variables for, 72–80

variety in, 359

warming up, 171, 184

women and, 299–304

workout clothes, 144–146

Actos, 41, 281

addictions, 341

adductors, 245

adenosine triphosphate (ATP), 66

Adho mukha svanasana (Downward-facing dog pose), 248

adipocytes, 70

adjusting medications, 279–281

adrenaline, 64

adult, *vs.* kids, 306

adult onset diabetes (type 2)

about, 12–13

diagnosing, 17

misdiagnosing, 18

preventing with activity, 270

weight gain with, 278

advanced glycation end products, 118

aerobic system, 68–70

aerobic (cardio) training

about, 165–166, 181, 194–201

aerobic exercise, 194–201

choosing, 270

combining with resistance training, 263

getting started, 182–184

indoor cardio machines, 191–194

interval training, 189–191

jogging, 186–189

during pregnancy, 303

running, 186–189

for seniors, 316

walking, 184–186

Afrezza, 53

age, as a cardiovascular risk, 38

aging

about, 29–30

assessing, 320–322

effect on balance of, 226–227

maximizing protein for, 132–133

in seniors, 311–315

alpha-glucosidase inhibitors, 43, 45, 48

alpha-lipoic acid, 123–124

Amaryl, 281

American Diabetes Association (website), 286

amount, of cardio training, 182

amylin, 45–46, 49

anaerobic glycolysis, 68

anaerobic system, 67

analogs, 52

angina, 290

ankle sprain, 175

antioxidants, 122–124

anxiety, 282

Apidra, 51, 52, 334

Ardha matsyendrasana (Half lord of the fishes pose), 249

arm stretches, 244

arthritis, 272–274, 319

assessing

aging, 320–322

barriers to activity, 151–156

athletes

about, 323

activity for, 323–326

carb loading for, 326–327

low-carb diet, 327–328

troubleshooting exercise blood glucose, 328–335

ATP (adenosine triphosphate), 66

ATP-CP (glycolytic system), 67

autonomic neuropathy, 76, 138, 288–289

Avandia, 41, 281

average glucose

A1C equivalent to, 36

recommended goal for, 35

avoiding
    early-onset fatigue, 331–332
    excessive fatigue, 331–332
    fat gain, 314–315
    muscle wasting, 314–315
    weight gain, 277–281

B

B vitamins
    about, 117–118
    deficiencies in, 333
back of upper-leg stretch, 256–257
balance
    checking, 227
    improving, 227–231
balance training
    about, 168–169, 225
    effects of aging and diabetes on balance, 226–227
    exercises for, 232–237
    for seniors, 317
    Tai Chi, 231–232
    yoga, 231–232
balance/reach exercise, 234, 235
Balasana (Child's pose), 247
barriers, to activity, 151–156
Basaglar, 51
basal insulins, 50–52
BBT (Big Blue Test), 72–73
belly fat, 268–269
beta blockers, 58
beta cells, 12
Bhujangasana (Cobra pose), 246–247
Big Blue Test (BBT), 72–73
biguanides, 43, 44, 48
biking, 195–196
biomechanics, as a common cause of injury, 177
Bitiliasana (Cow pose), 248
blood, directing flow of glucose in, 64–65
blood glucose
    about, 8–10, 83
    for athletes, 332
    checking, 89, 358
    directing flow of in blood, 64–65

effect of food on, 28–29
exercise and, 65–66, 83–84, 307
identifying hypoglycemia, 84–88
increasing, 260
managing, 73
managing hyperglycemia, 99–101
oral medications for lowering, 42–45
recommended goal for, 35
self-monitoring, 18–19
treating and preventing hypoglycemia, 88–99
blood glucose meters, 19–22
blood thinners, 58
body
    changes in seniors, 312
    composition of in seniors, 312
    concerns, as an exercise factor, 81
    listening to your, 343
    stretches for core, 243
body and mind, training your, 250–252
body fat, 99
body satisfaction, 342
body weight, for resistance training, 210
bodybuilding, 335
bolus (mealtime) insulin, 50–52
bone density, in seniors, 312
bone mineral density, aging and, 321
brain hormones, 341
breathing capacity, aging and, 321
bridging, 217, 351
burning calories, 276
buttock stretches, 245

C

caffeine, 135
calf raises, 230
calf stretch, 257–258
calories
    burning, 276
    counting, 115
    cutting, 276
carb loading
    about, 94–95
    for athletes, 326–327

carbohydrates
  about, 108–111, 126
  choosing, 89–91
  daily needs for, 127
  during exercise, 126–127
  exercise and, 128–130
  glycogen repletion and, 130–131
  role of, 28
  treating low blood glucose with, 89
  using as fuel, 70–71
cardiac autonomic neuropathy, 76, 288–289
cardio machines, 191–194
cardio (aerobic) training
  about, 165–166, 181, 194–201
  aerobic exercise, 194–201
  choosing, 270
  combining with resistance training, 263
  getting started, 182–184
  indoor cardio machines, 191–194
  interval training, 189–191
  jogging, 186–189
  during pregnancy, 303
  running, 186–189
  for seniors, 316
  walking, 184–186
cardiovascular function, aging and, 321
cardiovascular risks, 38–39
carnitine, 122
Cat pose (Majaryasana), 248
CDC quiz (website), 151
central nerve issues, 288–289
central nervous system, 288–289
CGMs (continuous glucose monitors), 21–22
Chair pose (Utkatasana), 249
chair push-ups exercise, 219–220
chair sit-ups exercise, 220–221
Cheat Sheet (website), 3
checking
  balance, 227
  blood glucose, 89, 358
chest discomfort, as a symptom of a heart attack, 291
chest pain, 290
chest/shoulder stretch, 254–255
Child's pose (Balasana), 247

chocolate milk, 91
cholesterol, 114
choosing
  activity, 358
  aerobic workouts, 270
  carbohydrates, 89–91
  exercises for resistance training, 215
  resistance training, 270
  training types, 164–170
cigarette smoking, as a cardiovascular risk, 38
Cobra pose (Bhujangasana), 246–247
coffee, 135
Colberg-Ochs, Sheri (author)
  contact information for, 3
  Diabetic Athlete's Handbook, 56
color, in food, 105
combination therapies, 45
continuous glucose monitors (CGMs), 21–22
cooling down, 171, 184
core ball transfers, 217
core muscle stretches, 244
core training
  abdominal squeezes, 348
  about, 167–168, 215–217, 347–348
  bridging, 351
  gym ball side plank, 350
  knee push-ups, 353
  lunges, 355–356
  modified plank, 349
  pelvic tilt, 351–352
  plank, 349
  raised side plank, 350
  for seniors, 316
  side plank pulse, 350
  side plank with lateral raise, 350
  side planks, 349–350
  squats with knee squeezes, 354–355
  suitcase lift, 353–354
  superhero pose, 352–353
Corgard, 58
cortisol, 64, 342, 343
cortisone, 59
cost, blood glucose meters and, 20
Coumadin, 58

counting calories, 115

Cow pose (Bitilasana), 248

CP (creatine phosphate), 67

creatine, 121

creatine phosphate (CP), 67

cross-country skiing, 194

cross-trainers, 192

cross-training

about, 169, 259

benefits of, 259–263

combining cardio training and resistance training, 263

with diabetes, 263–264

example exercise plan for, 262–263

crunches, 217

cutting calories, 276

cycling, 193, 195–196

D

Dandasana (Staff pose), 246

data storage, blood glucose meters and, 20

deep breathing, 251

delayed-onset muscle soreness (DOMS), 179

depression, 282

destressing, 250–252

dextrose, 89

DiaBeta, 281

diabetes. *See also specific topics*

about, 7

cross-training with, 263–264

diagnosing, 14–18

effect on balance of, 226–227

exercise and, 22–23

poorly controlled, as a cardiovascular risk, 38

risks for, 8

targets and goals, 35–37

testing for, 15–17

types of, 11–14

Diabetes Motion (website), 3

Diabetes Motion Academy (website), 3

Diabetes Prevention Program, 270

Diabetic Athlete's Handbook (Colberg-Ochs), 56

diabetic ketoacidosis (DKA), 19, 71, 100

Diabinese, 281

diagnosing

diabetes, 14–18

gestational diabetes, 17

prediabetes, 14–18, 17

type 1 diabetes, 17

type 2 diabetes, 17

diet

about, 103, 125

caffeine, 135

carbohydrates, 108–111, 126–131

cholesterol, 114

coffee, 135

fat and exercise, 133–134

healthy fats, 113–116

healthy foods, 103–117

hydration, 136–138

low-carb, 327–328

minerals, 117–120

protein, 112–113, 131–133

sugar, 111–112

supplements, 117–120, 120–124

training on a, 205–206

vitamins, 117–120

dietary fiber, 106–107

DigiFit iCardio, 150

discomfort

managing, 273

as a symptom of a heart attack, 291

diuretics, 58

DKA (diabetic ketoacidosis), 19, 71, 100

doctors, consulting, 33–34

DOMS (delayed-onset muscle soreness), 179

dopamine levels, 340–342

Downward-facing dog pose (Adho mukha svanasana), 248

DPP-4 inhibitors, 43, 44, 48

duration

as an exercise variable, 76–77

of cardio training, 182

of exercise during pregnancy, 303

for resistance training, 211–213

dynamic stretching, 241–242

E

early-onset fatigue, avoiding, 331–332

ease of use, blood glucose meters and, 20

Easy pose (Sukhasana), 246

elevated blood fats, as a cardiovascular risk, 38

elliptical machines, 192

emotional barriers, to activity, 155

emotional disorders, 282

emotional fitness, 144, 339–340

Endomondo Sports Tracker, 150

endorphin release, 340

endurance, in seniors, 312

Enduron, 58

energy systems, 66–70

environment

  as an exercise factor, 80

  as a common cause of injury, 177

environmental barriers, to activity, 154

epinephrine, 64

equipment, 144–146

essential amino acids, 121–122

estrogen, 299

excessive fatigue, avoiding, 331–332

exercise blood glucose, for athletes, 328–335

exercise buddy, 359–360

exercise(s)

  about, 63, 141, 161

  aerobic, 194–201

  for athletes, 323–326

  avoiding certain, 173–174

  avoiding certain activities, 173–174

  back of upper-leg, 256–257

  balance, 168–169, 225–237

  balance/reach, 234, 235

  barriers to, 151–156

  blood glucose and, 83–84, 307

  bodily concerns, 81

  calf raises, 230

  calf stretch, 257–258

  carbohydrates as fuel during, 70–71, 126–130

  cardio training, 181–201

  chair push-ups, 219–220

  chair sit-ups, 220–221

  chest/shoulder, 254–255

  choosing, 358

  choosing for resistance training, 215

  choosing training types, 164–170

  cooling down, 171, 184

  core, 347–356

  cross-training, 259–264

  diabetes and, 22–23

  effect of female hormones on, 299–301

  emotional fitness through, 144

  encouraging in kids, 307–311

  energy systems, 66–70

  environment, 80

  equipment, 144–146

  errors in, as a common cause of injury, 177

  excuses not to, 344

  exercise myths, 157–160

  fat as fuel during, 70–71, 133–134

  finding, 141–144

  flexibility, 239–258

  forward lean, 234, 235

  glucose and, 65–66

  glucose response, 71–72

  health complications and, 285–297

  heel raise, 236–237

  high blood pressure and, 291–292

  hormonal changes and, 301

  hormones, 64–66

  how it affects your body, 26–29

  hydration during, 136–137

  hypoglycemia-associated autonomic failure (HAAF), 82

  improving balance with, 229–231

  injuries, 174–180

  insulin action and, 313–314

  insulin needs for, 56

  insulin regimen changes, 80

  interactions with insulin, 53–54

  Kegel exercises, 170

  kidney disease and, 295–296

  in kids, 306

  managing with health complications, 296–297

  medications and, 46–49

  for mental health/function, 318–320

motivation for, 146–150, 357–361

myths about, 157–160

neck stretch, 253

with nerve damage, 286–289

peripheral artery disease (PAD) and, 293

planning, 345–346, 359

positive, stress-releasing, 251–252

during pregnancy, 301–304, 303–304

preventing hypoglycemia after, 93

preventing type 2 diabetes with, 270

as a punishment, 311

for resistance (strength) training, 203–224

retinopathy and, 293–295

routine for, 171–173

scheduling, 360

seated arm curls, 198, 199

seated foot drill, 197–198

seated march, 197

seated overhead punches, 198, 199

seniors and, 315–318

shoulder/upper-back, 253–254

side leg raises, 229

single leg balance, 232–233

sit-to-stand, 218–219, 230

spontaneity of, 98

spontaneous physical activity (SPA), 161–164, 360–361

standing calf raises, 223–224

standing leg curls, 222–223

standing march, 200

standing raise the roof, 200–201

starting with easier, 358

stretching, 252–258

three-way leg swing, 233–234

timing of, 346

toe raises, 229–230, 236

training effects, 79–80

travel backward, 231

tucking your chin, 231

upper-back/back of arm, 255–256

variables for, 72–80

variety in, 359

walk heel-to-toe, 231

wall push-ups, 221–222

warming up, 171, 184

women and, 299–304

workout clothes, 144–146

extensors, 245

F

"fake fiber" foods, 106

family activities, 309

family history, as a cardiovascular risk, 38

fasting plasma glucose, 15–16

fatigue, 331–332

fat(s)

avoiding gain of, 314–315

belly, 268–269

exercise and, 133–134

healthy, 113–116

highly processed, 114–115

plant, 113–114

role of, 28

subcutaneous, 268

trans, 114–115

using as fuel, 70–71

visceral, 268–269

features, of blood glucose meters, 20

feet, health complications with, 286–288

Fiasp, 51, 334

fiber, 106–107

fight-or-flight response, 64, 232, 251

finding activities, 141–144

Fitbit, 150

fitness, impact on insulin action of, 30–33

fitness goals, 37

flexibility training

about, 169, 239

basic stretches, 242–245

importance of, 240

improving, 231–232

muscles, 242–245

for seniors, 317

stretching, 240–242

stretching exercises, 252–258

whole-body approach for, 250–252

yoga, 245–249

flexors, 245

follicular phase, 300

foods

color of, 105

effect on blood glucose of, 28–29

how it affects your body, 26–29

for lowering inflammation, 104–106

footwear

as a common cause of injury, 177

for running, 187–188

forward lean exercise, 234, 235

free radicals, 122

frequency

as an exercise variable, 77

of exercise during pregnancy, 303

for resistance training, 211

fructose, 138

G

gastrocnemius, 179–180, 228, 245

gastroparesis, 289

gestational diabetes

about, 13

diagnosing, 17

managing, 304

testing for, 17

getting moving, importance of, 26

GI (glycemic index), 109–110, 127

GL (glycemic load), 110–111

glinides, 281

GLP-1 agonists (glucagon-like peptide-1 agonists), 45, 46, 49

glucagon, 9, 64, 91

glucagon-like peptide-1 agonists (GLP-1 agonists), 45, 46, 49

gluconeogenesis, 70

glucose

about, 8–10, 83

for athletes, 332

checking, 89, 358

directing flow of in blood, 64–65

effect of food on, 28–29

exercise and, 65–66, 83–84, 307

identifying hypoglycemia, 84–88

increasing, 260

managing, 73

managing hyperglycemia, 99–101

oral medications for lowering, 42–45

recommended goal for, 35

self-monitoring, 18–19

treating and preventing hypoglycemia, 88–99

glucose response, predicting, 71–72

glucose tablets, 90

Glucotrol, 281

glutathione, 123

gluteals, 228, 245

gluteus medius, 228

Glyburide, 41

glycated hemoglobin (A1C)

to average glucose equivalent, 36

recommended goal for, 35

test for, 16

glycemic index (GI), 109–110, 127

glycemic load (GL), 110–111

glycogen

about, 9, 313

carbohydrates and repletion of, 130–131

increasing use of, 260

stores of, for athletes, 332

glycogenolysis, 68

glycolytic system (ATP-CP), 67

Glynase, 281

goals, setting, 34–37, 360

growth hormone, 64

gut microbiome, 107

gym ball side plank, 350

H

HAAF (hypoglycemia-associated autonomic failure (HAAF)), 82, 96

Half lord of the fishes pose (Ardha matsyendrasana), 249

hamstrings, 245

hand weights, 208, 209

health
  boosting, 339–346
  in seniors, 311–315
health complications
  about, 285
  exercise and, 285–297
  kidney disease, 295–296
  managing, 286, 344–345
  managing exercise with, 296–297
  retinopathy, 293–295
  vessel disease, 289–293
health goals, 37
healthy fats, 113–116
healthy foods
  about, 103–104
  carbohydrates, 108–111
  color, 105
  fiber, 106–107
  for lowering inflammation, 104–106
heart attack, 290–291
heart disease, 290–291
heart rate reserve (HRR), 73, 75–76
heel raise exercise, 236–237
heel spur, 175
hemoglobin, 332–333
high blood pressure, 291–292
high-intensity activities, 183
high-intensity interval training (HIIT), 191
highly processed fats, 114–115
HIIT (high-intensity interval training), 191
hip stretches, 245
home training machines, 194
hormonal swings, 300–301
hormones
  about, 64
  directing glucose flow in blood, 64–65
  effect on insulin and exercise of, 299–301
  glucose and, 65–66
household items, for resistance training, 209–210
HRR (heart rate reserve), 73, 75–76
Humalog, 51, 52, 334
Humulin N, 51–52
hydration, 136–138

hyperglycemia
  managing, 99–101, 330–331
  symptoms of, 14
hypertension (high blood pressure), as a
    cardiovascular risk, 38
hypoglycemia
  about, 19, 278
  identifying, 84–88
  managing, 329–330
hypoglycemia unawareness, 95–96
hypoglycemia-associated autonomic failure
    (HAAF), 82, 96
hyponatremia, 136

I

ibuprofen, 177
icons, explained, 2–3
identifying hypoglycemia, 84–88
IFG (impaired fasting glucose), 15
IGF (insulin-like growth factor), 334
IGT (impaired glucose tolerance), 16
iliotibial band (ITB), 245
illnesses, 81
impaired fasting glucose (IFG), 15
impaired glucose tolerance (IGT), 16
impaired thermoregulation, 289
improving
  balance, 227–229, 229–231
  insulin action, 206
inactivity, 29–30
Inderal, 58
indoor cardio machines, 191–194
indoor treadmills, 186–187
inflammation, lowering, 104–106
inhaled insulin, 53
injected (non-insulin) medications, 45–46, 49
injuries
  avoiding, 213
  overuse, 177–179
  preventing and managing, 174–180
  R.I.C.E, 176–177
  stretching and, 241–242

innate love of movement, in kids, 308–309

insulin

about, 8–10, 49–50

for athletes, 334

basal, 50–52

bolus (mealtime), 50–52

delivery methods for, 52–53

effect of female hormones on, 299–301

exercise interactions with, 53–54

inhaled, 53

intermediate-action, 51–52

long-acting, 279

lowering for physical activity, 54–56

needs for exercise, 56

short-acting, 279

types, 279

insulin action

activity and, 313–314

enhancing, 206

impact of fitness on, 30–33

women and, 300–301

insulin bodybuilding, 335

insulin pumps, 52–53

insulin regimen changes, as an exercise factor, 80

insulin resistance

about, 10, 11

avoiding excessive, 301

insulin sensitizers, 48

insulin-dependent diabetes. *See* type 1 diabetes

insulin-like growth factor (IGF), 334

insurance coverage, blood glucose meters and, 20

intense pain, 176

intensity

as an exercise variable, 73–76

of cardio training, 182

of exercise during pregnancy, 303

interesterified fat, 115

intermediate-action insulins, 51–52

Internet resources

American Diabetes Association, 286

CDC quiz, 151

Cheat Sheet, 3

Colberg-Ochs, Sheri (author), 3

Diabetes Motion, 3

Diabetes Motion Academy, 3

glycemix index (GI), 110

interpreting test results, 16–17

interval training

about, 165–166, 189–191

for athletes, 324

for seniors, 316

intramuscular triglycerides, 70

inversion ankle sprain, 175

iron levels, for athletes, 332–333

iron status (serum ferritin), 332–333

ischemia, 290

ITB (iliotibial band), 245

J

jogging, 186–189

joint damage, 178

joint issues, 272–274

juice, 138

juvenile onset diabetes. *See* type 1 diabetes

juvenile onset diabetes (type 1)

about, 11–12

diagnosing, 17

oral medications for, 41

weight gain with, 278

K

Kegel exercises, 170

kidney disease, 295–296

kids

about, 305

vs. adults, 306

encouraging activity in, 307–311

inactivity in, 306

safety of, 307–308

knee fold tucks, 217

knee injuries, 176

knee planks, 216

knee push-ups, 353

knee side planks, 217

L

lactic acid system, 68

Lantus, 51

Lantus/Basaglar, 334

Lasix, 58

leg lifts, 217

legs

  health complications with, 286–288

  stretches for, 245

leucine, 121

Levatol, 58

Levemir, 51

life span, 39–40

liver, storing less fat in, 269

long-acting insulin, 279

Lopressor, 58

low-carb eating, 327–328

lower back injuries, 176

lower body stretches, 243

Lozol, 58

lunges, 355–356

luteal phase, 300

M

macronutrients, 28

magnesium

  about, 119–120

  for athletes, 333

Majaryasana (Cat pose), 248

managing

  blood glucose, 73

  discomfort, 273

  effects of medications, 57–59

  exercise with health complications, 296–297

  gestational diabetes, 304

  health complication, 344–345

  health complications, 286

  hyperglycemia, 99–101, 330–331

  hypoglycemia, 329–330

  injuries, 174–180

  pain, 273

  weight gain, 270–272

maximal aerobic capacity, aging and, 322

maximizing

  muscle strength, 204–206

  protein for training and aging, 132–133

  resistance (strength) training, 207–213

maximum heart rate (MHR), 75

mealtime (bolus) insulins, 52

measuring

  aging, 320–322

  barriers to activity, 151–156

medications

  about, 41

  adjusting, 279–281

  exercise and, 46–49

  insulin, 49–56

  monitoring effects of, 57–59

  non-insulin (injected), 45–46, 49

  oral, 41–45

  weight loss and, 277–281

meglitinides, 43, 45, 47, 48, 281

menstrual cycle, 300

mental health/function

  about, 318–320

  aging and, 322

metabolic activity, aging and, 321

metabolic rate, in seniors, 312

Metformin, 41, 43

MHR (maximum heart rate), 75

Micronase, 281

micronutrients, 28

Microzide, 58

milk, 90–91

minerals, 117–120

misdiagnosing type 2 diabetes, 18

mobile technology, 150

moderate-intensity activities, 183

modified plank, 349

monitoring

  blood glucose, 73

  discomfort, 273

  effects of medications, 57–59

  exercise with health complications, 296–297

  gestational diabetes, 304

  health complication, 344–345

monitoring *(continued)*
  health complications, 286
  hyperglycemia, 99–101, 330–331
  hypoglycemia, 329–330
  injuries, 174–180
  pain, 273
  weight gain, 270–272
motivation
  for activity, 146–150
  for exercise, 357–361
Mountain pose (Tadasana), 245–246
movement, for seniors, 318
muscle cramps, 179–180
muscle endurance, 207
muscle fibers, 205
muscle glycogen, restoring, 94
muscle soreness, 179
muscle strength
  about, 207
  aging and, 322
  maximizing, 204–206
muscle wasting, avoiding, 314–315
muscles, 242–245
MyFitnessPal, 150
myoglobin, 264

N

N (NPH), 51
naproxen sodium, 177
neck stretch, 244, 253
nerve damage, exercising with, 286–289
nitroglycerin, 58
non-insulin (injected) medications, 45–46, 49
non-insulin-dependent diabetes. *See* type 2 diabetes
non-insulin-dependent dianetes (type 2)
  about, 12–13
  diagnosing, 17
  misdiagnosing, 18
  preventing with activity, 270
  weight gain with, 278
norepinephrine, 64
NovoLog, 51, 52, 334
NovoRapid, 52
NPH (N), 51

O

obesity, as a cardiovascular risk, 39
OGTT (oral glucose tolerance test), 16
omega-3/-6 fats, 113–114
oral contraceptives, 300
oral glucose tolerance test (OGTT), 16
oral medications, 41–42
orthostatic hypotension, 289
overcoming barriers to activity, 151–156
overhydrating, 136
overload principle, 324
overpronate, 145
overuse injuries, 177–179

P

PAD (peripheral artery disease), 292–293
pain
  intense, 176
  managing, 273
parasympathetic nervous system, 232, 251
pedometer, 147–148
pelvic tilt, 351–352
pens, 52
perceived exertion, 74
performance variables, for athletes, 332–334
peripheral artery disease (PAD), 292–293
phosphagens system, 67
physical activity, lowering insulin for, 54–56
physical health barriers, to activity, 154
physical inactivity, as a cardiovascular risk, 38
phytochemicals, 104
phytonutrients, 104
pick up the pace (PUP) training, 190
planks, 216, 349
planning exercise, 345–346, 359
plant fats, 113–114
plantar fasciitis, 175
Polar Beat, 150
polypharmacy, 314
portal vein, 22
positive, stress-releasing activity, 251–252
Prandin, 281

prediabetes
  about, 14
  diagnosing, 14–18, 17
  poorly controlled, as a cardiovascular
    risk, 38
  risks for, 17
  testing for, 15–17
Prednisone, 59
preeclampsia, 302
pregnancy
  activity during, 301–304
  gestational diabetes, 304
preventing
  hypoglycemia, 88–99
  injuries, 174–180
  type 2 diabetes with, 270
progesterone, 299
progress, tracking, 147–149
progression, of exercise during pregnancy, 303
proliferative retinopathy, 294–295, 349
pronators, 145
protein
  about, 112–113, 131
  intake of, 131–132
  intake of for insulin users, 132
  maximizing for training and aging, 132–133
  role of, 28
PUP (pick up the pace) training, 190

Q
quadriceps, 245

R
R (Regular), 51
raised side plank, 350
rapid glycolysis system, 68
reaction time, aging and, 322
Regular (R), 51
reps, for resistance training,
    210–211
resistance bands, 208
resistance machines, 209

resistance (strength) training
  about, 167–168, 203–204
  for athletes, 324–325
  choosing, 270
  combining with cardio training, 263
  core training, 215–217
  exercises for, 218–224
  maximizing, 207–213
  maximizing muscle strength, 204–206
  during pregnancy, 303
  safety for, 217–218
  for seniors, 316
  technique for, 213–214
  warming up, 207
  women and, 207
resources, Internet
  American Diabetes Association, 286
  CDC quiz, 151
  Cheat Sheet, 3
  Colberg-Ochs, Sheri (author), 3
  Diabetes Motion, 3
  Diabetes Motion Academy, 3
  glycemix index (GI), 110
rest time, for athletes, 332
resting heart rate (RHR), 75
restoring muscle glycogen, 94
retinopathy, 293–295
rewarding yourself for exercise, 360
RHR (resting heart rate), 75
R.I.C.E, 176–177
risks
  cardiovascular, 38–39
  for diabetes, 8
  for prediabetes, 17
routine, exercise, 171–173
rowing, 193
running, 186–189

S
safety, for resistance training, 217–218
scale weight, 277
scheduling exercise, 360
seated arm curls exercise, 198, 199

seated foot drill exercise, 197–198

seated march exercise, 197

seated overhead punches exercise, 198, 199

sedentary time, for seniors, 317–318

selecting

activity, 358

aerobic workouts, 270

carbohydrates, 89–91

exercises for resistance training, 215

resistance training, 270

training types, 164–170

self-monitoring blood glucose, 18–19

seniors

about, 305

activity and, 315–318

aging and health in, 311–315

assessing aging, 320–322

serotonin release, 341

sets, for resistance training, 210–211

setting

goals, 34–37, 360

SMART goals, 155–156

sex, as a cardiovascular risk, 38

SGLT-2 inhibitors, 41, 44, 45, 48

shin splints, 175

shoes, for foot issues, 287

short-acting insulin, 279

shortness of breath, as a symptom of a heart attack, 291

shoulder stretches, 244

shoulder/upper-back stretch, 253–254

side leg raises, 229

side plank pulse, 350

side plank with lateral raise, 350

side planks, 216, 349–350

silent ischemia, 288

single leg balance exercise, 232–233

SIT (sprint interval training), 191

sit-to-stand exercise, 218–219, 230

skin elasticity, aging and, 322

sleep, 173, 282–283

SMART goals, 155–156

socks, for foot issues, 287

soleus, 245

spontaneous physical activity (SPA), 161–164, 360–361

sports drinks, 138

sprint interval training (SIT), 191

sprinting, effects of, 97

squats with knee squeezes, 354–355

Staff pose (Dandasana), 246

stair-stepper, 192

standing calf raises exercise, 223–224

standing leg curls exercise, 222–223

standing march exercise, 200

standing on one leg, practicing, 228–229

standing raise the roof exercise, 200–201

Starlix, 281

static stretching, 241

statins, 57

step equivalency calculator, 149

strategies, for handling kids, 310–311

strength, in seniors, 312

strength (resistance) training

about, 167–168, 203–204

for athletes, 324–325

choosing, 270

combining with cardio training, 263

core training, 215–217

exercises for, 218–224

maximizing, 207–213

maximizing muscle strength, 204–206

during pregnancy, 303

safety for, 217–218

for seniors, 316

technique for, 213–214

warming up, 207

women and, 207

stretches/stretching

about, 240–242

arm, 244

back of upper-leg, 256–257

basic, 242–245

buttock, 245

calf, 257–258

chest/shoulder, 254–255

core muscle, 244

dynamic, 241–242

effectiveness of, 242

exercises for, 252–258

hip, 245

lower body, 243

neck, 244, 253

shoulder, 244

shoulder/upper-back, 253–254

static, 241

upper body, 243

upper-back/back of arm, 255–256

stroke, 291–292

subcutaneous fat, 268

sugar, reducing, 111–112

suitcase lift, 353–354

Sukhasana (Easy pose), 246

sulfonylureas, 42–43, 44, 47, 48, 281

"sunshine vitamin," 118–119

superhero pose, 352–353

supplements, 117–124

swimming, 194–195

Symlin (pramlintide), 45–46

sympathetic nervous system

about, 232, 251

peripheral artery disease (PAD), 292–293

symptoms

about, 14–15

heart attack, 291

hypoglycemia, 86–87

of low magnesium, 333

stroke, 292

syringes, 52

systemic inflammation, aging and, 322

T

Tadasana (Mountain pose), 245–246

tai chi, 231–232, 250, 317

talk test, 74

tapering, 326

Technical Stuff icon, 3

technique

for resistance (strength) training, 213–214

running, 187

tendinitis, 178

Tenormin, 58

testing

for diabetes, 15–17

for gestational diabetes, 17

interpreting results from, 16–17

for prediabetes, 15–17

Thiamin B1, 333

thiazolidinediones (TZDs), 41, 43, 44, 48, 281

three-way leg swing exercise, 233–234

thyroid issues, 334

tibialis anterior, 228

timing

of activity, 346

as an exercise variable, 77–79

toe raise exercise, 236

toe raises, 229–230

total insulin needs, 278–279

Toujeo, 51, 334

tracking progress, 147–149

training

choosing types, 164–170

cross-training, 169

on a diet, 205–206

effects of, 79–80

flexibility, 169

maximizing protein for, 132–133

order of, 98

training, aerobic (cardio)

about, 165–166, 181, 194–201

aerobic exercise, 194–201

choosing, 270

combining with resistance training, 263

getting started, 182–184

indoor cardio machines, 191–194

interval training, 189–191

jogging, 186–189

during pregnancy, 303

running, 186–189

for seniors, 316

walking, 184–186

training, balance
  about, 168–169, 225
  effects of aging and diabetes on balance, 226–227
  exercises for, 232–237
  for seniors, 317
  Tai Chi, 231–232
  yoga, 231–232
training, core
  abdominal squeezes, 348
  about, 167–168, 215–217, 347–348
  bridging, 351
  gym ball side plank, 350
  knee push-ups, 353
  lunges, 355–356
  modified plank, 349
  pelvic tilt, 351–352
  plank, 349
  raised side plank, 350
  for seniors, 316
  side plank pulse, 350
  side plank with lateral raise, 350
  side planks, 349–350
  squats with knee squeezes, 354–355
  suitcase lift, 353–354
  superhero pose, 352–353
training, cross-
  about, 169, 259
  benefits of, 259–263
  combining cardio training and resistance training, 263
  with diabetes, 263–264
  example exercise plan for, 262–263
training, flexibility
  about, 169, 239
  basic stretches, 242–245
  importance of, 240
  improving, 231–232
  muscles, 242–245
  for seniors, 317
  stretching, 240–242
  stretching exercises, 252–258
  whole-body approach for, 250–252

  yoga, 245–249
training, interval
  about, 165–166, 189–191
  for athletes, 324
  for seniors, 316
training, resistance (strength)
  about, 167–168, 203–204
  for athletes, 324–325
  choosing, 270
  combining with cardio training, 263
  core training, 215–217
  exercises for, 218–224
  maximizing, 207–213
  maximizing muscle strength, 204–206
  during pregnancy, 303
  safety for, 217–218
  for seniors, 316
  technique for, 213–214
  warming up, 207
  women and, 207
training state, for athletes, 325–326
trans fats, 114–115
travel backward exercise, 231
treadmills, 186–187
treating
  hypoglycemia, 88–99
  low blood glucose with carbohydrates, 89
Tree pose (Vrksasana), 249
Treisba, 51
tucking your chin exercise, 231
twists, 217
type
  as an exercise variable, 72–73
  of exercise during pregnancy, 303
type 1 diabetes
  about, 11–12
  diagnosing, 17
  oral medications for, 41
  weight gain with, 278
type 2 diabetes
  about, 12–13
  diagnosing, 17

misdiagnosing, 18

preventing with activity, 270

weight gain with, 278

TZDs (thiazolidinediones), 41, 43, 44, 48, 281

U

upper body stretches, 243

upper-back/back of arm stretch, 255–256

Utkatasana (Chair pose), 249

V

variables, for exercise, 72–80

variety, in exercise, 359

vasodilators, 58

vessel disease, 289–293

vigorous-intensity activities, 183

visceral fat, 268–269

visualization, 252

vitamin D, 118–119

vitamins, 117–120

Vrksasana (Tree pose), 249

W

walk heel-to-toe, 231

walking, 184–186

"The Walk," 150

wall push-ups exercise, 221–222

warming up, 171, 184, 207

water intoxication, 136

"water pills," 58

websites

American Diabetes Association, 286

CDC quiz, 151

Cheat Sheet, 3

Colberg-Ochs, Sheri (author), 3

Diabetes Motion, 3

Diabetes Motion Academy, 3

glycemix index (GI), 110

weight gain

arthritis, 272–274

avoiding, 277–281

joint issues, 272–274

limiting impact of, 268–269

losing weight, 274–277

managing, 270–272

pregnancy and, 302–303

sleep and, 282–283

training with extra, 267–283

with type 1 and type 2 diabetes, 278

weight loss, 274–281, 281–282

weight machines, 208

whey protein, 121–122

women

about, 299

female hormones, 299–301

pregnancy, 301–304

resistance (strength) training and, 207

workout clothes, 144–146

workout plan, for running, 188–189

workouts, aerobic (cardio)

about, 165–166, 181, 194–201

aerobic exercise, 194–201

choosing, 270

combining with resistance training, 263

getting started, 182–184

indoor cardio machines, 191–194

interval training, 189–191

jogging, 186–189

during pregnancy, 303

running, 186–189

for seniors, 316

walking, 184–186

workouts, balance

about, 168–169, 225

effects of aging and diabetes on balance, 226–227

exercises for, 232–237

for seniors, 317

Tai Chi, 231–232

yoga, 231–232

workouts, core
  abdominal squeezes, 348
  about, 167–168, 215–217, 347–348
  bridging, 351
  gym ball side plank, 350
  knee push-ups, 353
  lunges, 355–356
  modified plank, 349
  pelvic tilt, 351–352
  plank, 349
  raised side plank, 350
  for seniors, 316
  side plank pulse, 350
  side plank with lateral raise, 350
  side planks, 349–350
  squats with knee squeezes, 354–355
  suitcase lift, 353–354
  superhero pose, 352–353
workouts, cross-training
  about, 169, 259
  benefits of, 259–263
  combining cardio training and resistance
    training, 263
  with diabetes, 263–264
  example exercise plan for, 262–263
workouts, flexibility
  about, 169, 239
  basic stretches, 242–245
  importance of, 240
  improving, 231–232
  muscles, 242–245
  for seniors, 317
  stretching, 240–242

  stretching exercises, 252–258
  whole-body approach for, 250–252
  yoga, 245–249
workouts, interval training
  about, 165–166, 189–191
  for athletes, 324
  for seniors, 316
workouts, resistance (strength)
  about, 167–168, 203–204
  for athletes, 324–325
  choosing, 270
  combining with cardio training, 263
  core training, 215–217
  exercises for, 218–224
  maximizing, 207–213
  maximizing muscle strength, 204–206
  during pregnancy, 303
  safety for, 217–218
  for seniors, 316
  technique for, 213–214
  warming up, 207
  women and, 207

Y

yoga
  about, 231–232
  poses for, 245–249
  for seniors, 317

Z

Zebeta, 58

About the Author

Dr. Sheri R. Colberg, PhD, FACSM, is a world-renowned diabetes motion expert. She is a prolific author, exercise physiologist, lecturer, and professor emerita of exercise science (Old Dominion University, Norfolk, VA) who has helped countless people, with and without diabetes, live healthier lives and age successfully. In 2016, she was honored with the prestigious American Diabetes Association Outstanding Educator in Diabetes Award for all she has done to educate people worldwide about keeping fit and living well with diabetes.

A distinguished graduate of Stanford University (BA), University of California, Davis (MA), and University of California, Berkeley (PhD), she has authored more than 300 articles on exercise, diabetes, and health and 25 book chapters. Her numerous books include *Diabetes-Free Kids* (Avery), *The 7 Step Diabetes Fitness Plan* (Da Capo Press), *50 Secrets of the Longest Living People with Diabetes* (Da Capo Press), *The Science of Staying Young* (McGraw-Hill), *Diabetic Athlete's Handbook* (Human Kinetics), and *The Diabetes Breakthrough* (William Morrow Paperbacks), many of which have been translated into other languages. She has given hundreds of interviews that have appeared in magazines, on TV and radio, online in magazine and video blogs, and elsewhere worldwide.

A respected researcher and lecturer, Dr. Sheri has helped shape exercise and fitness guidelines for many professional organizations. She has consulted for the American Diabetes Association and the Juvenile Diabetes Research Foundation, as well as worked closely with the American College of Sports Medicine, American Association of Diabetes Educators, and Academy of Nutrition and Dietetics on diabetes-related topics and projects.

Her articles, columns, blogs, and more are available on her websites at www.shericolberg.com and www.diabetesmotion.com. If you're a fitness professional looking for continuing education in diabetes and fitness, visit her other website, Diabetes Motion Academy, at www.dmacademy.com. Follow Dr. Sheri on Twitter at @SheriColberg.

Dr. Sheri has been described by her colleagues, acquaintances, and friends as energetic, prolific, dynamic, motivated, intelligent, caring, collegial, goal-oriented, inspirational, fun, and funny. She has set the standard as the definitive source in her areas of expertise with high-quality work and attention to detail. And she has also chosen to live life to the fullest and embodies wholesome good health and fitness. With nearly 50 years of personal experience as an exerciser living well with type 1 diabetes, she enjoys working out regularly on conditioning machines, swimming, biking, walking, weight training, and hiking with her husband in coastal California.

Dedication

First and foremost, I dedicate this book to all the people out there struggling and desiring to live well with diabetes or prediabetes. I hope this book helps you find your way and makes that journey easier for you.

And, of course, I give my heartfelt thanks to my husband, Ray Ochs, for his unconditional love and support. Without his selfless backing, I would not be able to help others half as much as I do.

Publisher's Acknowledgments

Senior Acquisitions Editor: Tracy Boggier

Editorial Project Manager and Development Editor: Christina Guthrie

Copy Editor: Megan Knoll

Production Editor: G. Vasanth Koilraj

Cover Image: © ratmaner/iStockphoto

Take dummies with you everywhere you go!

Whether you are excited about e-books, want more from the web, must have your mobile apps, or are swept up in social media, dummies makes everything easier.

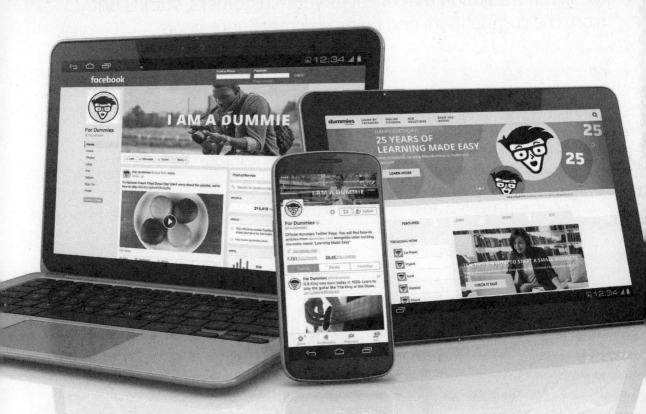

Find us online!

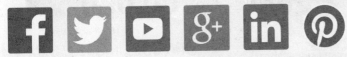

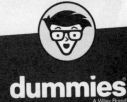

Leverage the power

Dummies is the global leader in the reference category and one of the most trusted and highly regarded brands in the world. No longer just focused on books, customers now have access to the dummies content they need in the format they want. Together we'll craft a solution that engages your customers, stands out from the competition, and helps you meet your goals.

Advertising & Sponsorships

Connect with an engaged audience on a powerful multimedia site, and position your message alongside expert how-to content. Dummies.com is a one-stop shop for free, online information and know-how curated by a team of experts.

- Targeted ads
- Video
- Email Marketing
- Microsites
- Sweepstakes sponsorship

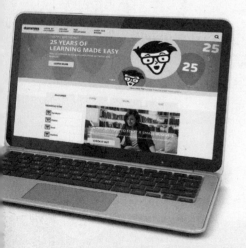

20 MILLION PAGE VIEWS EVERY SINGLE MONTH

15 MILLION UNIQUE VISITORS PER MONTH

43% OF ALL VISITORS ACCESS THE SITE VIA THEIR MOBILE DEVICES

700,000 NEWSLETTER SUBSCRIPTIONS TO THE INBOXES OF

300,000 UNIQUE INDIVIDUALS EVERY WEEK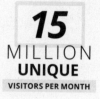

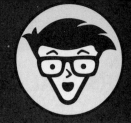

Custom Publishing

Reach a global audience in any language by creating a solution that will differentiate you from competitors, amplify your message, and encourage customers to make a buying decision.

- Apps
- Books
- eBooks
- Video
- Audio
- Webinars

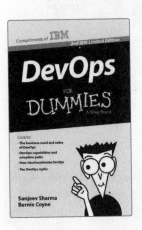

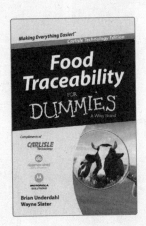

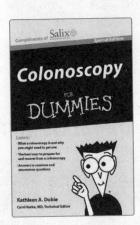

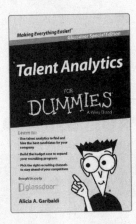

Brand Licensing & Content

Leverage the strength of the world's most popular reference brand to reach new audiences and channels of distribution.

For more information, visit **dummies.com/biz**

PERSONAL ENRICHMENT

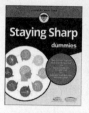 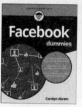 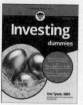 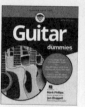 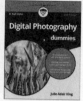 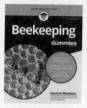

Staying Sharp
9781119187790
USA $26.00
CAN $31.99
UK £19.99

Facebook
9781119179030
USA $21.99
CAN $25.99
UK £16.99

Guitar
9781119293354
USA $24.99
CAN $29.99
UK £17.99

Investing
9781119293347
USA $22.99
CAN $27.99
UK £16.99

Beekeeping
9781119310068
USA $22.99
CAN $27.99
UK £16.99

Digital Photography
9781119235606
USA $24.99
CAN $29.99
UK £17.99

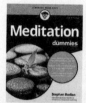 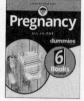 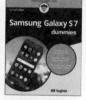 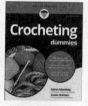 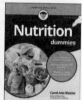

Meditation
9781119251163
USA $24.99
CAN $29.99
UK £17.99

Pregnancy
9781119235491
USA $26.99
CAN $31.99
UK £19.99

Samsung Galaxy S 7
9781119279952
USA $24.99
CAN $29.99
UK £17.99

iPhone
9781119283133
USA $24.99
CAN $29.99
UK £17.99

Crocheting
9781119287117
USA $24.99
CAN $29.99
UK £16.99

Nutrition
9781119130246
USA $22.99
CAN $27.99
UK £16.99

PROFESSIONAL DEVELOPMENT

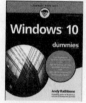 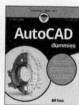 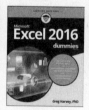 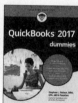 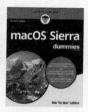 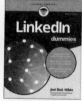 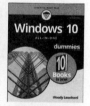

Windows 10
9781119311041
USA $24.99
CAN $29.99
UK £17.99

AutoCAD
9781119255796
USA $39.99
CAN $47.99
UK £27.99

Excel 2016
9781119293439
USA $26.99
CAN $31.99
UK £19.99

QuickBooks 2017
9781119281467
USA $26.99
CAN $31.99
UK £19.99

macOS Sierra
9781119280651
USA $29.99
CAN $35.99
UK £21.99

LinkedIn
9781119251132
USA $24.99
CAN $29.99
UK £17.99

Windows 10
9781119310563
USA $34.00
CAN $41.99
UK £24.99

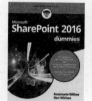 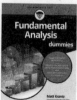 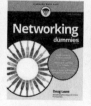 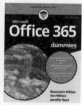 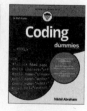

SharePoint 2016
9781119181705
USA $29.99
CAN $35.99
UK £21.99

Fundamental Analysis
9781119263593
USA $26.99
CAN $31.99
UK £19.99

Networking
9781119257769
USA $29.99
CAN $35.99
UK £21.99

Office 2016
9781119293477
USA $26.99
CAN $31.99
UK £19.99

Office 365
9781119265313
USA $24.99
CAN $29.99
UK £17.99

Salesforce.com
9781119239314
USA $29.99
CAN $35.99
UK £21.99

Coding
9781119293323
USA $29.99
CAN $35.99
UK £21.99

dummies.com

dummies
A Wiley Brand